PRACTICAL REVIEW
OF NEUROPATHOLOGY

PRACTICAL REVIEW OF NEUROPATHOLOGY

GREGORY N. FULLER, M.D., PH.D.

Associate Professor
Chief, Section of Neuropathology
Department of Pathology
The University of Texas MD Anderson Cancer Center
Houston, Texas

J. CLAY GOODMAN, M.D.

Professor
Neuropathology Program Director
Departments of Pathology, Neurosurgery, and Neurology
Baylor College of Medicine & The Methodist Hospital
Houston, Texas

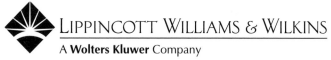

LIPPINCOTT WILLIAMS & WILKINS
A **Wolters Kluwer** Company
Philadelphia · Baltimore · New York · London
Buenos Aires · Hong Kong · Sydney · Tokyo

Acquisitions Editor: Ruth W. Weinberg
Developmental Editors: Cynthia Shepherd/Brian Brown
Production Editor: Patrick Carr
Manufacturing Manager: Benjamin Rivera
Cover Designer: Christine Jenny
Compositor: Maryland Composition
Printer: Edwards Brothers

© 2001 by LIPPINCOTT WILLIAMS & WILKINS
530 Walnut Street
Philadelphia, PA 19106 USA
LWW.com

Printed in the USA

Library of Congress Cataloging-in-Publication Data
Fuller, Gregory N.
      Practical review of neuropathology/Gregory N. Fuller, J. Clay Goodman.
          p. ; cm.
      Includes bibliographical references and index.
      ISBN 0-7817-2778-2
          1. Nervous system—Diseases. I. Goodman, J. Clay. II. Title.
      [DNLM: 1. Nervous System Diseases. WL 140 F9655p 2001]
      RC347 .F84 2001
      616.8—dc21
                                                                00-069010

Care has been taken to confirm the accuracy of the information presented and to describe generally accepted practices. However, the authors, editors, and publisher are not responsible for errors or omissions or for any consequences from application of the information in this book and make no warranty, expressed or implied, with respect to the currency, completeness, or accuracy of the contents of the publication. Application of this information in a particular situation remains the professional responsibility of the practitioner.

The authors, editors, and publisher have exerted every effort to ensure that drug selection and dosage set forth in this text are in accordance with current recommendations and practice at the time of publication. However, in view of ongoing research, changes in government regulations, and the constant flow of information relating to drug therapy and drug reactions, the reader is urged to check the package insert for each drug for any change in indications and dosage and or added warnings and precautions. This is particularly important when the recommended agent is a new or infrequently employed drug.

Some drugs and medical devices presented in this publication have Food and Drug Administration (FDA) clearance for limited use in restricted research settings. It is the responsibility of the health care provider to ascertain the FDA status of each drug or device planned for use in their clinical practice.

10 9 8 7 6 5 4 3 2 1

Dedication

This book is dedicated to my teachers: Frances Thomas, Jack Barcley, Arthur Harper,
John Lock, Harrell Odom, Jack Dobson, Richard Wiggins

—G.N.F.

This book is dedicated to my parents, who taught me all the essential principles of an honorable life;
to my wife, a beloved partner in the journey through that life; and to my teachers,
colleagues, patients, and students who make that journey meaningful.

—J.C.G.

CONTENTS

PREFACE

This book is designed to provide the reader with an up-to-date, practical, and succinct overview of contemporary neuropathology. Our intent specifically was not to produce yet another ponderous reference tome or colorfully illustrated atlas, but rather to emphasize key concepts and contemporary biomedical principles coupled with discussions of the essential elements of specific neuropathological disorders. This approach has been received enthusiastically for the past fifteen years in widely diverse venues from first year medical student courses to international course offerings for neuropathologists and neurologists. We also believe that this book will be useful to pathologists on the front lines of diagnosis by providing practical hints on reaching correct answers while avoiding pitfalls.

We are witnessing extraordinary growth in the scientific foundations of neuroscience with ever accelerating translation of basic insights into clinical practice. Far from being an arcane backwater, neuropathology is a vibrant wellspring and pivotal conduit for this new information, and we hope that our readers will be able to understand and perhaps actively participate in these exciting developments. Our intent is that the content of this book should be readily accessible to medical students, house officers, and practitioners; to this end we have provided early chapters delineating the biological underpinnings of modern neuropathology. Subsequent chapters focus on specific categories of neurological disease and frequently reprise the bedrock principles defined in earlier chapters.

We also believe that this review may be of interest to basic scientists seeking insights into disorders of the nervous system. It is absolutely essential that a dialogue occur between basic scientists and clinical investigators; in order for such a dialogue to be fruitful, each group must have an understanding of the other's intellectual world. Scientists cannot all receive medical training, nor can most physicians keep up with the rapid advances in scientific techniques and concepts, but all should strive to attain a sufficiently broad biomedical literacy so as to permit an appreciation of each other's efforts and thereby facilitate reciprocal contributions to each other's fields. We hope that this book will increase the neuropathological sophistication of a broad range of readers, and that this will ultimately lead to improved diagnosis and treatment of our patients.

Gregory N. Fuller, M.D., Ph.D.
J. Clay Goodman, M.D.

BIOLOGICAL BEDROCK

PERSPECTIVE

1. The unifying theme of contemporary neuropathology is the molecular regulation of cellular life and death.
2. Cellular division, growth, differentiation, and programmed cell death are under genetic control.
3. Cellular division is tightly controlled in order to assure genetic fidelity. Loss of genetic integrity leads to programmed cell death in normal cells.
4. The mature central nervous system has a small reserve of stem cells capable of limited division, differentiation, and repopulation of lost cells.

OBJECTIVES

1. Understand that neuropathological processes can broadly be divided into those involving disordered cellular growth and differentiation, and those involving cellular death.
2. Distinguish between programmed cell death (apoptosis) and necrotic cell death.
3. Appreciate the key features involved in cell division.
4. Learn about the recent recognition of neural stem cells that reside even in the mature nervous system and the triggers that may activate them.

A major theme which has emerged in modern neuropathology is the concept that pathological alterations reflect derangements of normal cellular processes, and that an understanding of these normal processes may in turn lead to a more insightful grasp of the pathological processes' underlying disease. Neoplasia at its most fundamental level is a molecular genetic abnormality of cellular growth and differentiation—cellular life. Diseases in which cells are lost are disorders of cellular death—a complex tightly regulated process (Fig. 1-1) . There are two major forms of cellular death—necrosis and apoptosis—each with dramatically different morphology, biochemistry, and potential therapeutic targets.

> **Key Concept:** Cell proliferation, differentiation, and programmed cell death are under genetic control.

There are genes that control entry into the cell cycle where cells synthesize DNA and undergo mitosis. Proliferation can be triggered by internal signals or in response to external growth factor stimulation. During the cell cycle, the cell's DNA content goes from the normal diploid amount in G0 and G1, to an incrementing amount during synthesis (S-phase), to twice the normal amount during G2 when the cell prepares to divide, and finally in the mitotic period (M-phase), two new cells are created having a diploid amount of

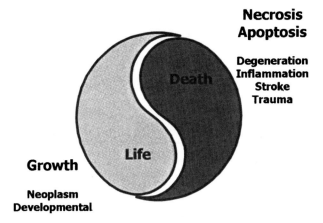

FIGURE 1-1. The Yin and Yang of cellular fate. Neuropathological processes can broadly be considered as those in which there is disordered cellular division and differentiation versus those where cellular death of either an apoptotic or necrotic nature occurs.

Principles of Flow Cytometric DNA Analysis

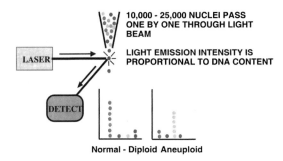

FIGURE 1-2. The proliferative fraction and the degree of aneuploidy in a population of cells can be measured using flow cytometry.

Nuclear DNA Content Increases During the Cell Cycle

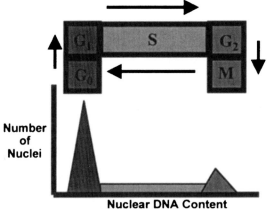

FIGURE 1-3. The cell cycle is a carefully controlled series of events that evolved to assure high fidelity genetic replication. At multiple points during the process, the integrity of the replication and the readiness of the cell to continue is assessed. The process moves forward only if all components are ready. If the cell is unable to proceed, programmed cell death is initiated. During normal cell division, the cell's DNA content progressively increases as two sets (one for each daughter cell) are generated.

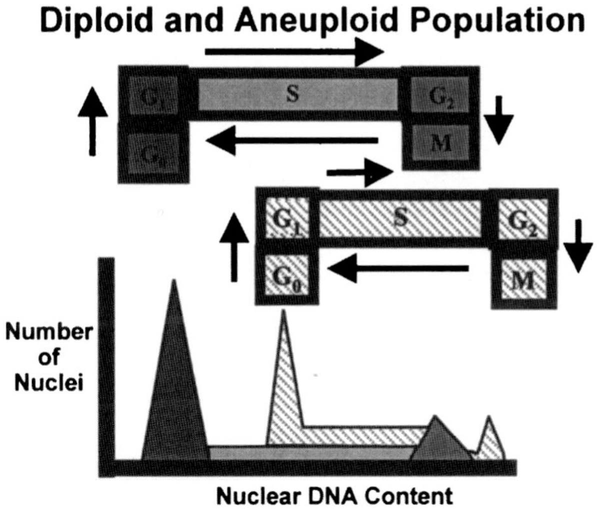

Diploid and Aneuploid Population

FIGURE 1-4. In cancer, there is genetic instability leading to the emergence of aneuploid populations of cells often having an increased proliferation fraction.

Pitfalls of Flow Cytometric DNA Analysis of Archival Material

- Intra-tumor heterogeneity

- Sample adequacy

- DNA preservation dependent on fixative

- DNA fragmentation

FIGURE 1-5. Flow cytometric analysis can be performed on archived paraffin embedded material so that the archives of tissue in pathology departments can be used to provide new genetic insights. There are limitations, however, on the use of this material.

DNA. These events can be measured in populations of cells by flow cytometry by measuring the amount of DNA in the nuclei of the cells (Fig. 1-2). From the amount of DNA contained, the fraction of cells at various points in the cell cycle are known (Fig. 1-3). Some normal cell populations such as bone marrow have a high proliferative fraction, but many tumors also have increased cell cycle activity. Tumor cells also are less careful about replicative fidelity and may accumulate abnormal amounts of DNA; this is called "aneuploidy" (Figs. 1-4 and 1-5).

Other genes regulate the expression of unique sets of proteins that give cells their differentiated features. Finally, during normal tissue development and maintenance, there is programmed cell death that is under genetic control. All of these genes controlling cell division, differentiation and death operate in concert, and there are counter-regulatory genes operating to fine-tune the process.

> **Key Concept:** At the most fundamental level, cancer is a set of disorders characterized by mutations of genes regulating cell growth, differentiation, and death.

Early explorations of viral-induced malignancies led to the discovery of viral oncogenes—genes carried by viruses, which, when expressed in the infected cells, resulted in cancer. Soon it was recognized that normal cells possess genes with structural similarities to these viral oncogenes, but that these genes have roles in cellular growth regulation. The cellular genes are known as proto-oncogenes. These cellular proto-oncogenes carry out normal and indeed essential regulatory functions, but if mutation arises in one of these genes, the stage is set for the evolution of a tumor. The classical chemical carcinogens and irradiation are now known to result in cancer by inducing mutations in any one of many potential proto-oncogenetic targets. Similarly, viruses may induce tumors by directly introducing oncogenes into the cell or by placing a regulatory gene near a proto-oncogene leading to abnormal production of that gene's protein product. Similarly, chromosomal rearrangements can lead to cancer by placing oncogenes under the control of inappropriate regulatory sequences. This occurrence of cancer-producing chromosomal rearrangements provides the link between molecular biology of tumors and cancer cytogenetics.

The mutation which changes a proto-oncogene into an abnormal cellular oncogene usually occurs in somatic cells, that is, the cells of the tissues of the nonreproductive organs. This may lead to the clonal expansion of that mutated cell to eventually form a tumor. In rare instances, mutations may occur in the germ cell lines so that the oncogenic mutation is passed to offspring, accounting for some familial cancer syndromes.

There is a set of genes that appear to inhibit cellular proliferation; they are the "brakes" of the cell cycle. Loss of these genes may lead to tumor growth. Since they can inhibit tumor growth, these genes are call antioncogenes or tumor suppressor genes. In the normal diploid state, each cell possesses two copies of these antioncogenes and one copy is usually sufficient to inhibit tumorogenesis; therefore, loss of both copies is required to produce a tumor. The mutation or chromosome break leading to loss of these alleles need not affect both genes in the same manner, but both genes must be rendered nonfunctional. Since both copies must be defective for carcinogenesis, these genes are also sometimes called "recessive oncogenes." In contrast, oncogenes which are tumorogenic when only one allele is defective are known as dominant oncogenes. Loss of antioncogenes may be detected cytogenetically as chromosomal deletions.

Conceptually, the normal function of the gene undergoing mutation may have important consequences in terms of tumor therapy. Mutations leading to increased proliferation (entry into the cell cycle), for example, would be expected to lead to a substantial population of cells vulnerable to cell cycle specific therapy. Conversely, some tumors are produced by mutations of genes which trigger programmed cell death; these cells are genetically immortalized and may infrequently enter the cell cycle, but when they do, their offspring join in their vampirish existence.

> **Key Concept:**   Tumor progression results from the sequential acquisition of new mutations which confer selective advantage.

The phenomenon of increasing tumor invasiveness, metastatic potential, and loss of differentiation ("dedifferentiation") reflects acquisition of additional mutations in the tumor cell line. A new mutation conferring selective advantage to a given cell line will result in the clonal expansion of that line in the tumor mass. Tumor progression represents a problem in population genetics in which cells initially freed of the shackles of growth regulation may evolve relentlessly with the emergence of clones with greater invasive potential, faster growth rate, or resistance to chemotherapy. In some tumors, progression is associated with a somewhat orderly acquisition of increasingly fearsome mutations.

> **Key Concept:**   Cellular death occurs by either necrosis or apoptosis. At the most fundamental levels these processes underlie diseases as diverse as stroke, trauma, demyelinating disorders, infections and neurodegenerative disorders. Different inciting events set into motion common mechanisms of cellular destruction.

Necrosis was the first form of cell death recognized. The cell undergoing necrosis exhibits cytoplasmic, mitochondrial and nuclear swelling as water flows into the cell along osmotic gradients. The cell membranes rupture spilling cellular and organelle chemical contents into the surrounding tissue. Pro-inflammatory signals are emitted from such necrotic cells inciting the entry of lymphocytes and polymorphonuclear cells into the area of injury with the potential for attendant secondary injury as these inflammatory cells engulf necrotic debris and release cytotoxic compounds.

Apoptosis (*apo-ptosis*) is a more discrete, orderly form of cellular death in which a cascade of genes is turned on leading to the activation of intracellular proteases. The mitochondria and nucleus condense, and fragments of the cytoplasm and nucleus bleb-off the dead cell to be discretely taken up by

Necrosis vs Apoptosis

• Passive • Swell and explode • Membrane leakiness • Random DNA breaks • Nuclear pycnosis	• Active • Cells fragment • Membranes intact • DNA laddering • Chromatin margination • Endonuclease activation

FIGURE 1-6. Cellular death occurs either by necrosis (bug on a windshield, passive, messy) versus apoptosis (carefully orchestrated, active, fulfilling the ancient covenant of multicellularity).

macrophages without inciting a frenzy of inflammatory activity. In addition to the activation of proteases, intranuclear nuclease is activated leading to degradation of the cell's DNA. The DNA is cut at the nucleosome leading to strands of DNA which are multiples of the internucleosomal distance in length; on a gel, these strands appear as rungs on a ladder rather than the smear of DNA seen with random nuclease degradation. Apoptosis normally occurs in development to eliminate unnecessary cells which are over-produced during normal organogenesis, to eliminate "forbidden clones" of lymphocytes directed at the self, and is a response that the cell can make to cellular injury. If a cell sustains genetic damage, entry into the cell cycle is arrested and the extent of the damage is assessed. If the genetic damage can be repaired, these repairs are effected and the cell is permitted to complete the cycle. If the damage is not repairable, the cell's apoptotic cascade is triggered, and the cell dies without creating a damaging local reaction which might endanger its neighbors. At the most fundamental level, apoptosis is one of the elements of the contract made by cells in cooperating to form a multicellular organism; when the cell can no longer contribute to the good of the organism, it agrees to commit suicide quietly and discretely (Fig. 1-6).

> **Key Concept:** The intensity of cellular injury determines whether the cell dies or is able to survive. Very severe injury leads to the passive process of necrosis, less severe but irreparable injury leads to the active process of apoptosis, and survivable injury leads to reactive changes such as gliosis and neuronal chromatolysis (Fig. 1-7).

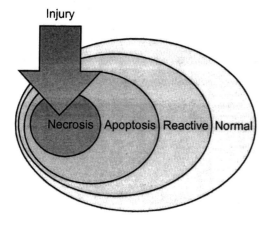

Injury

Necrosis | Apoptosis | Reactive | Normal

FIGURE 1-7. The severity of cellular damage may determine whether cellular death occurs by necrosis or apoptosis. Since apoptosis is an active cellular process, some level of cellular structural and functional integrity is required.

In some diseases, necrosis, apoptosis and reactive changes may coexist while in other diseases necrosis or apoptosis may dominate the picture.

> **Key Concept:** Neuronal loss in the mammalian brain has classically been regarded as a depressingly irreversible process with no prospect of reversal. In the past few years, evidence has accumulated that production of new neurons (neurogenesis) occurs even in the mature brain.

Subventricular zone (SVZ) cells are stem cells that spawn new glia and new neurons. This region immediately beneath the ependymal cell layer produces new cells at a very low rate compared to the prodigious neurogenesis that occurs in the germinal matrix during early development. Nevertheless, the new cells migrate widely throughout the brain and conform phenotypically to the regions where they ultimately end up. It is entirely possible that the brain is a self-repairing biological computer capable of replacing lost or defective "components." Harnessing this reparative potential is a major area of neurobiological investigation. As always, every silver lining has an accompanying cloud, the stem cells that make constructive neurogenesis possible may also be sources of brain tumors if stem cell maturational arrest analogous to leukemia occurs in the brain.

> **Key Concept:** Two major mechanisms of cellular injury—excitotoxicity and free radical injury—are at work in a number of neuropathological conditions (Fig. 1-8). These molecular mechanisms of cellular damage may lead to necrosis or apoptosis.

Excitotoxicity results from the inappropriate activation of excitatory amino acid receptors leading to entry of cations (calcium in particular) into the cell. The calcium activates intracellular proteases and disrupts mitochondrial function (Fig. 1-9).

Free radicals are generated by malfunctioning mitochondria predominantly and to some degree by nitric oxide synthesis. These highly reactive compounds disrupt membrane integrity by reacting with lipids, degrade enzymes, and react with DNA leading to genotoxicity. There is increasing evidence that free radical formation is an obligatory component of excitotoxicity.

Damaged cells unable to maintain amino acid homeostasis and necrotic cells release excitotoxins which in turn damage their neighbors.

These mechanistic considerations provide a framework from which the classic neurological disorders can be considered. Throughout this book, we will discuss major categories of neurological disease, and we will direct attention to the mechanisms of cellular death.

Evil Twins of Neuronal Death

- **Excitotoxicity**

- **Free Radical Injury**

FIGURE 1-8. The two major mechanisms of neuronal cellular damage leading to cellular death are excitotoxicity and free radical injury.

Excitotoxicity

- **Inappropriate activation of the NMDA receptor**

- **Membrane depolarization**

- **Influx of calcium**

- **Activation of hydrolytic enzymes and quenching of mitochondria**

FIGURE 1-9. One major means of cellular injury unique to the nervous system is excitotoxicity in which the most abundant endogenous neurotransmitters assume a toxic role.

2

CELLS OF THE NERVOUS SYSTEM AND SPECIALIZED REGIONAL ORGANS: NORMAL, AGED, AND PATHOLOGICAL

PERSPECTIVE

1. The nervous system is perhaps the most complex of all organs not only because of its anatomy but also in the diversity and uniqueness of its cellular constituents.
2. In addition to gray matter and white matter, there are several specialized regions in the CNS with their own distinctive tissue architecture found in no other location, such as the pineal gland, neurohypophysis, and circumventricular organs.
3. All of the many diverse cellular constituents and regional organs of the nervous system exhibit an equally complex spectrum of alterations produced by aging, disease, and neoplastic transformation.

OBJECTIVES

1. Learn the major morphological, ultrastructural, and immunohistochemical characteristics of the different neuroectodermal and mesenchymal cellular constituents of the nervous system.
2. Develop a knowledge of the histologic and cytologic structure of the specialized regional organs of the nervous system: the pineal gland, pituitary gland, circumventricular organs, optic nerves, olfactory tracts and bulbs, and filum terminale.
3. Become familiar with the principal reactions shown by each nervous system cell type to aging, disease, and neoplastic transformation.

INTRODUCTION

The nervous system is unparalleled among organ systems in terms of diversity of cellular constituents. The various elements may be divided into two broad groups based on embryologic considerations: neuroectodermal derivatives and mesenchymal derivatives (Table 2-1). The neuroectodermal constituents comprise the neurons and glia. Mesenchymal components are represented by an assortment of cell types composing the vasculature and meninges, and also include the microglia (in contrast to all of the other glia, which are derived

TABLE 2-1. CELLULAR CONSTITUENTS OF THE NERVOUS SYSTEM

Neuroectodermal elements
  Neurons
  Astrocytes
  Oligodendroglia
  Ependymocytes
Mesenchymal elements
  Meninges
  Blood vessels
  Adipose tissue
  Microglia

TABLE 2-2. METHODS BY WHICH CELLULAR CONSTITUENTS CAN BE DISTINGUISHED

Light microscopic morphology
Neuroanatomic distribution
Immunocytochemistry
Ultrastructure
Aging changes
Reactions to injury
Neoplastic counterparts

from the neural tube or neural crest, the microglia are the progeny of bone marrow–derived monocytes that subsequently colonize the CNS).

All of the many cell types that compose the nervous system participate in a wide variety of pathologic processes, which are discussed in the latter half of this book. The following sections provide a foundational review of the basic features of each cellular constituent, with particular attention to the distinguishing aspects of light microscopy, ultrastructure, immunocytochemistry, and the alterations produced by aging, injury, and neoplastic transformation (Table 2-2).

NEURONS

Light Microscopic Morphology

The basic functional unit of the nervous system is the neuron. While the stereotypical neuron is exemplified by large projection-class neurons such as the Betz cells of the cerebral cortex and the alpha-motor neurons of the spinal cord, the actual range of neuronal sizes and shapes is exceedingly broad. A striking comparison of the extremes of neuronal morphology is seen in sharp contrast in the cerebellar cortex, with the juxtaposition of Purkinje cells and granular cell neurons.

The prototypical neuronal morphologic features, as exemplified by Purkinje cells and motor neurons, are a large cell body (soma; perikaryon), a large nucleus with a single, prominent, centrally located nucleolus, and *conspicuous rough endoplasmic reticulum ("Nissl substance")* (Table 2-3; Fig. 2-1). Granular cell neurons, in contrast, are hardly recognizable as neuronal by these criteria; they appear to consist of only small naked nuclei by light microscopy (Fig. 2-2).

Between these two extremes exists a richly textured spectrum of morphologic subtypes, varying in the size and shape of the soma, number and type of cell processes, and length of axon. Notable specialized variants include the amacrine cells of the retina (amacrine: *a macros inos*, literally, "no long process"—from the lack of an axon in these neurons—a feature shared with the granular cell neurons of the olfactory bulb), and the neurons of the mesen-

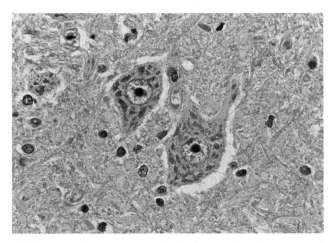

TABLE 2-3. LIGHT MICROSCOPIC FEATURES OF NEURONS

Large cell body
Nucleus with single prominent nucleolus
Nissl substance

FIGURE 2-1. Motor neurons. Classical "ganglion cell" neuronal features are characteristic of large projection-class neurons such as motor neurons and Purkinje cells, and include a large cell body (soma), nucleus with a single large nucleolus, and prominent basophilic Nissl substance (rough endoplasmic reticulum and polyribosomes) in the cytoplasm.

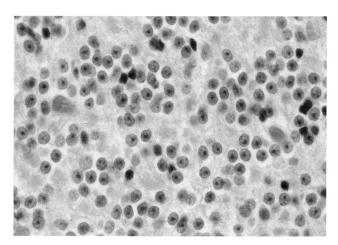

FIGURE 2-2. Granular cell neurons. Small "local circuit" neurons, such as those of the cerebellum and hippocampal formation, do not display prominent Nissl substance or the other features of large neurons and appear as only "naked nuclei."

cephalic nucleus of the trigeminal nerve (Fig. 2-3), which are true unipolar (or, from a developmental viewpoint, pseudounipolar) neurons, i.e., neurons which possess only a single cell process emanating from the cell body (this configuration is consistent with the unique status of these cells as the only primary [first order] sensory neurons whose cell bodies are located intraaxially; all other primary sensory neuronal perikarya are found in either the cranial sensory ganglia or the spinal dorsal root ganglia).

Distribution

Neurons are found in densest concentration in the gray matter of the cortices and deep nuclei of the cerebrum. It is not uncommon, however, to find isolated neuronal cell bodies in normal white matter. This fact is not of purely academic interest. One location that frequently exhibits neurons in white mat-

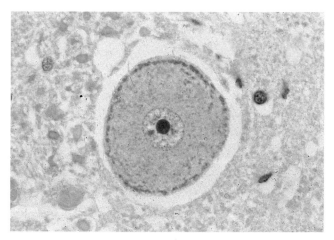

FIGURE 2-3. Unipolar neurons of the mesencephalic nucleus of the trigeminal nerve. Among the many varied morphologies exhibited by neurons, that of the mesencephalic nucleus of cranial nerve V is unique; these are the only primary sensory unipolar neurons with cell bodies located within the CNS rather than externally in cranial and spinal ganglia.

ter is the temporal lobe. This must be borne in mind to avoid diagnosing a neuronal migration disorder. As an additional example, when assessing neoplasms originating in this location, it is important to remember the normal presence of scattered neurons in temporal lobe white matter in order to avoid misdiagnosing a white matter glioma with entrapped neuronal cell bodies as a ganglioglioma. The broader problem of distinguishing entrapped neurons from neoplastic neurons in tumors that infiltrate gray matter structures is discussed later.

Immunocytochemistry

Neuron-specific immunochemical markers have long been sought to aid in tumor diagnosis, imaging, and treatment (Table 2-4). One such marker introduced early on was neuron-specific enolase (NSE). Unfortunately, despite the optimistic name, the *non*-specificity of anti-NSE antibodies for neuronal differentiation has achieved wide notoriety. Currently, *the most useful and widely used neuronal marker is synaptophysin* (Fig. 2-4). Synaptophysin is a major integral membrane protein of synaptic vesicles and antibodies directed against synaptophysin have so far proved quite useful in detecting neuronal differentiation in a wide variety of neoplasms. Most importantly, synaptophysin expression is relatively independent of the degree of neuronal morphologic differentiation exhibited by the tumor as assessed by light microscopy, thus providing a useful diagnostic adjunct applicable to neuronal neoplasms as histologically and biologically diverse as gangliogliomas and primitive neuroectodermal tumors. *NeuN is a recently introduced neuronal marker that has the advantage of nuclear localization* (Fig. 2-5), rather than the exclusive cell membrane or cytoplasmic staining that is seen with synaptophysin, thus providing unambiguous identification of individual cell positivity. An additional neuronal marker, alpha-synuclein, is widely employed to facilitate visualization of inclusion bodies, as discussed in later chapters.

Ultrastructure

The most informative ultrastructural features of neurons are dense-core ("neurosecretory") vesicles, clear ("presynaptic") vesicles, synaptic junctions, and neuro-

TABLE 2-4. IMMUNOHISTOCHEMICAL MARKERS FOR NEURONAL DIFFERENTIATION

Synaptophysin
NeuN
Neurofilament proteins
Neuron-specific enolase[a]

[a] *Not* specific for neurons!

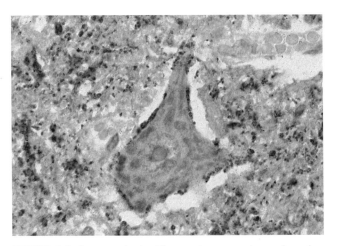

FIGURE 2-4. Synaptophysin. The most commonly used marker for neuronal differentiation is synaptophysin, which labels neuropil with a diffuse punctate granular pattern and also decorates large neuronal cell bodies as seen here.

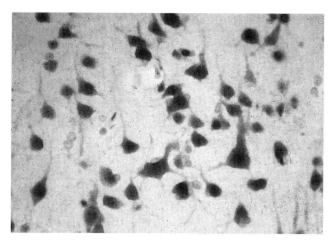

FIGURE 2-5. NeuN. In contrast to synaptophysin, NeuN strongly labels neuronal nuclei.

tubule bundles (Table 2-5; Figs. 2-6 and 2-7). These signatures are retained to a greater or lesser extent in many tumors of neuronal lineage. In general, synaptic junctions are found only in the most differentiated lesions (i.e., in tumors that are clearly recognizable as neuronal by routine H&E histology, such as ganglion cell tumors), whereas dense-core granules and neurotubule bundles may be present in more primitive neuronal neoplasms (i.e., in tumors in which the differentiation status is not clearly discernible by routine histology and, hence, ultrastructural help is needed) and are therefore often more useful markers.

Aging Changes

Although arguably the single most common and pronounced aging effect on neurons is simple death and subsequent dropout, many neurons undergo a variety of other changes that are far more visually striking (Table 2-6). The most frequently encountered of these are the aging inclusions, of which the most common is *lipofuscin* (lipochrome; "wear and tear" pigment). Lipofuscin accumulates in many neuronal populations, but is most obvious in large, pro-

TABLE 2-5. ULTRASTRUCTURAL FEATURES OF NEURONS

Dense-core ("neurosecretory") vesicles
Neurotubule bundles
Clear ("presynaptic") vesicles
Synaptic junctions

TABLE 2-6. AGING CHANGES SEEN IN NEURONS

Simple loss
Lipofuscin accumulation
Neuromelanin
Marinesco bodies
Hyaline ("colloid") inclusions
Alzheimer's changes

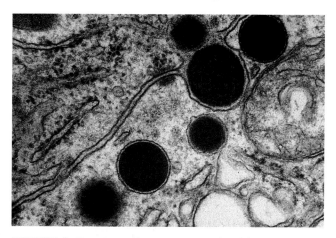

FIGURE 2-6. Dense core ("neurosecretory") vesicles. Neurosecretory vesicles are an ultrastructural hallmark of neuronal or neuroendocrine differentiation.

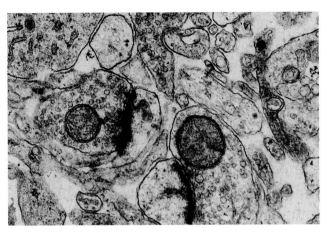

FIGURE 2-7. Synapses and clear synaptic vesicles. Although extremely specific for neuronal differentiation, synapses and synaptic vesicles are generally only seen in very mature neuronal neoplasms, such as ganglion cell tumors. Identification of these structures played a major role in the discovery of central neurocytoma.

jection-class neurons, where it displaces cytoplasmic organelles, often to the point of mimicking central chromatolysis (other mimics of central chromatolysis are discussed below). The lateral geniculate body provides an example of a densely populated nucleus whose neuron's prominent accumulation of lipofuscin is often discernible macroscopically at autopsy in the form of a subtle but distinctly mahogany hue compared to adjacent cortex.

The pigmented nuclei of the brain stem owe their unique cognomen to the accumulation of "*neuromelanin*," which is a by-product of catecholaminergic neurotransmitter synthesis that gradually accumulates with age. Neuromelanin is a bona fide member of the loosely defined melanin congener family, but is distinctly different from other classes of melanins, including "melanocytic" melanin, in terms of its synthetic pathway, biochemical composition, precursor organelle scaffolding, and various measurable physicochemical properties. Parenthetically, true "melanocytic" melanin is also an autochthonous intracranial constituent: it is found in leptomeningeal melanocytes.

Intranuclear inclusions, termed "Marinesco bodies," may also be seen in neurons with a frequency directly related to increasing age (Fig. 2-8). These are largely confined to specific neuronal populations; in this case to the pigmented brain stem nuclei, principally the substantia nigra and locus ceruleus. Marinesco bodies are brightly eosinophilic, about the size of a nucleolus, and may be single or, not infrequently, multiple with up to four to five per nucleus. Marinesco bodies provide the most frequently encountered example of Cowdry type B intranuclear inclusions. The importance of recognizing Marinesco bodies lies in avoiding their potential misidentification as intranuclear viral inclusions! Marinesco bodies are not viral in origin, and, although their significance has yet to be fully (or, in truth, even partially) elucidated, they have so far not been definitively linked with any pathological process. It is also important not to confuse the *intranuclear Marinesco body* with the *cytoplasmic Lewy body*, which is seen in the same population of neurons in Parkinson's disease (Fig. 2-9).

Another cytoplasmic inclusion that is often striking is the *hyaline (colloid) inclusion, which is seen predominantly in the motor neurons of the hypoglossal nucleus* and, less often, in the ventral horn motor neurons of the spinal cord (Fig.

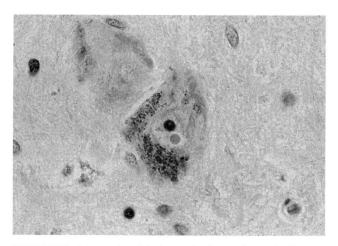

FIGURE 2-8. Intranuclear Marinesco body. Marinesco bodies are brightly eosinophilic intranuclear inclusions most commonly seen in the pigmented neurons of the substantia nigra and locus ceruleus. There may be from one to four or five per nucleus. Marinesco bodies are seen in increasing numbers with increasing age, have no pathologic significance, and should not be mistaken for intranuclear viral inclusions.

2-10). These intensely eosinophilic inclusions have been shown to consist of dilated endoplasmic reticulum cisternae by electron microscopy, and, although visually arresting, have no proven pathologic correlation.

Among aging inclusions in neurons, one unique group warrants special consideration—those associated with *Alzheimer's disease: neurofibrillary tangles, granulovacuolar degeneration (of Simchowitz), and Hirano bodies* (Table 2-7; Figs. 2-11 through 2-13). Sparse numbers of all of these structures may be found in aged individuals with no history of altered mentation. The presence of more than an occasional inclusion, however, should sound the tocsin and prompt a thorough dementia evaluation.

TABLE 2-7. ALZHEIMER'S DISEASE INCLUSIONS SEEN IN NEURONS

Neurofibrillary tangles
Granulovacuolar degeneration (of Simchowitz)
Hirano bodies

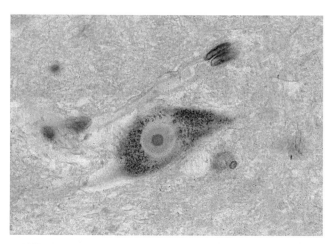

FIGURE 2-9. Intracytoplasmic Lewy body. Lewy bodies, the characteristic inclusions of Parkinson's disease, like Marinesco bodies are brightly eosinophilic and occur in the same populations of pigmented neurons; however, Lewy bodies are intracytoplasmic, whereas Marinesco bodies are intranuclear. Among the many inclusion bodies that can be seen in neurons in various diseases, Lewy bodies are probably the most conspicuous because of the way they are highlighted by the surrounding neuromelanin of their host cells, reminiscent of the former use of India ink as a "negative stain" to highlight crytococcus in the cerebrospinal fluid.

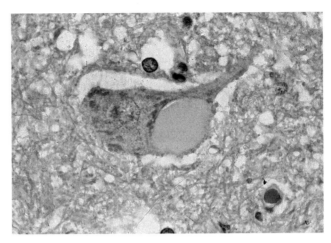

FIGURE 2-10. Hyaline (colloid) inclusion. Hyaline inclusions are seen in only two populations of neurons: the hypoglossal nucleus in the floor of the medullary fourth ventricle, in which they are quite common, and, more rarely, in the motor neurons of the anterior horns of the spinal cord. They consist of dilated cisternae of endoplasmic reticulum and have no known pathologic significance.

TABLE 2-8. CONDITIONS IN WHICH NEUROFIBRILLARY TANGLES CAN BE SEEN

Aging
Dementing diseases
Tuberous sclerosis
Meningioangiomatosis
Ganglion cell tumors

An additional note with respect to neurofibrillary tangles: they may also be *rarely* encountered in a few conditions other than aging and the various dementing diseases, namely, tuberous sclerosis, meningioangiomatosis, and in occasional ganglion cell tumors (Table 2-8). It is likely that neurofibrillary tangles are the end product of a final common pathway of neuronal demise shared by many different disease entities.

Pathologic Reactions

Simple Dropout

One of the most common reactions of neurons to a wide variety of insults—particularly those of a chronic, subacute nature—is simple loss. As with aging

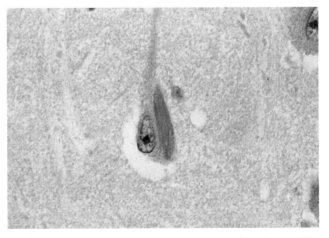

FIGURE 2-11. Neurofibrillary tangle. Intracytoplasmic neurofibrillary tangles take on the shape of the neuron's cell body. In this example, a pyramidal cell of the hippocampal formation, the tangle extends from the cell body into the large apical dendrite giving it the classical "flame" shape characteristic of this neuronal population. In neurons with round somas, such as those of the locus ceruleus, the tangles are globoid in shape.

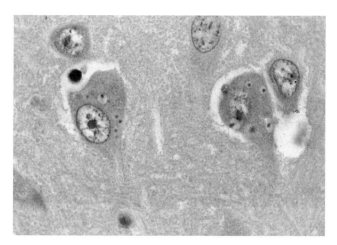

FIGURE 2-12. Granulovacuolar degeneration (of Simchowitz). As the name states, GVD consists of small cytoplasmic vacuoles that each contain a granule. The number of these inclusions varies from one to dozens that literally fill the cytoplasm.

changes, under certain conditions more picturesque (and informative!) cellular alterations may be seen, as detailed below (Table 2-9).

Ischemic Change

Ischemic/hypoxic damage to the nervous system is manifested in the acute stage by the appearance of "red neurons"—neurons that display conspicuous, brightly eosinophilic cytoplasm (with concomitant loss of the basophilic Nissl substance) and dark, pyknotic nuclei in which the typically prominent nucleolus is not discernible (Fig. 2-14). *The "red neuron" is the sine qua non of ischemic/hypoxic insult to the CNS.* Although most commonly encountered in the setting of acute cerebral infarction, ischemic change is nonspecific and may

TABLE 2-9. THE SPECTRUM OF REACTIONS OF NEURONS TO DISEASE

Simple loss
Ischemic change
Central chromatolysis
Mineralization ("ferruginization")
Pathologic inclusions

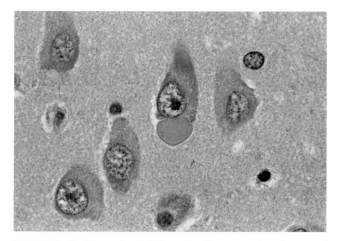

FIGURE 2-13. Hirano body. Hirano bodies are oval to elongated rod-shaped eosinophilic inclusions that on routine H&E-stained sections appear either to be free in the neuropil or nestled up in close apposition to neuronal cell bodies. Ultrastructural studies have shown them to be located within neuronal cytoplasmic processes. Hirano bodies are composed of a mixture of cytoskeletal elements including alpha-actinin.

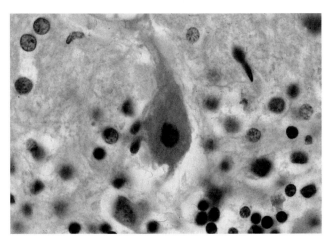

FIGURE 2-14. Red neuron. As illustrated by this Purkinje neuron, the hallmark of hypoxic/ischemic insult to the nervous system is the "red neuron." Red refers to the pronounced eosinophilia of ischemic neuron's cytoplasm, which normally should be studded with basophilic Nissl substance. The other characteristic features are a shrunken cell body and a shrunken, darkly pyknotic nucleus in which the normally prominent large nucleolus can no longer be seen. These ischemic changes are obviously more readily seen in large neurons like pyramidal cells and Purkinje cells as compared to small neurons like granular cells.

TABLE 2-10. HISTOLOGIC FEATURES OF CENTRAL CHROMATOLYSIS

Margination of the Nissl substance
Margination of the nucleus
Swelling of the cell body
Rounding off of the soma

be seen in the vicinal gray matter of a wide variety of lesions, including, for example, malignant gliomas! *Caveat medicus*: the presence of ischemic neurons in a neurosurgical biopsy does not exclude the possibility of an underlying malignancy!

Central Chromatolysis

Damage to an axon in relative proximity to the neuronal cell body characteristically results in a distinctive constellation of morphologic changes referred to as central chromatolysis (Table 2-10; Figs. 2-15 and 2-16).

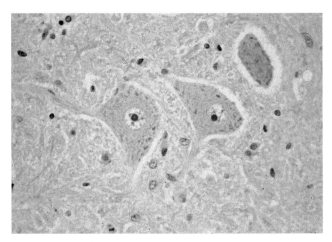

FIGURE 2-15. Healthy motor neurons. Central chromatolysis is best appreciated by direct comparison with normal neurons in which robust angular dendritic branches and evenly distributed Nissl substance are seen.

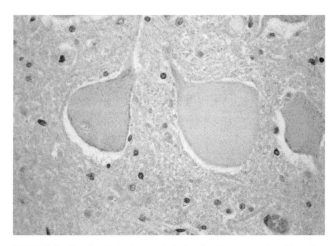

FIGURE 2-16. Central chromatolysis. As the name implies, the hallmark of central chromatolysis is loss of the basophilic Nissl substance in the central part of the cell body. The nucleus is also marginated to the periphery of the soma and there is swelling of the cell body with resultant rounding off of the soma contour.

When compared to normal neuronal morphology, the *principal feature of central chromatolysis, as the name implies, is peripheral margination of the Nissl substance*, with resultant central homogeneous eosinophilic clearing of the cell body. This conspicuous alteration is accompanied by peripheral displacement of the nucleus, perikaryal swelling, and general rounding off of the normally angular cell body profile.

In the setting of axonal damage, the central chromatolysis response is often appropriately referred to as "axonal reaction." Central chromatolysis, however, is not strictly pathognomonic of axon injury *per se*; it is also a feature of other, more specific, pathologic entities—most notably *pellagra* and *Wernicke's encephalopathy*.

Peripheral chromatolysis, i.e., loss of Nissl substance from only the periphery of the soma with central preservation, is much more rarely encountered than central chromatolysis and has been ascribed by some investigators to a stage of recovery from the latter process.

There are numerous *mimickers of central chromatolysis* that lie in wait for the unwary (Table 2-11). For example, some neuronal populations display Nissl substance that is normally preferentially distributed peripherally in the soma. Other neurons, such as the unipolar neurons of the mesencephalic nucleus of the trigeminal nerve, mentioned above, have large, exquisitely rounded somas, thus mimicking that aspect of central chromatolysis. Additionally, a variety of substances may accumulate within the cell body, displacing the Nissl substance to the periphery and thereby mimicking central chromatolysis. The most common such substance is lipofuscin, which may accumulate to a truly impressive extent in some populations of large neurons, such as the anterior horn motor neurons of the spinal cord, the inferior olivary neurons of the medulla, the cerebellar dentate nuclei neurons, and the lateral geniculate nuclei neurons. (Interestingly, although lipofuscin accumulation is usually confined to large neurons, it is not simply a function of cell size as some classes of very large neurons appear comparatively immune to significant accumulation, such as the cerebellar Purkinje cells.) Additional substances that may accumulate in the cell body and displace the Nissl substance peripherally, thus mimicking central chromatolysis, include those of the broad spectrum of hereditary storage disorders.

TABLE 2-11. NORMAL CELLS AND DISEASES THAT MIMIC CENTRAL CHROMATOLYSIS

Normal Cells	Feature
Betz cells	large size
Mesencephalic nucleus of cranial nerve V	rounded soma
Lipofuscin	displaced nucleus and Nissl
Clarke's nucleus	eccentric nuclei
Paraventricular and supraoptic nuclei	eccentric nucleus and Nissl
Diseases	
Storage disorders	displaced nucleus and Nissl
Ganglion cell tumors	eccentric nucleus and Nissl

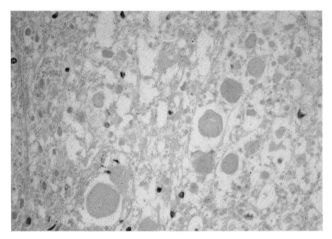

FIGURE 2-17. Axonal spheroids. Axonal injury is frequently manifest as swollen dilatations termed "axonal spheroids" or "axon retraction balls." Axonal spheroids can be seen in many disease states but are very characteristic of a few such as radiation necrosis of the pons and traumatic diffuse axonal injury.

Axonal Spheroids

A commonly encountered reaction to injury exhibited by axons is the formation of localized dilatations known as axonal spheroids (also called "axonal retraction balls"; Fig. 2-17). Ultrastructural examination shows greatly distended axons filled with neurofilament bundles and subcellular organelles. A regional variant of this process is often observed in the granular layer of the cerebellar cortex where focal dilatations of Purkinje cell axons have historically been termed "*axon torpedoes.*" These structures are seen in a variety of cerebellar degenerative diseases as well as in normal aging.

Another site where axonal spheroids are commonly seen as an incidental finding in aged individuals is in the fasciculus gracilis in the vicinity of nucleus gracilis of the brain stem medulla. Spheroids in this location often undergo secondary mineralization (Fig. 2-18).

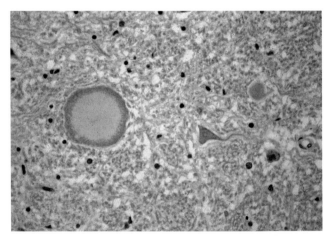

FIGURE 2-18. Mineralized axonal spheroid in fasciculus gracilis. Experienced neuropathologists are familiar with seeing scattered axonal spheroids in the most rostral part of the fasciculus gracilis near its termination in the nucleus gracilis in the medulla. Axonal spheroids at this location are frequently mineralized and are a very common incidental finding at autopsy in asymptomatic older individuals.

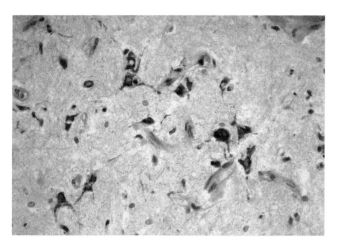

FIGURE 2-19. Ferruginized neurons. Mineral-encrusted cell bodies of expired neurons are commonly seen adjacent to healed infarcts.

Caveat: Not all axonal dilatations are pathological or degenerative in nature! Prominent axonal swellings are routinely encountered in the infundibulum and neurohypophysis; these structures are specialized storage sites for the hormones of the hypothalamo-hypophyseal tract, oxytocin and vasopressin, and are termed "*Herring bodies.*"

Mineralization ("Ferrugination")

While the vast majority of neurons that succumb to various nefarious insults to the nervous system pass quietly unnoticed into oblivion, a privileged few are immortalized as mineral-encrusted statues—historical monuments to an epic struggle that transpired in earlier times. Such "ferruginized" neurons are most frequently encountered in the neural parenchyma adjacent to the cystic cavities of remote infarcts (Fig. 2-19). *Damaged axons, as well, may acquire a patina of iron and mineral salts*; such clusters may be mistaken for fungal hyphae by the inexperienced or diagnostically challenged (Fig. 2-20).

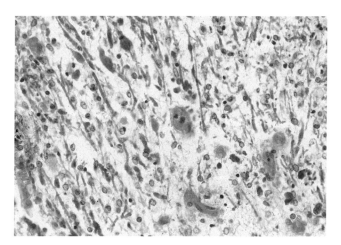

FIGURE 2-20. Ferruginized axon cluster. Clusters of axons in white matter can also become fossilized through mineral salt deposition. Care must be taken not to misinterpret these for fungal hyphae.

TABLE 2-12. PATHOLOGIC INCLUSIONS SEEN IN NEURONS IN VARIOUS DISEASES

Intracytoplasmic		Intranuclear	
Inclusion	**Disease**	**Inclusion**	**Disease**
Neurofibrillary tangles	Alzheimer's disease	Cowdry type A	Cytomegalovirus; herpes; subacute sclerosing panencephalitis
Pick bodies	Pick's disease		
Lewy bodies	Parkinson's disease Lewy body disease		
Negri bodies	Rabies	Cowdry type B	Acute polio
Polyglucosan bodies	PGB disease		
Lafora bodies	Myoclonic epilepsy	Intranuclear inclusions	Huntington's disease
Bunina bodies	Amyotrophic lateral sclerosis		

Pathologic Inclusions

In addition to normally occurring nonpathologic substances such as lipofuscin, neuromelanin, and Marinesco bodies, a wide variety of abnormal intranuclear and intracytoplasmic inclusions may be encountered in neurons (Table 2-12). Already mentioned in this regard are the intracytoplasmic inclusions of storage disorders and Alzheimer's disease. Other degenerative/dementing illnesses that are accompanied by characteristic intracytoplasmic inclusions are Pick's disease (Pick's bodies), Parkinson's disease (Lewy bodies), Lewy body disease (Lewy bodies), and polyglucosan body disease (polyglucosan bodies). Still further examples of intracytoplasmic inclusions include Lafora bodies (myoclonic epilepsy) and Bunina bodies (first described in amyotrophic lateral sclerosis); the latter inclusion is frequently encountered only on board examinations.

Intranuclear inclusions may be divided into two classes based purely on morphologic criteria: Cowdry type A and Cowdry type B. The salient characteristics of these eosinophilic inclusions were delineated by E. V. Cowdry in 1934 (Table 2-13). By far the most commonly encountered in pathologic conditions are the type A inclusions, which are typified by those seen in viral encephalitis produced by Herpes simplex, Herpes simiae Varicella zoster, cytomegalovirus, measles virus (in subacute sclerosing panencephalitis), and, occasionally, JC virus (in progressive multifocal leukoencephalopathy; although "ground glass" inclusions are much more typical of JC virus) (Fig. 2-21). *Type B inclusions*, in contrast, are more limited in distribution. An example is provided by the inclusions observed in anterior horn cells in *acute* poliomyelitis. Despite the frequent association with viral encephalitides, neither type of intranuclear inclusion is pathognomonic of viral infection. In fact, the quotidian Marinesco bodies that are routinely observed in the neurons of the pigmented brain stem nuclei are sterling examples of the Cowdry type B *beau idéal* (Fig. 2-22).

Not all viral intranuclear inclusions are of either classic Cowdry type A or type B morphology: witness the homogeneous *"ground glass" inclusions produced in oligodendroglial nuclei by JC virus in progressive multifocal leukoencephalopathy*, which are far more prevalent in this disease than are type A inclusions (Fig. 2-23 and 2-24).

Neoplastic Counterparts

Neuronal neoplasms display a wide range of morphologies, from the primitive, embryonic features of neuroblastoma to the mature lineaments of gan-

TABLE 2-13. COWDRY INCLUSIONS

Cowdry type A
  Large
  Solitary
  Surrounded by halo
  Effacement of nucleus
Cowdry type B
  Small
  Multiple
  No halos
  No effacement of nucleus

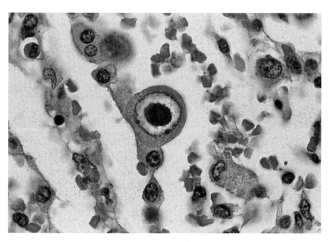

FIGURE 2-21. Cowdry type A inclusion. Intranuclear inclusions can take one of three morphologic patterns: Cowdry A, Cowdry B, or ground glass. Cowdry A inclusions, as exemplified here by cytomegalovirus, are large, solitary, and surrounded by a clear halo secondary to peripheral margination of the nuclear chromatin.

gliocytoma. All, however, have in common the expression of one or more phenotypic traits characteristic of neurons in general. Thus, *the hallmark of "ganglionic" differentiation at the light microscopic level is the presence of Nissl substance.* Reactive or neoplastic astrocytes may mimic many of the features of ganglion cells, such as a large prominent solitary nucleolus, but they do not possess the abundant rough endoplasmic reticulum and polyribosomal aggregates that form the Nissl substance of large neurons and neoplastic ganglion cells. This observation was exploited in former times with the use of "Nissl stains"—basophilic stains such as Cresyl violet—that highlighted nucleic acids and thus helped to distinguish neuronal differentiation. With the advent of immunohistochemistry and the ready availability of many antibodies that rec-

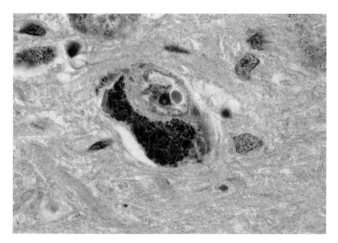

FIGURE 2-22. Cowdry type B inclusions. In contrast to Cowdry A inclusions, Cowdry B inclusions, as exemplified here by Marinesco bodies in the nucleus of a pigmented neuron of the substantia nigra, are small and multiple. The only viral infection in which Cowdry B, rather than Cowdry A, inclusions are seen is acute polio. No inclusions are seen in survivors with post-polio syndrome as the infected neurons have long since died and disappeared.

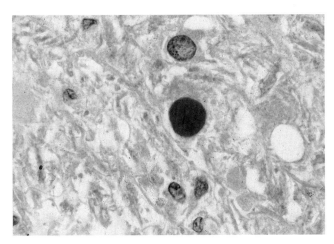

FIGURE 2-23. "Ground glass" inclusion. The third type of intranuclear viral inclusion is termed "ground glass" because of the homogenized appearance. As seen here in progressive multifocal leukoencephalopathy (PML), oligodendrocytes infected with the JC virus have enlarged nuclei with a homogenous smudging of the chromatin. On H&E-stained tissue sections, the ground glass nuclei are also purplish compared to the normal dark blue.

TABLE 2–14. TYPES OF ROSETTES SEEN IN NEURONAL AND GLIAL TUMORS

Neuronal	Glial
Homer Wright (neuroblastoma type)	Ependymomatous Perivascular pseudorosettes
Flexner-Wintersteiner (retinoblastoma type)	
Pineocytomatous	

ognize neuron-associated antigens, the use of Nissl stains has largely been supplanted.

Evidence for neuronal differentiation in neoplasms that are less well-differentiated than ganglion cell tumors is sometimes provided by the presence of tumor cell rosettes. Several types of rosettes may be formed by neuronal tumors; others are more typical of glial tumors (Table 2-14). Although somewhat pedantic, some authors distinguish between so-called "true" rosettes and "pseudo" rosettes based on the presence or absence of a central lumen; examples of the former include *Flexner–Wintersteiner (retinoblastoma type) rosettes* (Fig. 2-25) and "true" ependymoma rosettes, and of the latter: *Homer Wright (neuroblastoma type) rosettes* (Fig. 2-26) and the perivascular pseudorosettes of ependymomas.

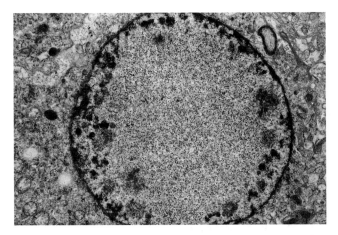

FIGURE 2-24. Ultrastructure of ground glass inclusions. As illustrated in this electron micrograph of an oligodendroglial cell infected with JC virus, ground glass nuclei result from intranuclear replication of the virions that fill the nucleus and displace the chromatin peripherally.

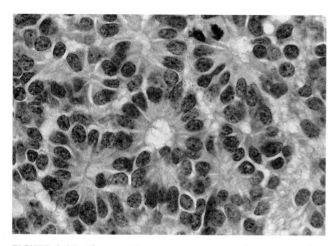

FIGURE 2-25. Flexner–Wintersteiner rosettes. These are called "true rosettes" because a central lumen is formed by the tumor cells in the center of the rosette. Flexner–Wintersteiner rosettes are characteristic of retinoblastoma and can also be seen in other types of primitive neuroectodermal tumors (PNETs).

For more "primitive" and problematic tumors, *evidence of neuronal differentiation may be sought in the form of immunohistochemical positivity for synaptophysin, NeuN* or other neuronal markers. By electron microscopy, the presence of dense-core vesicles, neurotubule bundles, presynaptic vesicles or synapses provide evidence of neuronal differentiation.

One footnote on "differentiation" in neuronal neoplasms: the end point of "maturation" is not always typified by large "ganglion cells" with features that resemble motor neurons or Purkinje cells. The granular cell neurons of the cerebellum, for example, are fully differentiated neurons that do not display prominent Nissl substance (or even cytoplasm!) by routine H&E microscopy. Thus, by analogy, some CNS neoplasms that are composed of small, ostensibly "poorly differentiated" cells that evince neuronal pheno-

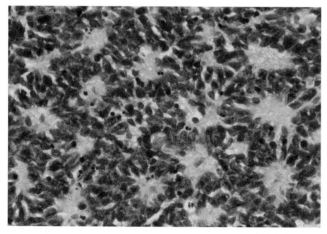

FIGURE 2-26. Homer Wright rosettes. Homer Wright rosettes differ from Flexner–Wintersteiner rosettes in that there is no central lumen; rather, the center of the rosette is filled with the intertwined cytoplasmic processes of the tumor cells. Homer Wright rosettes are characteristic of neuroblastoma and medulloblastoma, and can also be seen in other PNETs.

typic characteristics only by immunochemistry or electron microscopy may not be "primitive" neuronal tumors (with the attendant implication of aggressive behavior), but rather may be comparatively "mature" (and potentially more indolent) tumors that have differentiated along the morphologic lines of the smaller neuronal subtypes indigenous to the nervous system. An example of this type of neuronal tumor is provided by central neurocytoma.

ASTROCYTES

Light Microscopy

Astrocytes (literally "star cells") have traditionally been divided on the basis of morphologic criteria into two main categories: the protoplasmic astrocytes of gray matter and the fibrous astrocytes of white matter. The principal difference between these two groups being degree of cytoplasmic process branching; fibrous astrocytes show relatively more numerous and extensive processes compared to protoplasmic astrocytes.

Consonant with their more robust arborization, fibrous astrocytes also exhibit more abundant glial intermediate filaments by electron microscopy and more prominent labeling with antibodies directed against glial fibrillary acidic protein (GFAP) epitopes. There are other, specialized, astrocytic variants in some regions of the nervous system (Table 2-15); the most prominent example being the Bergmann glia of the cerebellum.

Immunochemistry

Antibodies directed against glial fibrillary acidic protein (GFAP) constitute an invaluable diagnostic aid in identifying cells of glial lineage, and are of particular importance in the evaluation of neoplasms that exhibit complex mixed or ambiguous cellular constituents (Fig. 2-27). Astrocytes and their reactive and neoplastic progeny also exhibit strong immunopositivity for S-100 protein (as do the other glial cell types: oligodendroglia, the ependyma, and the choroid plexus epithelium).

TABLE 2-15. SPECIALIZED SUBTYPES OF ASTROCYTES

Fibrous (Fibrillary)
Protoplasmic
Bergmann
Velate

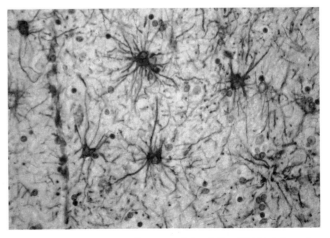

FIGURE 2-27. Astrocytes immunostained for GFAP. Astrocytes are characterised by many delicately radiating cytoplasmic processes that are exquisitely visualized by immunostaining for glial fibrillary acidic protein (GFAP).

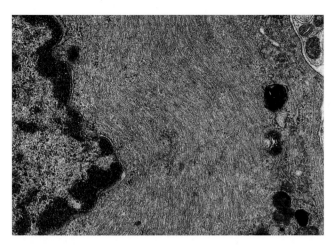

FIGURE 2-28. Astrocytic intermediate filaments (ultrastructure). The immunopositivity of astrocytes for GFAP is due to their content of glial filaments composed of that protein. Ultrastructurally, glial filaments are indistinguishable from the other types of intermediate diameter filaments.

Ultrastructure

The most salient distinguishing feature of astrocytes is their content of glial filaments, which are visualized at the ultrastructural level as *"intermediate filaments"* (Fig. 2-28). The propensity to extend cytoplasmic processes with "end feet" that form junctions with blood vessels and at the nervous system parenchymal periphery with the pia mater are also typical of astrocytic ultrastructure.

Caveat: With regard to the ultrastructural identification of intermediate filaments, under the electron microscope filaments are traditionally categorized by cross-sectional diameter into thin, intermediate, and thick (Table 2-16). The various members of the intermediate filament group (GFAP, desmin, cytokeratins, neurofilament proteins, vimentin, and nestin) exhibit identical ultrastructural features and are indistinguishable from one another; immunohistochemistry performed with specific antibodies is required for definitive identification.

Aging Changes

The principal light microscopic manifestation of aging in astrocytes is the accumulation of cytoplasmic inclusions termed *"corpora amylacea"* (Fig. 2-29).

TABLE 2-16. CLASSIFICATION AND COMPOSITION OF CYTOPLASMIC CYTOSKELETAL FILAMENTS AND TUBULES

Thin (5–7 nm)	Intermediate (10–12 nm)	Thick (16 nm)	Microtubules (24 nm)
Actin	Glial fibrillary acidic protein Neurofilament proteins Cytokeratins Desmin Vimentin Nestin	Myosin	Tubulin

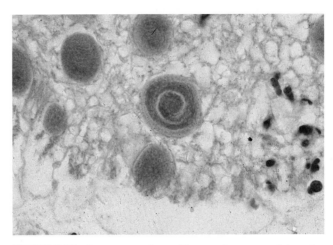

FIGURE 2-29. Corpora amylacea. The most common intracytoplasmic inclusions seen in astrocytes are corpora amylacea. These concentrically laminated spheres increase with advancing patient age.

These spherical bodies are composed of glucose polymers ("polyglucosan bodies") and, although they may be found in virtually any CNS location, exhibit a distinct proclivity for perivascular and subpial locations (Figs. 2-30 and 2-31). Their numbers increase with advancing age. Although there is a specific illness associated with polyglucosan bodies (Polyglucosan Body Disease), there is no convincing evidence of any deleterious effect of normal corpora amylacea, which may be present in striking numbers in the predilection areas in some people.

Corpora amylacea pose one potential hazard to the diagnostician unaccustomed to their appearance and characteristic anatomic distribution; they can be mistaken for fungal yeast, particularly when found in large numbers in the subpial vicinity where *they not infrequently are artifactually dislodged during tissue sectioning and may thereby appear to be freely disseminating within the subarachnoid space.* To make the possibility of diagnostic error even greater, corpora amylacea are strongly positive for all of the most commonly employed

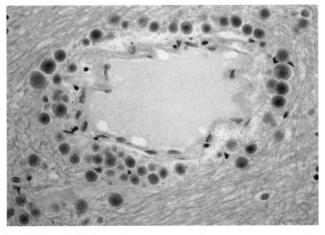

FIGURE 2-30. Perivascular corpora amylacea. Corpora amylacea are often found in highest concentration in astrocytic cell processes around blood vessels, as seen here, and beneath the pia.

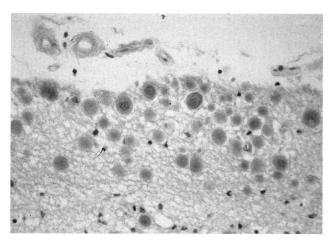

FIGURE 2-31. Subpial corpora amylacea. The subpial corpora amylacea are often artifactually dislodged during tissue sectioning and can appear to be floating in the subarachnoid space, mimicking cryptococcus or other fungal yeast.

fungal stains, including PAS, Alcian blue, and Gomori methenamine silver (GMS) (Fig. 2-32). Upon close scrutiny, however, the singular concentric multilaminar structure is usually apparent, and is quite distinctive *vis-a-vis* cryptococcus and other fungal pathogen yeast forms; moreover, in contrast to cryptococcus, corpora amylacea have never been observed to reproduce by budding!

Pathologic Reactions

Gliosis

Astrocytes serve as sentinels for the CNS, always on the qui vive for insult of any stripe. While normally among the most morphologically demure of ner-

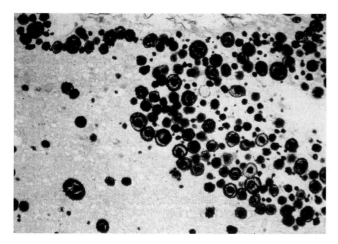

FIGURE 2-32. Corpora amylacea: fungal stain. Corpora amylacea stain intensely with all of the commonly employed fungal stains, including Alcian blue, periodic acid–Schiff (PAS), and, as illustrated here, Gomori methenamine silver (GMS). Thus, if corpora are initially mistaken for yeast on H&E-stained tissue sections and confirmation is sought through use of a fungal stain, the potential for diagnostic misadventure is obvious!

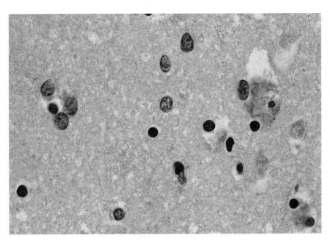

FIGURE 2-33. Cell types and neuropil of the CNS. All of the principal cell types of the CNS are seen in this photomicrograph: a neuron with its large cell body, prominent nucleolus and abundant cytoplasm; the small, dark and perfectly round nuclei of oligodendrocytes; and the larger, more oval nuclei of astrocytes. The background substance between the cells, which by electron microscopy is found to be composed of axons, dendrites, and glial cell processes, is called "neuropil."

vous system constituents, with only "naked nuclei" typically visible by routine H&E morphology (Fig. 2-33), astrocytes respond rapidly and dramatically to CNS injury. The astrocytic response typically consists of two components: hypertrophy and hyperplasia. The initial hypertrophic response, an increase in cell size and cytoplasmic prominence, occurs rapidly following CNS damage. In fact, *the observable presence of well-defined astrocytic cytoplasm on routine H&E tissue sections per se usually indicates reactive gliosis and is prima facie evidence of CNS injury* (Fig. 2-34).

Reactive astrocytes display a range in the amount of cytoplasm present, from just barely discernible to strikingly embonpoint. The latter cells are known as *"gemistocytes"* (literally, "stuffed cells") (Fig. 2-35), and have neo-

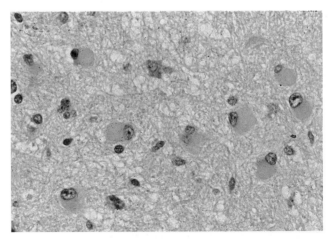

FIGURE 2-34. Reactive astrocytosis. Reactive astrocytes are identified on H&E-stained sections by the conspicuous presence of their cytoplasm; in the absence of any noxious stimulation, normal astrocytes display only naked nuclei.

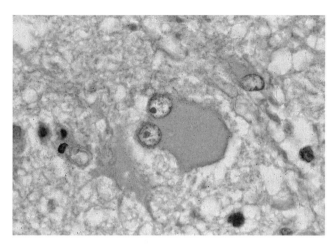

FIGURE 2-35. Gemistocytic astrocytosis. Large reactive astrocytes with cell bodies greatly distended with glial intermediate filaments are termed "reactive gemistocytes."

plastic counterparts that may be observed in astrocytic tumors as occasional scattered elements or, more impressively, constituting the bulk of the neoplasm in gemistocytic astrocytomas.

The end result of chronic astrogliosis is frequently a dense fibrillary gliosis (Fig. 2-36), which is classically described as exhibiting one of two configurations: isomorphic (organized parallel bundles of filaments, which is most often seen in subacutely damaged CNS structures that possess a preexisting linear scaffolding to which the gliosis conforms, such as in the corpus callosum and internal capsule), or anisomorphic (disheveled gliosis with no discernible organizational pattern). The often drawn analogy of the astrocyte as the "fibroblast of the CNS"—i.e., a cell with mitotic potential that responds with alacrity to deleterious stimuli—is quite apposite.

The term "gliosis" can have different meanings depending on the context (Table 2-17). For example, the term "myelination gliosis" refers to the normal proliferation of oligodendroglia during development in preparation for myeli-

TABLE 2-17. TYPES OF GLIOSIS

Astrogliosis
Alzheimer gliosis
Bergmann gliosis
Chaslin gliosis
Microgliosis
Myelination gliosis

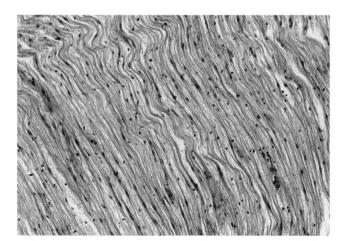

FIGURE 2-36. Fibrillary astrocytosis (isomorphic). Old healed infarcts and other remote CNS injuries are surrounded by dense glial "scars" composed of elongated astrocyte processes filled with GFAP-positive intermediate filaments.

nation. The most common usage of "gliosis," however, is to denote reactive astrogliosis.

An increase in astrocytic cell number also may accompany diverse insults to the CNS. Nonneoplastic astrocytic mitotic figures are occasionally observed, but a hyperplastic response is more often typified by the presence of so-called "mirror nuclei"—astrocytic nuclei occurring in physically contiguous matched pairs, presumably the result of prior mitotic division. In later stages, particularly in chronic disorders, an increase in the number of astrocytic nuclei may be obvious, but more often special procedures (such as anti-GFAP immunochemistry) are required for confirmation and quantitation.

One regionally specialized subtype of astrocyte warrants brief mention: the *Bergmann glia*. These astrocytes have cell bodies that are located in the Purkinje cell layer of the cerebellar cortex and extend long cytoplasmic processes through the molecular layer to the subpial surface. These processes serve an important function during development as guides for migrating granular cell neurons during the diaspora from the fetal external granular layer. In the adult nervous system, the Bergmann glia are inconspicuous unless stimulated by local injury to the cerebellum, at which time they proliferate in a similar fashion to astrocytes in other parts of the nervous system. This process, termed "*Bergmann gliosis*," is routinely observed in the zone immediately adjacent to remote cerebellar infarcts, where the Bergmann glia and vascular elements are often virtually the only surviving cellular constituents (Figs. 2-37 and 2-38).

TABLE 2-18. MORPHOLOGIC SUBTYPES OF REACTIVE ASTROCYTES SEEN IN HYPERAMMONEMIC CONDITIONS

Alzheimer type II astrocytes
Alzheimer type I astrocytes
Opalski cells (*Grammatici certant!*)[a]

[a] As suggested by the warning in the table, the lineage of the Opalski cells has been disputed, but a subset, at least, appear to be astrocytic based on immunopositivity for glial fibrillary acidic protein.

Alzheimer Type II Astrocytosis

Specific types of astrocytic reaction to injury are seen in certain metabolic disorders, particularly in hyperammonemic states that accompany a variety of hepatic diseases (Table 2-18). The most common reaction consists exclusively of nuclear changes: swelling, contortion, central clearing with margination of the chromatin, and the development of one or two prominent nucleoli. In sharp contrast to all of the various gliotic states described above, these "Alzheimer type II astrocytes" fail to exhibit prominent (or even subtle!) cytoplasm by routine H&E microscopy (Fig. 2-39). This unusual response may be

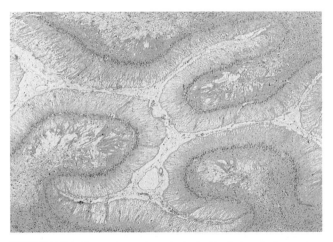

FIGURE 2-37. Bergmann astrocytosis. In the ischemic penumbra that immediately surrounds an area of cerebellar infarction, the degree of insult is sufficient to kill all of the neurons but the hardy glia survive. In this low power view the cerebellar folia are readily recognizable by the Bergmann astrocytes that form a narrow layer where the Purkinje cells used to be.

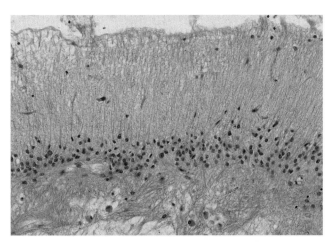

FIGURE 2-38. Bergmann astrocytosis. At higher magnification, the Bergmann glia nuclei are seen with their apical cytoplasmic processes extending upward to the pial surface. No neurons remain.

explained in part by the fact that the culpable noxious agent—*ammonia*—is thought to function as a glial toxin; thus, the primary CNS damage is to the astrocytes themselves. Alzheimer type II astrocytes may be seen throughout the neuraxis, but typical locations (such as the globus pallidus) have been described in which they are particularly prominent. *Alzheimer type I astrocytes* are also occasionally seen in diverse hyperammonemic states, but are especially typical of Wilson's disease. They differ from type II astrocytes in displaying abundant eosinophilic cytoplasm and also have hyperchromatic, multilobulated nuclei rather than the cleared nuclei that are characteristic of type II astrocytes (Fig. 2-40). As the names imply, *both types of pathologic astrocytic changes were described by Alois Alzheimer, and are, of course, totally unrelated to the dementing disease also investigated by Dr. Alzheimer.*

Parenthetically, an additional cell type—the *Opalski cell*—is also seen in the hyperammonemic state accompanying Wilson's disease. The Opalski cell

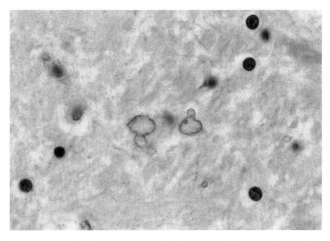

FIGURE 2-39. Alzheimer type II astrocytes. This type of reactive astrocyte, which is seen in hyperammonemia, is characterized by an open, clear nucleus and irregular nuclear contour. In contrast to other types of reactive astrocytes, no cytoplasm is seen.

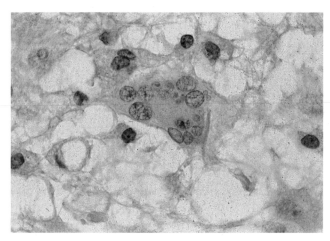

FIGURE 2-40. Alzheimer type I astrocytes. Type I astrocytes are also associated with hyperammonemia, but are significantly less common than type II astrocytes and are most strongly associated with hepatolenticular degeneration (Wilson's disease). In contrast to type II astrocytes, type I cells have abundant eosinophilic cytoplasm and either multiple nuclei or an irregular hyperchromatic nucleus.

TABLE 2-19. EPONYMIC DESIGNATIONS OF A VARIETY OF REACTIVE ASTROCYTE POPULATIONS ASSOCIATED WITH DIFFERENT DISEASES OR REGIONS OF THE CENTRAL NERVOUS SYSTEM

Alzheimer type I astrocyte
Alzheimer type II astrocyte
Bergmann gliosis
Chaslin's gliosis
Creutzfeldt astrocyte

lineage remains disputed; some investigators favor a neuronal or macrophage derivation, while those championing the astrocytic hypothesis point to reported GFAP-immunopositivity.

From the foregoing discussion, it is apparent that a number of eponyms have historically been associated with various types of reactive astrocytosis (Table 2-19).

Additional examples include Chaslin's gliosis (subpial astrogliosis) (Fig. 2-41) and *Creutzfeldt astrocytes* (Fig. 2-42), which are multinucleated reactive astrocytes seen in a variety of conditions but particularly characteristic of the demyelinating diseases.

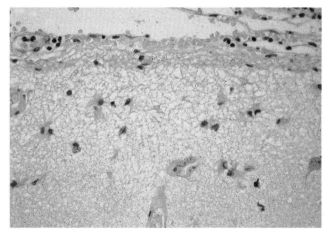

FIGURE 2-41. Chaslin's subpial gliosis. Reactive astrocytosis of the subpial glia, resulting in a dense eosinophilic band of glial cell processes immediately subjacent to the pia, is termed "Chaslin's gliosis" and can be elicited by either intraparenchymal or subarachnoid space disease processes.

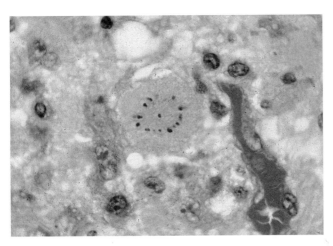

FIGURE 2-42. Creutzfeldt astrocytes and granular mitoses. Reactive astrocytes with multiple small nuclei ("micronuclei") are termed "Creutzfeldt astrocytes," and their precursors with tiny chromatid bodies are called "granular mitoses." Although not pathognomonic, both of these cell types are very common in demyelinating diseases and their conspicuous presence serves as a "red flag" to the surgical pathologist to consider demyelinating disease high in the differential diagnosis.

Astrocytic Reaction in Progressive Multifocal Leukoencephalopathy

Among astrocytic reactions to injury, none is more striking than that observed in progressive multifocal leukoencephalopathy (PML). In fact, *not infrequently the most eye-catching aspect of PML lesions is the alarming nuclear pleomorphism exhibited by the astrocytes*, which has on more than one occasion elicited a mental frisson from even the most experienced observer (Fig. 2-43). Although the pathophysiology of this phenomenon has not been elucidated, the fact that there are only two case reports in the pertinent literature of gliomas occurring in association with PML militates against an interpretation of neoplastic trans-

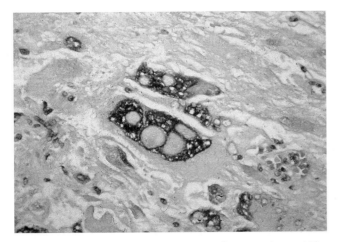

FIGURE 2-43. Bizarre reactive astrocyte of progressive multifocal leukoencephalopathy (PML). In PML, scattered highly atypical reactive astrocytes with bizarre, pleomorphic, hyperchromatic nuclei can be seen. The degree of atypia is so extreme as to suggest malignant astrocytoma.

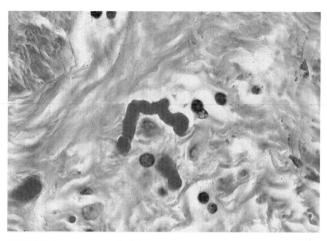

FIGURE 2-44. Rosenthal fiber. Rosenthal fibers are brightly eosinophilic irregularly elongated inclusions in astrocyte cell processes. They are associated with a range of reactive, neoplastic and metabolic diseases, but all share in common significant chronicity.

formation and in favor of a reactive response. Awareness of this unusual astrocytic reaction lessens the chance of rendering an erroneous diagnosis of malignant astrocytoma.

Inclusions

The two most commonly observed intracytoplasmic inclusions in astrocytes are the corpora amylacea, mentioned above in connection with aging changes, and *Rosenthal fibers* (Fig. 2-44). The latter are brightly eosinophilic (actually slightly magenta-hued compared to the orange-red of erythrocytic rouleau with which they may be mistaken), and exhibit elongated, anfractuous ("corkscrew" or "lumpy-bumpy") profiles.

Rosenthal fibers are observed in a wide variety of reactive states, most often in those associated with significant chronicity. They are also a morphologic hallmark of *Alexander's disease (of which some forms are now known to arise from mutations of the gene encoding glial fibrillary acidic protein)* (Fig. 2-45). Rosenthal fibers are frequently identified as a "normal" finding in the pineal gland where they are seen in the gliotic mural tissue surrounding small intrinsic pineal cysts. Like the gemistocytic astrocytes mentioned above, Rosenthal fibers also have counterparts that may be encountered in neoplasia. Although found as occasional constituents in a wide variety of gliomas, Rosenthal fibers are most characteristic of pilocytic astrocytoma—a distinctive low-grade glioma that occurs with highest frequency in the cerebellum (but which can also frequent other locales, including the cerebral hemispheres, optic nerves, diencephalon, brain stem, and spinal cord). The importance of recognizing these structures in an astrocytic neoplasm cannot be overemphasized. The nuclear pleomorphism of most pilocytic astrocytomas is more than sufficient to suggest anaplastic astrocytoma; the identification of Rosenthal fibers significantly mitigates the risk of this potential overdiagnosis. Again, *it should be stressed that Rosenthal fibers may be particularly abundant in the vicinity of chronic benign conditions (such as syringomyelia) and around the margins of nonglial, slow-growing tumors (such as craniopharyngioma and hemangioblastoma),* and the differential diagnosis of Rosenthal fibers in a biopsy must include all of the entities in

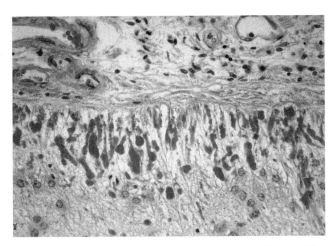

FIGURE 2-45. Rosenthal fibers in Alexander's disease. The largest numbers of Rosenthal fibers are seen in Alexander's disease in which they are present throughout the CNS in both gray and white matter, but are particularly dense around blood vessels and beneath the pia as seen here.

which they are commonly found as either intrinsic principal players in the primary disease process (such as Alexander's disease and pilocytic astrocytoma) or as prominent components of the surrounding parenchymal reaction (Table 2-20).

Neoplastic Counterparts

The most distinguishing feature of astrocytic neoplasms by both immunohistochemistry and electron microscopy, as might be expected, is their content of glial filaments. The light microscopic appearance of the gliomas (and especially glioblastoma) varies widely; individual neoplastic glia may even mimic ganglion cells. In the face of such variegation, *immunohistochemical detection of GFAP epitopes remains the most reliable indicator of glial lineage*, usually unmasking even the most artful poseurs.

OLIGODENDROGLIA

Light Microscopy

Oligodendroglia are usually associated with white matter, where, in fortuitous longitudinal sections of white matter tracts, coffles of oligocytes may be seen queuing up between fascicles of myelinated axons (*interfascicular oligodendroglia*) (Fig. 2-46). Oligodendrocytes are responsible for the formation and continual maintenance of the myelin sheath in the CNS. Additionally, it may be remembered that they are integral constituents of the optic nerves (these structures are, of course, not really "nerves" *sensu stricto,* but rather erumpent CNS tracts). Oligodendroglia also myelinate the proximal segments of cranial nerve roots for variable distances outside the neuraxial pial surface. For most roots this is only a millimeter or two; however, in the eighth nerve they extend to the vicinity of the internal acoustic meatus. One practical clinical consequence of oligo anatomic distribution is that, by virtue of their very presence, oligodendrocytes confer upon the host structure vulnerability to CNS demyelinating diseases. For example, witness the frequency of optic nerve lesions in multiple sclerosis.

TABLE 2-20. THE THREE ETIOLOGIES OF ROSENTHAL FIBERS

Reactive
Neoplastic
Genetic/metabolic

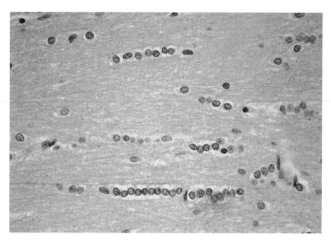

FIGURE 2-46. Interfascicular oligodendroglia. Interfascicular oligodendroglia form the myelin sheaths of CNS white matter tracts and are seen here in queues between bundles of myelinated axons.

Besides their well-known role in fabricating and maintaining CNS myelin, oligodendrocytes are also found in gray matter where they serve as "satellite cells" to neuronal cell bodies (Fig. 2-47). The putative trophic role of these "perineuronal oligodendroglia" is largely conjectural at present. It should be noted that astrocytes and microglia can also assume a "satellite" position with respect to neuronal somas, with equally obscure significance. Oligodendroglial "satellitosis" is most conspicuous in the deeper cortical layers around the cell bodies of large, projection-class neurons.

Normal satellitosis is to be distinguished from a similar phenomenon exhibited by infiltrating glioma cells ("neoplastic satellitosis"), which also often display an affinity for the neuronal cell body. Neoplastic satellitosis is one type of "*secondary structure of Scherer.*"

As the name implies, oligodendroglia ("few branch glia") have fewer cytoplasmic processes than astrocytes. In fact, by light microscopy, processes are

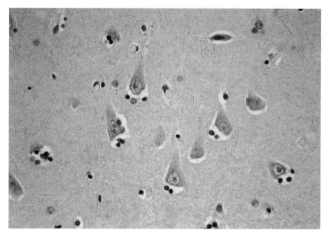

FIGURE 2-47. Satellite oligodendroglia. In the gray matter, oligodendrocytes, called "satellite cells," are found closely apposed to neuronal cell bodies.

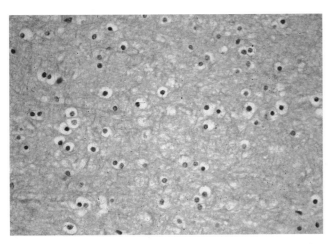

FIGURE 2-48. Normal oligodendroglia: perinuclear halos. The signature feature of oligodendrocytes is the perinuclear halo ("fried egg artifact"). This hydropic swelling and clearing of the cytoplasm is a reproducible and useful artifact of delayed fixation that is retained by the neoplastic oligodendrocytes of oligodendrogliomas.

not discernible at all, with only "naked nuclei" being apparent. The most characteristic morphologic feature of oligodendroglia is the delayed fixation artifact referred to as a *"perinuclear halo" or "fried egg" appearance* (Fig. 2-48). This cytoplasmic vacuolation is not seen in intraoperative frozen sections or in surgical specimens in which the transit time from excision to fixation is comparatively brief. Nevertheless, it is routinely encountered in formalin-fixed permanent tissue sections and, when present, *is a useful corroborative artifact that typifies not only normal oligodendrocytes (or "oligos") but also the tumor cells of oligodendroglial neoplasms* (Fig. 2-49). Perinuclear halo artifact is of considerable utility in the evaluation of CNS tumors in which the presence of an oligodendroglial component is suspected (for example, mixed oligoastrocytomas). The nuclei of oligos are also fairly distinctive—small, dark, and uniformly rounded compared to the larger, more oval or mildly irregular, and less hyperchromatic nuclei of astrocytes.

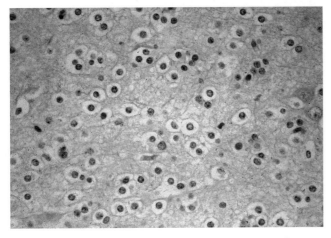

FIGURE 2-49. Oligodendroglioma. Note the presence of prominent perinuclear halos in this oligodendroglioma.

Immunochemistry

Antisera raised against a number of specific compounds, most notably myelin-associated glycoprotein (MAG) and myelin basic protein (MBP), have been used for the experimental investigation of developing oligodendroglia; however, these antibodies have so far not proven reliably and reproducibly useful in the routine evaluation of neoplastic tissues. Oligo nuclei are immunopositive for S-100 protein, but this attribute is shared with astrocytes. In contrast to the excellent antibodies widely employed for assessing neuronal and astrocytic differentiation (antisynaptophysin and anti-GFAP, respectively), a sensitive and reliable immunohistochemical marker specific for oligodendroglial differentiation is not currently available.

Ultrastructure

In brain tissue that has been rapidly and appropriately fixed for ultrastructural examination, oligodendroglia may be distinguished from astrocytes by virtue of a nearly complete lack of cytoplasmic fibrils and glycogen, and by the prominent microtubule content of the sparse cell processes. The dense nuclei are typically surrounded by only a thin rim of cytoplasm. Examination of specimens deliberately delayed in fixation reveals the morphologic basis for the characteristic "fried egg" perinuclear halos: hydropic cytoplasmic swelling and vacuolation.

Pathologic Reactions and Inclusions

Oligodendroglia are susceptible to a wide variety of pathologic conditions. A reactive proliferation of oligos with pronounced satellitosis can be seen in a number of pathologic states, such as chronic seizure disorders, and may give the impression of oligodendroglioma.

In that a myelin internode is not static and inert, but is rather a dynamic living extension of the oligodendrocyte, *the most morphologically striking (and physiologically deleterious) result of oligo compromise is demyelination* (Fig. 2-50).

Pathologic changes in oligo nuclei may be observed as well, as illustrated by the characteristic lesions of progressive multifocal leukoencephalopathy

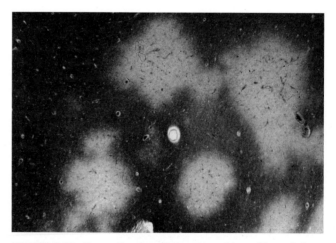

FIGURE 2-50. Demyelination. The most striking effect of damage to oligodendrocytes is demyelination, as seen here in a case of PML. The Luxol fast blue stain seen here stains intact myelin dark blue whereas areas of demyelination are seen in sharp contrast as the pale zones.

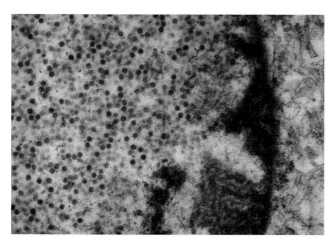

FIGURE 2-51. JC virus particles in oligo nucleus. Oligodendroglia are vulnerable to JC viral infection, resulting in intranuclear propagation of the virus seen in this electron micrograph. Subsequent lysis of the cell results in loss of the myelin sheaths that it maintains and thus demyelination.

(PML) in which oligos adjacent to foci of demyelination exhibit characteristic "ground glass" intranuclear inclusions produced by JC virus. The ground glass appearance is produced by massive viral replication within the nucleus as clearly seen by electron microscopy (Fig. 2-51).

Intracytoplasmic inclusion bodies in oligodendrocytes have recently been recognized to be a constant feature of some degenerative diseases such as *multiple system atrophy*. The inclusions are best visualized through the use of special procedures such as silver stains or immunohistochemistry for ubiquitin or alpha-synuclein.

Neoplastic Counterparts

Oligodendroglia may participate in the neoplastic process alone (oligodendrogliomas) or in collaboration with other glial elements (e.g., mixed oligoastrocytoma). In all cases, *identification of an oligo component is greatly facilitated by the presence of characteristic perinuclear halos.* As noted previously, this useful artifact is frequently exhibited by neoplastic as well as normal oligodendrocytes.

Caveat: The cytologic and tissue architectural features of the oligodendroglioma, including the characteristic perinuclear halos, can be mimicked to a remarkable extent by several other tumor types, particularly the clear cell variant of ependymoma and central neurocytoma.

Secondary Structures of Scherer

The neoplastic satellitosis observed in oligodendrogliomas and astrocytomas is perhaps the most commonly encountered example of what are termed "secondary structures of Scherer." In an extensive study of the morphological features of gliomas (*Am J Cancer* 1938;34:333–351), Dr. Scherer categorized the many patterns he observed into three major categories: proper (which we now call primary), secondary, and tertiary (Table 2-21 and Table 2-22). Primary structures are those that the tumor can form spontaneously out of its own innate genetic programming, such as true ependymal rosettes. Secondary structures, in contrast, are dependent upon the interaction of infiltrating tumor

TABLE 2-21. DEFINITION OF THE THREE CATEGORIES OF SCHERER STRUCTURES (IN SCHERER'S OWN WORDS)

Category	Definition
Proper (primary)	Structures in a glioma which do not depend on preexisting tissue but are an expression of the intrinsic architectural potentialities of the tumor cells.
Secondary	All those structures formed by the cells of the glioma which depend on the preexisting tissue elements.
Tertiary	Formations which are brought about by the interaction of the glioma with the proliferating mesenchymal tissue of the tumor (vascular proliferation excluded).

Data from Scherer (*Am J Cancer* 1938;34:333–351).

TABLE 2-22. SPECIFIC EXAMPLES OF THE THREE CATEGORIES OF SCHERER STRUCTURES (FROM SCHERER'S ORIGINAL PAPER)

Category	Examples
Proper (primary)	Canalicular or glandular structures (e.g., ependymal true rosettes)
	Papillary structures (e.g., perivascular pseudo-rosettes)
	Fascicular "fibrosarcoma" growth pattern
	Symplastic formations (spheres, bands, whorls)
	Heaps, bands, palisades
Secondary	Perineural (perineuronal) satellitosis
	Surface growth (subpial accumulation)
	Perivascular satellitosis
	"Elective" growth in gray matter
	Perifascicular growth
	Intrafascicular growth
	Interfibrillary growth
	"Elective" growth in white matter
Tertiary	Meningeal invasion
	Organization of necrosis (vascular proliferation excluded)

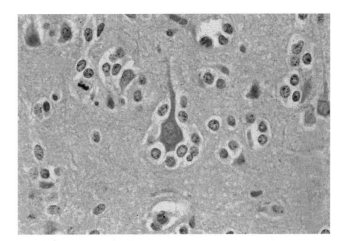

FIGURE 2-52. Neoplastic satellitosis. Neoplastic oligodendrocytes frequently infiltrate the cortex where they are drawn to neuronal cell bodies just like their normal counterparts. Perineuronal satellitosis is one of the secondary structures of Scherer that are very useful to the surgical pathologist in identifying the presence of an infiltrating glioma on frozen tissue sections performed for intraoperative diagnosis.

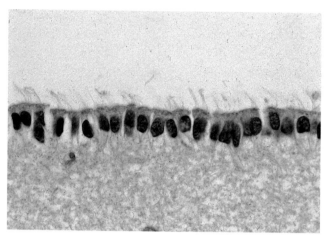

FIGURE 2-53. Ciliated columnar ependyma. In some parts of the ventricular lining the ependyma forms a tall ciliated columnar epithelium.

cells with normal host tissue elements, such as neuronal cell bodies, blood vessels, and the pial membrane, which results in perineuronal satellitosis, perivascular satellitosis, and subpial tumor growth, respectively (Fig. 2-52). Tertiary structures of Scherer result from proliferating connective tissue elements, such as the desmoplastic reaction elicited by tumor invasion of the leptomeninges and the organization of necrotic tumor foci by fibroblasts and vascular elements.

EPENDYMA

Light Microscopy and Distribution

The ependyma constitutes an epithelial surface that provides a lining for the ventricular system. The ependymal lining varies from *robust ciliated columnar to flattened cuboidal* (Figs. 2-53 and 2-54). In the fetal and infant nervous system, the ependyma is profusely ciliated; with increasing age, cilia become less

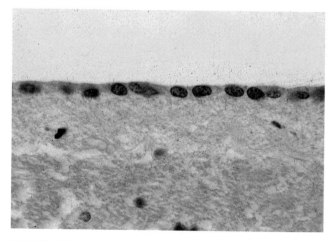

FIGURE 2-54. Flat cuboidal ependyma. With increasing age or chronic ventricular dilatation the ependyma assumes a flat cuboidal to almost squamous morphology.

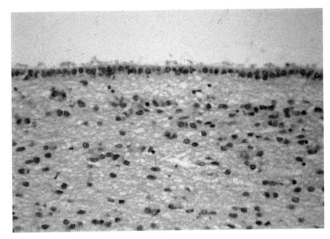

FIGURE 2-55. Subependymal plate. The zone immediately beneath the ependyma is very sparsely cellular and is called the "subependymal plate." The few glial cells that reside in this region are termed "subependymal glia" and are capable of reactive proliferation (ependymal granulations) and neoplastic proliferation (subependymomas).

conspicuous. The initially columnar ependyma also becomes progressively flattened in many parts of the ventricular system in older individuals.

The neuropil that is immediately subjacent to the ependyma forms a relatively hypocellular zone known as the *subependymal plate* in which are found sparsely scattered cells termed "*subependymal glia*" (Fig. 2-55). These cells, together with the overlying ependyma, occasionally give rise to tumors called "subependymomas." In the reactive arena, the ependyma and subependymal plate often form small excrescences into the ventricular cavity termed "*plicae*" (Fig. 2-56). These normal protrusions should not be mistaken for granular ependymitis (compare with Figs. 2-61 and 2-62).

In addition to forming the ventricular lining, scattered ependymal nests and rosettes are also found throughout the neuraxis in the parenchyma subja-

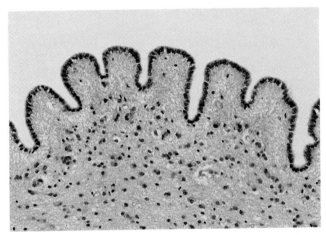

FIGURE 2-56. Ependymal plicae. The ependymal lining is normally thrown into undulating folds, called "plicae," at various ventricular locations such as the lateral walls of the third ventricle. Note the intact ependymal lining and normal hypocellular subependymal plate. Plicae should not be mistaken for the ependymal granulations of granular ependymitis.

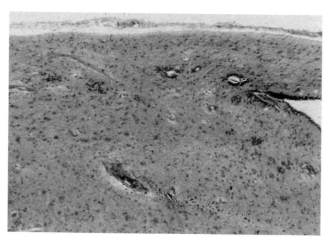

FIGURE 2-57. Ependymal nests. At any site near the ventricular system, small nests and rosettes can be found, such as those illustrated here just lateral to the fourth ventricle.

cent to the ventricular system. Such nests are especially frequent in locations where developmental fusion of juxtaposed ependymal surfaces has occurred, such as at the tips of the frontal and occipital horns, and the lateral angles of the fourth ventricle (Figs. 2-57 and 2-58). This fusion of adjacent ependymal surfaces at the angles of the ventricles is often referred to by the overly erudite with such learned terms as "goniosynapsis," "coaptation," or "coarctation."

The ependyma-lined central canal of the spinal cord is typically *patent in infants and young children* (Fig. 2-59), but is *discontinuous in adults* in which it consists of clustered ependymal nests and rosettes interspersed with short stretches of residual canal (Fig. 2-60).

Immunochemistry and Ultrastructure

Normal ependymal cells (excluding tanycytes) are negative for GFAP but strongly positive for vimentin. The most singular morphologic property of

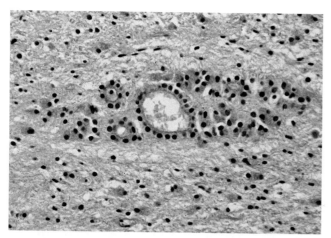

FIGURE 2-58. Ependymal rosettes of the occipital horn. The caudal tips of the occipital horns of the lateral ventricles almost always fuse during development to form a string of ependymal nests and rosettes as seen here. These small rosettes are not infrequently encountered in surgical specimens and should be recognized as a normal finding.

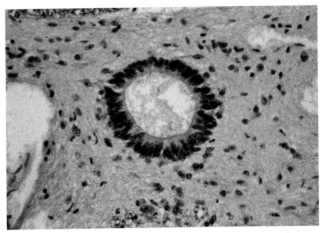

FIGURE 2-59. Patent spinal cord central canal of a child. In the fetus and young child, the central canal of the spinal cord is an open tube lined by columnar ependymal cells.

ependymal cells is their ventricular display of cilia (which, as noted above, gradually decrease in prominence with increasing age). Ultrastructurally, cilia are anchored in conventional *apical cytoplasmic basal bodies*. The light microscopic manifestations of basal bodies are termed *"blepharoplasts,"* which appear as minute punctate dots that are just resolvable under the light microscope with an oil-immersion lens (×1,000) and best seen in tissue sections stained with phosphotungstic acid–hematoxylin (PTAH). By electron microscopy, ependymal cells are seen to contain bundles of intermediate filaments. These filaments are composed of vimentin and account for the strong reactivity of the ependyma with antivimentin antibodies.

Pathologic Reactions

The ependyma is susceptible to injury by a wide variety of insults and does not appear capable of responding in any way except by simple loss. The resultant

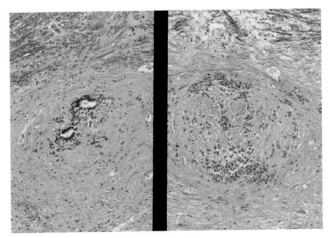

FIGURE 2-60. Gliotic spinal cord central canal of an adult. In adults, the central canal is not a continuously patent tube, but rather the fetal canal is replaced by a series of ependymal nests and rosettes as shown here at two cord levels.

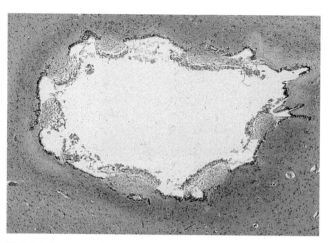

FIGURE 2-61. Cerebral aqueduct with ependymal granulations (granular ependymitis). In contrast to the normal ependymal folds (plicae) that can be seen in many parts of the ventricular system, ependymal granulations, as seen here in the cerebral aqueduct, are a reaction to ependymal injury and loss.

denudation of the ventricular lining elicits a proliferative response known as *granular ependymitis* (Figs. 2-61 and 2-62). The proliferating cells, however, are not ependymocytes, but rather the glia of the subependymal plate. On very rare occasions, granular ependymitis of the cerebral aqueduct may be so severe as to compromise CSF flow, resulting in obstructive hydrocephalus.

Ependymal granulations are a nonspecific marker of CNS injury, and while quite common in CNS viral infections, they may also be observed in longstanding mechanical hydrocephalus and other noninfectious conditions—in short, in virtually any pathologic process that results in ependymal loss.

Neoplastic Counterparts

Although fibrillary eosinophilic perivascular anuclear zones (known as *perivascular pseudorosettes or gliovascular rosettes*) (Fig. 2-63) are the most consistent feature of ependymomas, *true ependymal rosettes* (Fig. 2-64), which may be in-

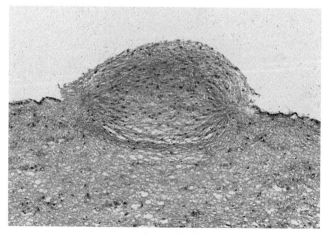

FIGURE 2-62. Ependymal granulation. At high power, an ependymal granulation is seen to consist of a hypercellular fusiform proliferation of the subependymal plate glia.

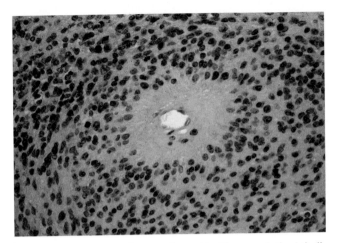

FIGURE 2-63. Perivascular pseudorosette. The morphologic hallmark of ependymomas is the perivascular pseudorosette (gliovascular pseudorosette), in which neoplastic ependymal cells surround a blood vessel but leave a nucleus-free zone around the vessel that is filled with the cytoplasmic processes of the tumor cells radiating to the vessel wall.

TABLE 2-23. TANYCYTE^a TYPES AND CHARACTERISTICS

Two distinctive categories
    Fetal nervous system
    Adult nervous system

Two major features
    Greatly elongated cell body
    GFAP immunopositive

^a Greek *tanyein,* "to stretch."
GFAP, glial fibrillary acidic protein.

terpreted teleologically as attempted neoventricular construction, provide totemic identification of ependymal lineage in a minority of cases. The identification of blepharoplasts by light microscopy using the PTAH stain, although infrequently performed today, reinforces the diagnosis of ependymoma and is certainly nothing to wink at.

Tanycytes: Specialized Cellular Constituents of the Ependyma

Before leaving the ependyma, brief mention needs to be made of one specialized cellular constituent—the tanycyte (Table 2-23). The term tanycyte (literally, "stretched cell") *per se* does not specify a single cellular entity, but is applicable to several cell populations of the developing and adult nervous system

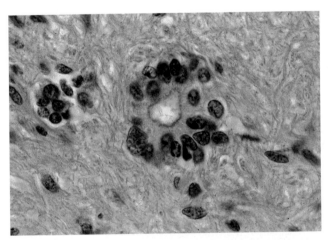

FIGURE 2-64. "True" ependymal rosette. Less commonly seen than the perivascular pseudorosette but very esthetic, the true rosette has at its center not a blood vessel but a well-defined lumen.

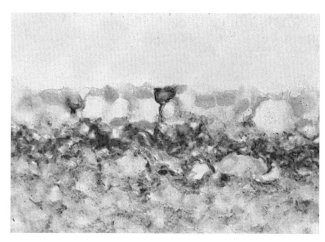

FIGURE 2-65. Tanycytes are GFAP-positive. As seen in this section of ependyma and subependymal plate, most cells of the ependyma are negative for GFAP (the glial subependymal plate is positive). The strong immunopositivity for GFAP of the single cell in the long row of ependymal cells identifies it as a tanycyte.

that share a highly elongated shape and which span the entire thickness of the ependyma from the ventricular surface to the subependymal CNS parenchyma. Multiple subclasses of tanycytes have been described in the developing ventricular wall, which vary with respect to position of the nucleus in the cell, type of cell processes (unipolar versus bipolar forms), and temporal longevity (a large percentage of fetal tanycytes do not persist as such into adulthood). The potential functional significance and relationships of these developmental tanycytes to common ependymal cells and to the radial glia (which in general span the *entire* cerebral wall, not just the ependymal layer) remain disputed at present and constitute an area of active investigation.

In the adult nervous system, a specific class of tanycytes is located in the floor of the third ventricle (median eminence). These cells have received much attention as potential neuroendocrine modulators that putatively sample CSF hormone levels via their ependymal processes and transmit information through their basal processes to the hypothalamic portal system. Again, this interesting hypothesis—as well as most other issues concerning tanycytes—awaits clarification.

The tanycyte can be distinguished from other ependymal cells by immunostaining for GFAP. Whereas *normal ependymal cells are GFAP-negative, tanycytes are strongly GFAP-positive* (Fig. 2-65).

The tanycyte has been implicated in the genesis of two CNS tumors that exhibit a tumor cell morphology with a tanycytic flavor: *tanycytic ependymoma* and a tumor of questioned authenticity, *astroblastoma*. Both of these malignancies display neoplastic glia that have elongated cytoplasmic processes, and each shares some ultrastructural features with the fetal tanycyte.

CHOROID PLEXUS

Light Microscopy and Neuroanatomic Distribution

Choroid plexus consists of *papillary tufts of epithelium-covered fibrovascular connective tissue* that project into the ventricles and produce cerebrospinal fluid (Fig. 2-66). The choroid plexus is a composite organ formed by the invagination of the vascular pia mater into the ventricular space. By this process, a cov-

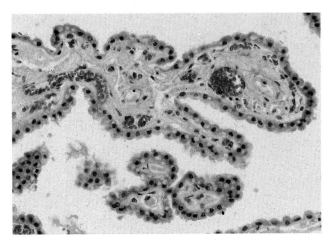

FIGURE 2-66. Choroid plexus. The choroid plexus consists of a highly vascular core of blood vessels and connective tissue covered by a cuboidal epithelium called "choroid plexus epithelium."

TABLE 2-24. THE NORMAL NEUROANATOMIC DISTRIBUTION OF CHOROID PLEXUS

Lateral ventricle (body, atrium, temporal horn)
Interventricular foramen (Monro)
Roof of third ventricle
Fourth ventricle[a]
Cerebellopontine angle (foramina of Luschka)

[a] Roof and lateral recesses.

ering of specialized ependyma is thus acquired. The choroid plexus epithelium exhibits distinctive features compared to nonchoroidal ependyma: in contrast to the flattened cuboidal ependyma, choroid cells are larger, plumper, and present a "cobblestoned" surface.

In terms of neuraxis distribution (Table 2-24), it should be noted that, like ependyma, choroid plexus is also a normal denizen of the CPA cistern, and is visible on the ventral aspect of the brain stem as small bilateral tufts protruding through the lateral foramina of Luschka covered by a delicate row of vagus nerve rootlets. Choroid is normally visible in the cisterna magna external to the median foramen of Magendie only in the fetus; persistence of this "fetal position" of the choroid at this site is sometimes associated with regional disturbances such as the Chiari malformations. *The largest masses of choroid plexus are found in the lateral ventricle atria (junction of the body, occipital, and temporal horns) and are called the "glomera choroidea" (s. glomus choroideum).*

Immunochemistry and Ultrastructure

Similar to other members of the glial family, choroid plexus epithelium is immunopositive for S-100 protein. It is negative for GFAP. Strong positivity for transthyretin (prealbumin) makes this a useful marker that has been exploited to confirm the presence of a choroid plexus component in a number of disease conditions, such as in teratomas and malformations.

Aging Changes

The choroidal matrix is composed of a fibrovascular stroma that undergoes progressive mineralization with age. Two distinct forms of calcification occur in the choroid plexus: nonspecific deposition of mineral salts in the collagenous stroma (Fig. 2-67), and *psammoma bodies* (Fig. 2-68), which arise from meningothelial cell whorls.

The presence of meningothelial (arachnoidal) cells in normal choroid plexus is a logical consequence of the choroid's invaginative mode of genesis during development, in which arachnoid cells are drawn into the forming plexus along with the pia. *Meningothelial nests and whorls are, in fact, common habitués of normal choroid plexus*, especially in the glomera choroidea of the lateral ventricle atria (Fig. 2-69). This observation has clinical relevance: it ex-

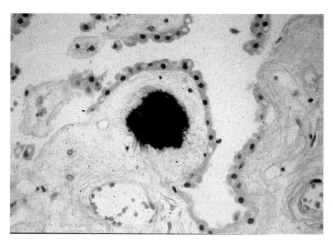

FIGURE 2-67. Nonspecific mineral deposition in choroid plexus. The most common form of calcification of the choroid plexus is simple nonspecific deposition of mineral salts onto the collagenous stroma.

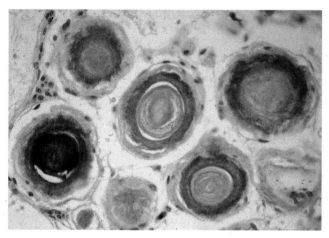

FIGURE 2-68. Psammoma body formation in choroid plexus. In contrast to nonspecific mineral deposition, psammoma bodies have a more interesting mode of genesis; they form in the center of arachnoid cell whorls.

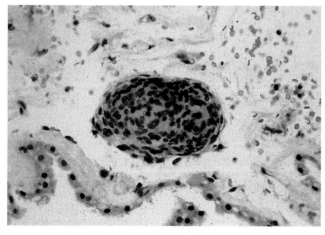

FIGURE 2-69. Arachnoid (meningothelial) nest in choroid plexus. Because the choroid plexus forms as an invagination of the vascular pia-arachnoid into the ventricle, arachnoid cell nests are normally found here in all people. In addition to fostering the development of psammoma bodies, the meningothelial nests also occasionally spawn intraventricular meningiomas.

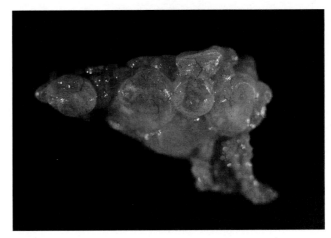

FIGURE 2-70. Cystic choroid plexus. Cystic change of the choroid plexus is a visually striking but asymptomatic accompaniment of aging in some people.

plains the existence of *"intraventricular" meningiomas* (which might be more precisely described as "intrachoroidal" meningiomas!).

In addition, *with age, choroid epithelial cells are prone to develop a single large intracytoplasmic lipid-containing vacuole.* Another intracytoplasmic inclusion occasionally noted in choroid plexus epithelial cells with aging is the Biondi ring, which is best visualized with silver stains and consists of filament bundles by electron microscopy. The significance of Biondi rings is uncertain.

Striking macroscopic *cystic change* is another finding often observed in the choroid plexus of adults and is thus associated with aging but otherwise without known pathologic significance (Figs. 2-70 and 2-71). A similarly impressive condition on gross examination is the *choroid plexus xanthogranuloma* (Figs. 2-72 and 2-73). As the name implies, xanthogranulomas are typically yellowish masses that, on microscopic examination, show granuloma formation; the granulomas are actually a giant cell reaction to cholesterol and other cellular debris, often including by-products of hemorrhage. Xanthogranulomas are frequently bilateral, and are more readily correctly identified on gross examination and on neuroradiologic imaging studies when occurring as pairs;

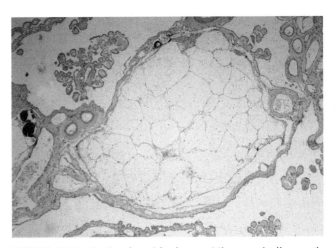

FIGURE 2-71. Cystic choroid plexus. Microscopically, cystic change consists of bland thin-walled fluid-filled sacs.

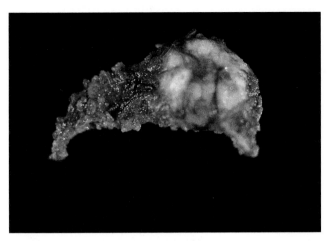

FIGURE 2-72. Xanthogranuloma of the choroid plexus. Xanthogranulomas are usually asymptomatic but can raise suspicion of metastatic carcinoma radiologically and grossly. They can arise unilaterally or bilaterally.

however, they may also arise unilaterally, and in such cases may be suspected to be of neoplastic origin. In cancer patients who are being evaluated for CNS metastatic disease, incidental xanthogranulomas have been biopsied as suspected choroid plexus metastases.

Neoplastic Counterparts

The choroid plexus gives rise to a range of neoplasms. *Choroid plexus papillomas* are benign tumors that closely mimic the characteristic papillary structure of normal choroid plexus (Fig. 2-74). The distinctive papillary architectural motif is significantly effaced in malignant tumors, *choroid plexus carcinomas* (Fig. 2-75).

Similar to normal choroid plexus, papillomas frequently display immunopositivity for transthyretin (prealbumin) and also for S-100 protein;

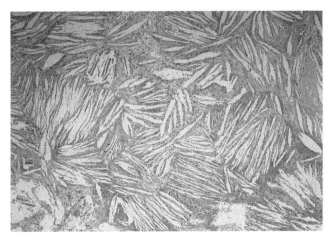

FIGURE 2-73. Xanthogranuloma of the choroid plexus. Microscopically, xanthogranulomas show a farrago of degenerative and reactive changes in which cholesterol clefts are usually prominent.

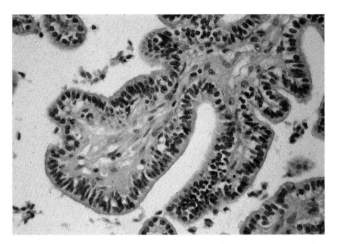

FIGURE 2-74. Choroid plexus papilloma. The papilloma retains the papillary architecture of normal choroid plexus but the lining cells are more crowded and columnar compared to normal choroid plexus epithelium.

however, the extent of positivity, and therefore clinical utility, of these markers is significantly reduced in the carcinomas. By ultrastructural examination, choroid plexus papillomas exhibit profuse numbers of apical microvilli and often cilia as well (Fig. 2-76).

MESENCHYMAL COMPONENTS OF THE CENTRAL NERVOUS SYSTEM

Microglia / Monocytes / Macrophages

Light Microscopy

Microglia are now generally accepted as monocyte-derived resident constituents of the reticuloendothelial system in the nervous system and thus arise from a com-

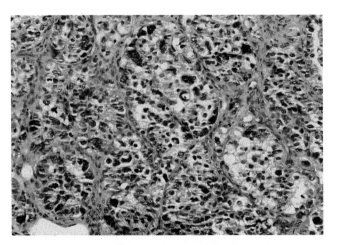

FIGURE 2-75. Choroid plexus carcinoma. In contrast to papillomas, choroid plexus carcinomas display solid tumor areas, as seen here, in which the papillary architecture is completely effaced. In most cases, carcinomas also show more nuclear and cellular pleomorphism than papillomas.

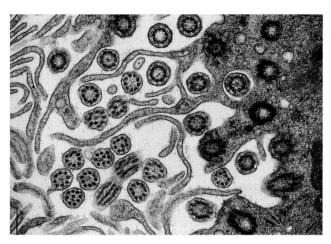

FIGURE 2-76. Papilloma with microvilli and cilia. Ultrastructurally, choroid plexus papillomas recapitulate the apical microvilli and cilia seen in the normal epithelium.

pletely separate cell lineage compared to the other glia. Historically, the designation "microglia" was coined to contrast with "macroglia"—an old term for all of the comparatively larger glia (astrocytes, oligodendroglia, and ependymocytes) that has fallen into desuetude. So-called "resting" microglia blend inconspicuously into the neuropil throughout the CNS (Fig. 2-77). A number of special histologic procedures, including *lectin histochemistry and a number of immunostains, permit visualization of the microglia and their cell processes*, which may be bipolar, tripolar, or more extensively branched (Fig. 2-78). Microglia can be identified in routine H&E tissue sections only with very close scrutiny and are seen as mildly elongated oval "naked nuclei."

Closely related to microglia are the tissue macrophages of the CNS, which are still occasionally referred to as Gitter cells (literally, "lattice cells") in the literature (Fig. 2-79). An even more obscure cognomen—*compound granular corpuscle*—appears now only in the abstruse musings of neurohistorians and neuroetymologists.

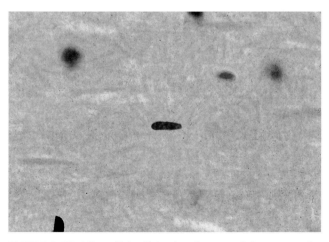

FIGURE 2-77. Microglial cell. In the absence of damage to the CNS, microglia are very inconspicuous, showing only oval-to-elongated nuclei, as seen in the center of this micrograph.

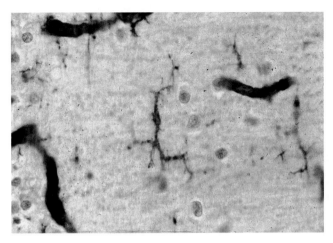

FIGURE 2-78. Microglia: lectin histochemistry. Many special procedures are available to identify "resting" microglia, including lectin histochemistry as seen here, and a variety of antibodies. Note the bipolar branching cytoplasmic processes, not usually seen with the H&E stain, are well visualized with special stains.

It is currently believed that CNS macrophages responding to injury derive from two sources: from the bloodstream via diapedetic monocytes, and by transformation of indigenous microglia (macrophages qua corpulent microglia). The concept of systemic monocyte influx in response to various forms of CNS injury has acquired added clinical significance with the adduction of data showing that this mechanism constitutes a primary route of CNS entry for the HIV virus (the "Trojan Horse" hypothesis).

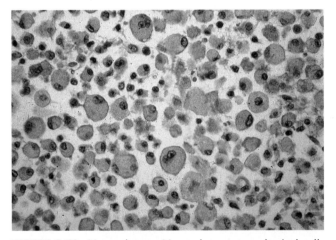

FIGURE 2-79. Macrophages. Macrophages are spherical cells with well-defined cell borders. In large clusters, as seen here in an infarct, they are usually easily identified, but as scattered cells that infiltrate the neuropil, they can mimic glioma by blending into the parenchyma and producing hypercellularity. They also constitute an actively cycling cell population so that mitotic figures will usually be seen; moreover, proliferation marker studies will show an increase in labeling index. Many antibodies are available to unmask lurking macrophages.

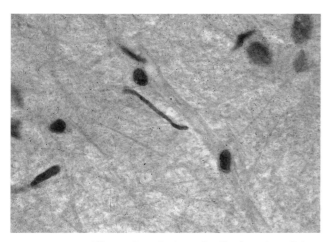

FIGURE 2-80. Diffuse microgliosis: rod cell. The microglial response to CNS injury can take one of two forms: diffuse microgliosis or multifocal microglial nodules. In either situation, microglia can be identified by their exceptionally elongated nuclei ("rod cells") as seen here in a case of ischemic injury.

Immunochemistry

As mentioned above, microglia have long been identified by lectin histochemistry and a host of antibodies are also available. Macrophages, in contrast, are often easily recognized in large tissue specimens without the aid of special stains. However, in the surgical pathology arena, particularly with the minute samples obtained by stereotactic needle biopsy, determination of macrophage participation in a pathologic process can be problematic and critical to the decision making process. In such situations, a variety of commercially available antibodies may be employed to confirm macrophage presence. Commonly employed antibodies include HAM-56 and KP-1.

Pathologic Reactions

Microglia respond to CNS insult both by diffuse proliferation and infiltration of CNS parenchyma *(diffuse microgliosis)* (Fig. 2-80) and by converging on specific foci of damage to form *microglial nodules*(Fig. 2-81) (also referred to as microglial stars, microglial shrubs, or Babes' nodes). Despite the exclusionary name, microglial nodules are generally acknowledged to consist of astrocytes as well as microglia. Microglial nodule formation is a nonspecific response to any number of pathologic conditions, although they typify the CNS response to viral and rickettsial infection. Diffuse microgliosis, likewise, constitutes a nonspecific response, and may be seen in a spectrum of illnesses ranging from hippocampal ischemia to general paresis of the insane ("general paresis" is an old term for CNS parenchymal syphilis; knowledge of past medical *causes célebrès* is forgotten at the diagnostician's peril!).

Meninges

The meninges consist of three layers of connective tissue that serve to cover and protect the nervous system: the dura mater, arachnoid, and pia mater. Only two layers were known to ancient scholars, a tough, thick outer pachymeninx and a delicate, thin inner leptomeninx (Table 2-25).

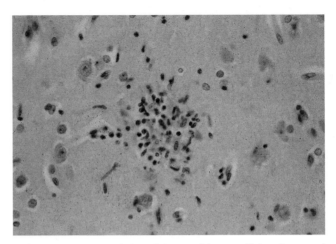

FIGURE 2-81. Microglial nodule. Focal hypercellular clusters of microglia and reactive astrocytes, termed "microglial nodules," can be seen in a number of diseases, including viral infections of the CNS from which this tissue was taken.

The Dura Mater (Pachymeninx)

The dura consists predominantly of dense connective tissue. Scattered amid the collagen bundles are resident mesenchymal elements—the fibroblasts. These unassuming spindle cells have small round-to-oval nuclei and elongated eosinophilic cytoplasmic processes. Occasional blood vessels and small peripheral nerve fascicles complete the rather bland landscape. These visual longueurs are intermittently punctuated by endothelium-lined dural venous sinuses that introduce welcome relief, particularly in areas where the arachnoid villi effloresce.

Based on descriptive and experimental ultrastructural observations, it has recently been generally accepted that *the dura and subjacent arachnoid exist in vivo as a physically continuous tissue*, with sparse—but unequivocal—intercellular junctions that link these two membranes that were formerly considered discrete and separated by a "potential space." *The storied "subdural space" has now taken its rightful position in the pantheon of neuromythology* alongside brain lymphatics and the syncytial theory of the neural net. Consequently, it has

TABLE 2-25. A BRIEF HISTORY OF THE MENINGES

Only two nervous system coverings were known to the ancient anatomists:
    Greek terms (Galen, A.D. c. 130 to c. 200)
        Meninx sklera pacheia (hard thick membrane)
        Meninx lepto (thin membrane)
    Arabic terms (Ali Abbas, A.D. 930–944)
        Umm al-dimagh (thick mother)
        Umm al-raqiq (thin mother)
    Latin equivalents of Arabic terms
        Crassa mater (thick mother)
        Tenuis mater (thin mother)
    Stephen of Antioch's translation of Ali-Abbas (A.D. 1127)
        Dura mater (hard mother)
        Pia mater (soft mother)
The arachnoid wasn't discovered until the 17th century:
    Frederick Ruysch (Dutch anatomist, 1638–1731)
        Arachnoid (1664)

been proposed that the term *spatium subdurale* be eliminated from the standardized nomenclature of Nomina Anatomica (Table 2-26).

Nevertheless, there is no disputing the fact that the interface between dural border cells and arachnoid barrier cells constitutes the "weak link" or "path of least resistance" for pathologic processes tending to disrupt the meninges, and it seems unlikely that such venerable terms as "subdural hematoma" will soon be cashiered for suggested alternatives such as "intradural hematoma" or "dural border cell hematoma." Time will judge.

Neoplastic Counterparts

The dura is a site of origin of comparatively rare, but well-recognized, primary intracranial sarcomas, which arise from the abundant population of dural fibroblasts and other mesenchymal elements. Meningiomas, despite the generic name, are generally considered to arise from arachnoid cells.

The Leptomeninges (Pia Mater and Arachnoid)

The arachnoid barrier cell layer mentioned above continuously bounds the subarachnoid space and is united with the pia by the delicate arachnoid trabeculae. Developmentally, the leptomeninges constitute a single layer that is subsequently driven by the flow of CSF, which occurs when the outlet foramina of the fourth ventricle become patent.

The arachnoid is by nature an investing epithelial tissue, and arachnoidal cells (also termed "meningothelial cells") are prone to express this intrinsic architectural property by forming cellular whorls that often mineralize to produce the psammoma bodies so characteristic of both normal and neoplastically transformed arachnoid (Fig. 2-82). Although arachnoid cell clusters, whorls, and psammoma bodies may be encountered anywhere along the arachnoid membrane, they are especially prominent over the apices of the arachnoid granulations, at which site they have received a special name, arachnoid cap cells (Fig. 2-83 and 2-84). Arachnoid granulations, in turn, are found in all of the major dural venous sinuses (although admittedly most numerous in the superior sagittal sinus and its lateral lacunae).

TABLE 2-26. THERE IS NO SUBDURAL SPACE

It is concluded that there is no evidence of a subdural space (actual or potential) in the region of the dura-arachnoid junction and it is suggested that the term *"spatium subdurale"* be removed from *Nomina Anatomica*.

—D.E. Haines, *Anat. Rec.* 230–233 (1991)

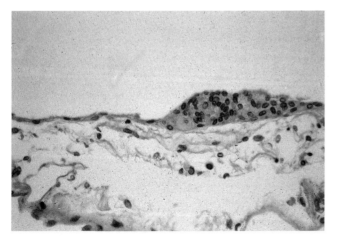

FIGURE 2-82. Arachnoid membrane. The arachnoid membrane forms a continuous layer around the CNS. Small clusters of arachnoid (meningothelial) cells, as seen here, are ubiquitously distributed throughout the membrane.

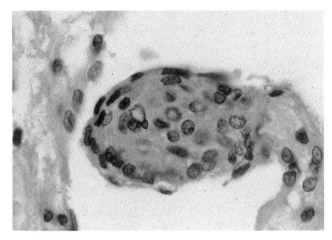

FIGURE 2-83. Arachnoid whorl. Larger clusters of normal arachnoid cells show the characteristic tendency to form whorls; this property is often expressed in the tumors of arachnoid cells: meningiomas.

With age, the subarachnoid space overlying the superior parasagittal cerebral convexities tends toward progressive fibrosis; this commonly observed process also prominently involves the neighboring arachnoid granulations, producing a collagenous hypertrophy of the villi that are then referred to eponymically as *Pacchionian granulations* (after Antonio Pacchioni, Italian anatomist, 1665–1726). These enlarged, botryoid villi gradually erode and sculpt the overlying inner table of the calvarium and the resultant pits are termed "foveoli granulares" or "Pacchionian foveoli."

Meningothelial cell clusters are also normally present in the stroma of the choroid plexus (accounting for intraventricular meningiomas, as mentioned above), in the arachnoid sheath of the optic nerves (another well-known site for meningiomas), in the spinal arachnoid, where they are preferentially located at the exit sites for spinal nerve roots (accounting for the predilection of spinal meningiomas for a lateral location), and in the subarachnoid space cisterns (such the CPA cistern and the superior cistern-velum interpositum that surrounds the pineal gland, accounting for the occurrence of meningiomas in these locations).

Immunochemistry and Ultrastructure

Consistent with their epithelial function, *arachnoidal cells are strongly positive epithelial membrane antigen (EMA)* (Fig. 2-84). At the ultrastructural level, the most striking features are the intricately interlaced cell processes and the abundance of *intercellular desmosomes* (Fig. 2-85), again reflecting the epithelial nature of this distinctive cell.

Neoplastic Counterparts

The most common neoplasms of meningothelial cells—meningiomas—frequently display of morphologic characteristics typical of their progenitors. The most salient of these are: (1) *cellular whorls and psammoma bodies* at the light microscopic level, (2) a surfeit of *desmosomes* that spot-weld together a Byzantine maze of intertwined cell processes at the ultrastructural level (which accounts for the inability to distinguish individual cell borders by light microscopy—leading to the technical misnomer "syncytial meningioma"), and

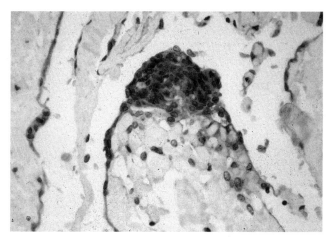

FIGURE 2-84. Arachnoid cap cells: epithelial membrane antigen (EMA). Clusters of arachnoid cells crown the apices of the arachnoid villi (arachnoid granulations) that project into the dural venous sinuses and are descriptively termed "arachnoid cap cells." All arachnoid cells are strongly immunopositive for EMA, a feature that is retained by meningiomas and often used as an aid to diagnosis.

(3) *immunopositivity for EMA*. Although a variety of maverick meningiomas may assume a remarkably impressive array of morphologic appearances, retention of the signal arachnoidal cell features of EMA immunopositivity and abundant desmosomes by most tumors regardless of subtype greatly facilitates diagnosis.

Leptomeningeal Melanocytes

True melanocytes like those of the skin are normal constituents of the intracranial cavity where they are found predominantly in the pia of the ventral-medial neuraxis—in particular, the ventral aspect of the upper cervical spinal cord and medulla (Fig. 2-86). In individuals with an abundant melanocytic presence,

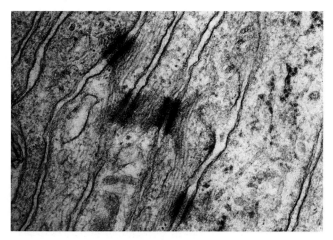

FIGURE 2-85. Desmosomes. The ultrastructural hallmark of arachnoid cells, including their neoplastic counterparts, is the presence of large numbers of desmosomes that tightly join the elongated cytoplasmic processes.

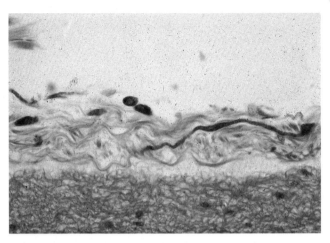

FIGURE 2-86. Leptomeningeal melanocytes. Melanocytes are normal cellular constituents of the CNS and reside in the leptomeninges (pia-arachnoid).

TABLE 2-27. TYPES OF PIGMENT SEEN IN THE CENTRAL NERVOUS SYSTEM

Normal
   Lipofuscin (aging pigment in neurons)
   Neuromelanin (catecholaminergic neurons)
   Melanocytic melanin (leptomeningeal melanocytes)

Abnormal
   Hemosiderin/hematoidin
   Melanin of metastatic melanoma
   Melanin of pigmented primary CNS neoplasms
   Pigmented fungi
   Malaria pigment

Artifact
   "Formalin pigment"

the distribution territory extends upward through the pontine and mesencephalic interpeduncular cisterns, lateral to the mesial aspects of the temporal lobes, and as far rostrally as the gyri recti of the orbitofrontal cortex.

It is not unusual for melanocytes to follow the investing leptomeninges of the perivascular Virchow–Robin spaces around large penetrating arteries for short distances into the CNS parenchyma. They may also be found in the cerebellar leptomeninges. Leptomeningeal melanocytes are seen, with considerable individual variation, in both fair and dark-skinned people. The melanin found in leptomeningeal melanocytes is identical to that of skin melanocytes, in contradistinction to the neuromelanin of catecholaminergic neurons. Melanocytic melanin is but one of many different "brown pigment" substances that may be encountered in the nervous system (Table 2-27).

Immunochemistry and Ultrastructure

As would be expected, CNS melanocytes are immunopositive for melanocytic markers such as HMB-45 and S-100 protein (immunoidentification is facilitated by the use of a *red* chromogen rather than the ubiquitous "brown stain"). By electron microscopy, typical melanosomes are seen.

Neoplastic Counterparts

The intrinsic melanocytes of the leptomeninges are involved in a spectrum of proliferative conditions, ranging from benign focal *melanocytoma* (Fig. 2-87) to the rare primary CNS melanoma.

Primary CNS melanoma is a diagnosis of exclusion that is difficult—some would argue virtually impossible—to prove conclusively even with thorough autopsy examination, due to several factors, including (1) the wide systemic distribution of possible primary origin sites, (2) the potential for even very small primary tumors to give rise to metastatic disease, (3) the possibility of primary lesion regression, and (4) the notorious vicissitudes of patient anamnesis, particularly with respect to minor dermatological excisions that may have occurred decades prior to presentation.

From a different perspective, the normal presence of melanocytes in the leptomeninges must be borne in mind when examining surgical biopsies ob-

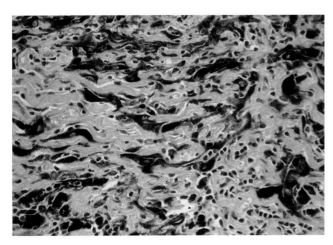

FIGURE 2-87. Melanocytoma. Leptomeningeal melanocytes can give rise to several different types of neoplasms, from benign focal melanocytomas, as seen here, to primary CNS melanoma. All of these tumors, however, are very rare compared to metastatic melanoma.

tained from CNS sites that are known to be inhabited by melanocytes; otherwise, these benign but distinctive cells might be misconstrued as evidence of a melanocytic tumor or mistaken for hemosiderin-laden macrophages.

Adipocytes

Fat does not usually come to mind when one thinks of the various normal cellular constituents of the CNS (at least for most people). It is, however, nonetheless present in a significant percentage of normal individuals in the filum terminale (Fig. 2-88) where small clusters of mature adipocytes may be found admixed with the abundant dense connective tissue of this locale, and may occasionally be encountered as focal nodules in the *glomera choroidea* as well (Fig. 2-89).

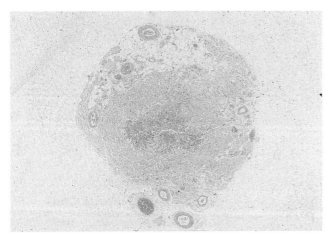

FIGURE 2-88. Adipose tissue in filum terminale. Fat cells are present in small clusters within the CNS of many normal people in two locations: the filum terminale, as seen here, and the choroid plexus. Larger collections that form mass lesions—lipomas—also occur in the CNS and show a predeliction for midline locations such as the corpus callosum and suprasellar region.

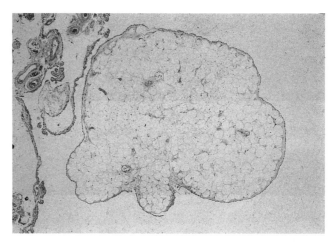

FIGURE 2-89. Adipose tissue in choroid plexus. Small clusters of fat cells are occasionally encountered in the choroid plexus as an incidental finding.

SPECIALIZED ORGANS AND REGIONS OF THE CENTRAL NERVOUS SYSTEM

The Pineal Gland

Light Microscopy

The pineal gland (Fig. 2-90) is unique among specialized CNS organs in terms of its anatomy, function, and primary neoplasms. The pineal parenchymal cells are organized into lobules, thus imparting a *distinctively glandular appearance* (Fig. 2-91). So pronounced is this attribute that pineal tissue could be mistaken on superficial examination for metastatic adenocarcinoma by the tyro.

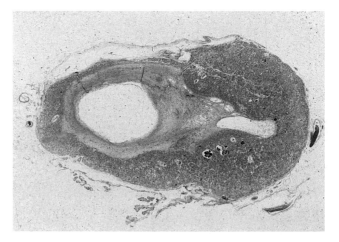

FIGURE 2-90. Pineal gland. The pineal gland commonly exhibits two features that can be seen on MRI and CT scans as well as grossly: calcification and cysts. Pineal cysts are sometimes biopsied under clinical suspicion of pineal tumor; the surgical pathologist must therefore be very familiar with the normal histologic features of the cysts (such as the common presence of Rosenthal fibers in the gliotic cyst wall) and of the surrounding normal pineal parenchyma that will inevitably be sampled in the biopsy as well.

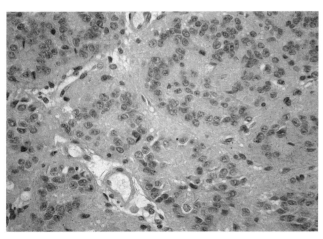

FIGURE 2-91. Pineal gland. Histologically, the pineal has a unique architecture unlike that of any other site in the CNS. A prominent lobular arrangement is seen, with clusters of pineal parenchymal cells forming rosette-like structures.

The aging pineal, like choroid plexus, is prone to both calcification and cystic change. As noted previously, this is one of the few sites in the normal CNS where Rosenthal fibers are commonly found (in the gliotic neuropil around small incidental pineal cysts).

Calcification occurs as both nonspecific mineral salt deposition and as psammoma body formation (arachnoidal cells are abundant in the leptomeninges that surround the pineal; these meninges are termed the "velum interpositum"). The older literature is replete with descriptive terms for pineal calcifications, most notably "*corpora arenacea*" (literally, "sand bodies") and "*acervuli cerebri*" (literally, "little heaps of the brain"). In addition to pineocytes, fibrillary astrocytes also populate the pineal and account for the occurrence of primary pineal gliomas. An ependyma-lined recess of the third ventricle extends for a short but variable distance into the pineal parenchyma and accounts for the occasional occurrence of ependymomas of the pineal region. The suprapineal recess of the third ventricle contains choroid plexus and accounts for the occurrence of choroid plexus papillomas in this vicinity. The pineal is innervated by the *nervi conarii* ("conarium"—literally, "cone"—is a superannuated term for the pineal), which are small nerve fascicles that contain sympathetic nervous system axons whose cell bodies are located in the superior cervical ganglion. Small clusters of arachnoid cells in the velum interpositum surrounding the pineal, which occasionally give rise to meningiomas, complete the pineal *tableau vivant* (Table 2-28).

TABLE 2-28. CELLULAR CONSTITUENTS OF THE PINEAL GLAND

Pineocytes
Astrocytes
Nerve fascicles *(nervi conarii)*
Ependyma (recess of 3rd ventricle)
Arachnoid cells (in velum interpositum)

Immunochemistry and Ultrastructure

Pineocytes may be regarded as a specialized type of neuron. By ultrastructural examination neurosecretory granules are seen. Immunohistochemically, pineocytes are strongly positive for neuronal and neuroendocrine markers, including synaptophysin and chromogranin. Pineocytes are also positive for retinal S-antigen, a rhodopsin-binding protein found in photoreceptor cells. As expected, the astrocytic constituents of the pineal are strongly positive for *GFAP*.

Neoplastic Counterparts

Benign tumors of pineal parenchymal cells, called "pineocytomas," generally retain the morphologic characteristics of pineocytes, with occasional frank neuronal (ganglion cell) differentiation. The most characteristic feature is *"pineocytomatous" rosettes*, which have been likened to hypertrophied Homer Wright (neuroblastoma-type) rosettes. The more "primitive" pineal neoplasms, pineoblastomas, can also exhibit neuronal differentiation in the form of classic Homer Wright rosettes and, in keeping with the developmental and phylogenetic kinship with the retina, can occasionally display retinoblastic differentiation in the form of Flexner–Wintersteiner (retinoblastoma-type) rosettes and fleurettes. Fleurettes (literally, "little flowers") are distinctive focal arrangements of tumor cells in a pattern resembling the heraldic *fleur-de-lis* ("flower of the lily"), and have been postulated to represent abortive attempts at photoreceptor differentiation.

Given the diversity of cellular constituents of the pineal and its environs, it is not surprising that a number of other tumors besides pineal parenchymal tumors can arise here. In particular, astrocytomas arise from the indigenous astrocytes of the pineal and meningiomas occasionally arise from the arachnoid nests in the velum interpositum. Note, however, that the most common tumor of the pineal gland is germinoma! Germinomas and other germ cell neoplasms of the pineal are postulated to arise from embryonic germ cell rests.

The Pituitary Gland

The *pituitary gland* is composed of two components, the larger adenohypophysis (anterior pituitary), which is a derivative of the embryonic Rathke's pouch, and the smaller neurohypophysis (posterior pituitary; *pars nervosa*), which arises as a direct evagination of the central neuraxis (Fig. 2-92). The infundibular stalk and pituitary gland are surrounded by leptomeninges in which arachnoid cell nests are not uncommonly seen. The sella turcica, which houses the pituitary, is lined with dura.

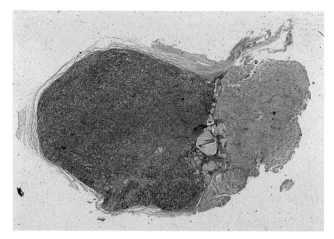

FIGURE 2-92. Pituitary gland. The pituitary gland is composed of three major components: anterior pituitary (adenohypophysis), posterior pituitary (neurohypophysis) and the pars intermedia. The latter middle component frequently contains small cystic remnants of Rathke's cleft, as can be seen in this autopsy specimen, which occasionally can enlarge to a size sufficient to cause symptomatic compression.

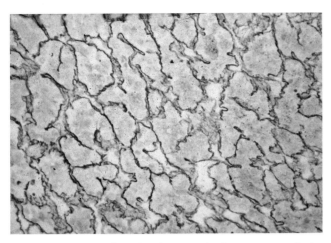

FIGURE 2-93. Reticulin stain. The normal acinar structure of adenohypophyseal tissue that is formed by parcellating fibrovascular septa is exceptionally well visualized with a reticulin stain; this stain is often employed to aid diagnosis of pituitary adenoma in which the normal pattern is destroyed by expansion of the adenoma.

Adenohypophysis

The adenohypophysis is composed of three parts: (1) the large *pars distalis*, (2) the pars intermedia, which is juxtaposed between the pars distalis and neurohypophysis, and (3) the *pars tuberalis*, which is a thin layer of adenohypophysial tissue that extends superiorly around the infundibulum. The adenohypophysis is a neuroendocrine organ composed of tight clusters of cells bounded by delicate fibrovascular septa. This lobular parcellation is best appreciated by application of a *reticulin stain* (Fig. 2-93).

Historically, adenohypophysial cells were classified into three groups based on the cytoplasmic tinctorial properties on H&E-stained tissue sections: (1) *acidophiles* (orange-red), (2) *basophiles* (purplish), and (3) *chromophobes* (pale-to-clear cytoplasm). The same classification was applied to neoplasms of the adenohypophysis (pituitary adenomas) and a crude correlation between staining properties and hormonal expression was established. However, *the H&E-based classification of anterior pituitary cell types and adenomas is notoriously imprecise and has been completely supplanted by immunohistochemistry performed for the various pituitary hormones.* Contemporary immunohistochemical studies have demonstrated considerable overlap in hormone expression when adenomas are classified according to the old H&E scheme.

The pars intermedia in normal individuals often exhibits multiple small cystic remnants of Rathke's pouch (*Rathke cleft cysts*; mucinous cysts) (Fig. 2-94). The lining of these cysts consists of a columnar ciliated epithelium with scattered mucin-producing goblet cells (note: a virtually identical lining is seen in colloid cysts of the third ventricle and neurenteric cysts of the spinal canal). Rarely, such cysts may attain sufficient size to exert a compressive mass effect. Although the vast majority of mucinous cysts are found in the pars intermedia within the sella, rare examples involving the infundibular stalk have been reported.

Occasionally, simple glands that share characteristics with salivary glands are found in association with Rathke cysts. Such *salivary gland rests* are usually seen in the posterior pituitary adjacent to Rathke cysts with which their lumina sometimes communicate. These interesting structures have been found

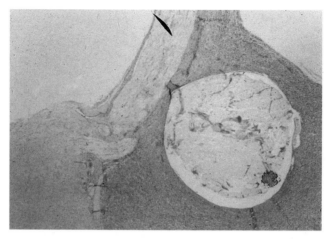

FIGURE 2-94. Rathke cleft cyst. Rathke cleft cysts are usually an incidental finding noted on MR scan or at autopsy, as was this case; however, some will compress the infundibulum, thereby compromising dopamine transport to the pituitary and result in mildly elevated serum prolactin ("stalk effect"), necessitating surgical decompression.

to be quite common if serial sections are employed in an assiduous search for their presence.

The *pars tuberalis* forms a thin layer around the infundibulum. A unique change commonly seen in glandular clusters of the pars tuberalis is squamous metaplasia. The resulting nests of squamous cells are known as *Erdheim's rests* (Fig. 2-95) and were observed as early as 1860 by Luschka. They are commonly observed in adults but are much less frequent in youth and virtually never seen in children less than 10 years of age.

The pars tuberalis, which extends along the infundibular stalk superior to the diaphragma sellae, occasionally serves as the site of origin of a primary suprasellar pituitary adenoma. Rare case reports of other extrasellar pituitary adenomas in such locations as the third ventricle and interpeduncular fossa are attributed to pituitary cell rests.

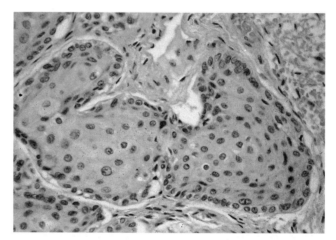

FIGURE 2-95. Erdheim's rests. Focal squamous metaplasia of adenohypophyseal acini, which is particularly common in the pars tuberalis, is a histologic oddity that should not be misinterpreted by the pathologist as abnormal.

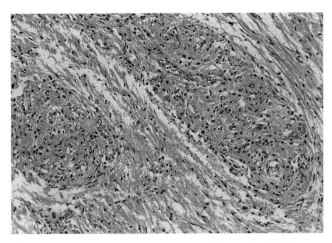

FIGURE 2-96. Gomitoli. Prominent vascular tangles in the neurohypophyseal component of the infundibulum resemble somewhat the glomeruloid vascular proliferation seen in gliomas.

Neurohypophysis

The neurohypophysis is a direct extension of the central neuraxis, but is composed of highly specialized neuronal, glial, and vascular elements. Prominent glomeruloid-like tangles of capillaries, termed *"gomitoli"* (Fig. 2-96), are present in the upper infundibulum and surround terminal arterioles of the superior hypophyseal arteries. Vessels arising from the gomitoli lead to portal vessels in the adenohypophysis.

The primary neuronal constituents are tracts of axons originating from the supraoptic and paraventricular nuclei of the hypothalamus. These axons are engaged in the transport of oxytocin and vasopressin. Specialized granular body storage vesicles for these hormones, termed *"Herring bodies"* (Fig. 2-97), are often seen in tissue sections of the infundibulum and posterior pituitary.

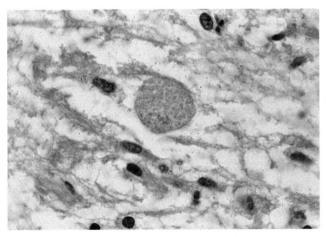

FIGURE 2-97. Herring body. Spherical eosinophilic granular bodies, termed "Herring bodies," are normally present in the neurohypophysis and constitute the storage structures for oxytosin and vasopressin. These should not be confused with other types of granular bodies seen in various CNS diseases, such as the eosinophilic granular bodies (EGBs) associated with low-grade tumors (pilocytic astrocytoma, ganglioglioma, pleomorphic xanthoastrocytoma) or the degenerative granular bodies found in the gliotic parenchyma around vascular malformations.

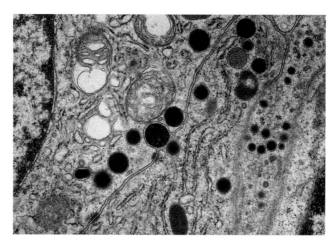

FIGURE 2-98. Dense core ("Neurosecretory") Vesicles. Dense core vesicles, as seen here in a pituitary adenoma, are an ultrastructural hallmark of neuroendocrine differentiation.

Specialized spindled astrocytes, termed "pituicytes," are also present in the neurohypophysis and occasionally give rise to pituicytomas. The overall morphologic appearance of the infundibulum and posterior pituitary is highly spindled and quite distinctive. The constellation of elongated fascicles of pituicytes, glomeruloid vascular tangles, and Herring bodies (qua eosinophilic granular bodies) exhibits a more than passing resemblance to pilocytic astrocytoma. The surgical pathologist must be aware of this fact when dealing with biopsies obtained from the sellar or suprasellar region.

An additional finding occasionally encountered in the infundibulum are *granular cell tumorlets.* These distinctive cell clusters are most often seen incidentally at autopsy; however, similar to the Rathke's cleft cysts mentioned above, they may rarely attain sufficient size to exert mass effect.

Immunochemistry, Ultrastructure, and Neoplastic Counterparts

As mentioned above, classification of pituicytes and their neoplasms according to hormonal product based on immunohistochemical methods has now completely supplanted the imprecise and antiquated classification based on H&E-stain tinctorial properties. Thus, for example, prolactin-producing adenomas are readily identified by application of antiprolactin antibodies, etc. By ultrastructural examination, pituitary adenomas exhibit characteristic *dense-core "neurosecretory-type" vesicles* (Fig. 2-98) that are typical of neuroendocrine cells and their neoplasms.

The Circumventricular Organs

TABLE 2-29. THE CIRCUMVENTRICULAR ORGANS

Pineal gland
Median eminence, infundibulum, and neuro-hypophysis
Subfornical organ
Organum vasculosum of the lamina terminalis
Subcommissural organ (vestigial in humans)
Area postrema (paired)

The circumventricular organs (CVOs; Table 2-29) are a heterogeneous group of six specialized CNS centers (pineal gland; median eminence, infundibulum and neurohypophysis; subfornical organ; organum vasculosum of the lamina terminalis; subcommissural organ; area postrema) that share several features. All of the CVOs have a periventricular location and all except for the subcommissural organ *lack a blood–brain barrier (BBB)* that is characteristic of the vasculature of all other regions of the CNS. All of the CVOs except for the area postrema of the medulla are unpaired midline structures associated with the diencephalon and third ventricle. The area postrema is a paired organ located in the caudal floor of the fourth ventricle.

Concerning the subcommissural organ (SCO), which is located on the ventral surface of the posterior commissure, three facts should be noted: (1) it is the only CVO that is not highly vascularized and the vessels that are present do possess a BBB, (2) in nonhuman mammals, the SCO secretes a mucopolysaccharide string (*Reissner's fiber*) into the cerebral aqueduct, which extends caudally all the way through the fourth ventricle to the end of the spinal cord central canal, and 3) in humans, although present in the developing fetus, the subcommissural organ is only identified as occasional vestigial remnants in adults and no Reissner's fiber is present in the adult human brain.

The lack of the BBB in most CVOs is presumed to play an integral part in the various functions of these organs; all are postulated to "sample" or "monitor" various blood components. The histology of the CVOs reflects this physiological attribute in that they exhibit a highly vascularized stroma (except for the above-noted SCO). The periventricular location of the CVOs also suggests a possible cerebrospinal fluid "monitoring" function. Some evidence has been adduced to support the idea that serotonin may serve as a neurohormone that modulates CVO function by direct innervation of the organs (by neurons of the dorsal raphe nuclei) and also perhaps by release of serotonin directly into the cerebrospinal fluid.

Optic Nerve

The optic "nerves" are not part of the peripheral nervous system, but rather are direct extensions of the CNS analogous to the olfactory tracts. Thus, *oligodendrocytes rather than Schwann cells constitute the myelin-forming elements* and the optic apparatus is therefore susceptible to CNS demyelinating illnesses, such as multiple sclerosis. The optic nerves are completely surrounded by leptomeninges (arachnoid, subarachnoid space, and pia) and a rigid pachymeningeal sheath that is continuous with the rest of the cranial dura (Fig. 2-99). Because of the investing dura, the optic nerves are vulnerable to compression by any expanding, space-occupying mass located within the sheath. The most common example is optic sheath meningioma. As in other locations throughout the CNS, these tumors arise from the arachnoid (meningothelial) cells of the arachnoid membrane.

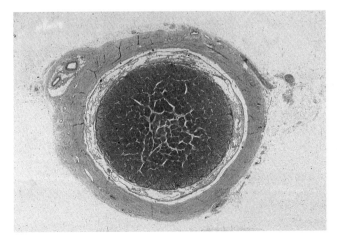

FIGURE 2-99. Optic nerve. The optic "nerve" is really a CNS tract whose myelin is formed by oligodendrocytes rather than Schwann cells. The optic nerve is surrounded by all three meningeal layers, including the subarachnoid space.

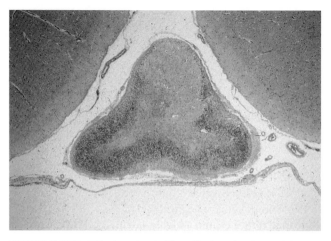

FIGURE 2-100. Olfactory tract. The olfactory tracts are triangular in cross section and contain myelinated axons and, in the adult, oftentimes large numbers of corpora amylacea in astrocyte cell processes.

Olfactory Tracts and Bulbs

The olfactory tracts and bulbs are direct extensions of the CNS. The tracts course rostrally from the basal forebrain in the olfactory sulci just lateral to the gyri recti. They are triangular in cross section and, in addition to myelinated axons, often contain large numbers of corpora amylacea in adults (Fig. 2-100). *The olfactory bulbs have a very distinctive laminated architecture* (Fig. 2-101). Starting from the most superficial layer, which is in contact with the cribriform plate of the ethmoid bone, the laminae are as follows: olfactory nerve layer, glomerular layer, external plexiform layer, mitral cell layer, and granule cell layer. Beneath these strata, the deep nuclei of the olfactory bulb are found surrounded by a white matter core of myelinated axons. The *glomeruli* are specialized synaptic zones where the terminals of afferent olfactory nerve fibers

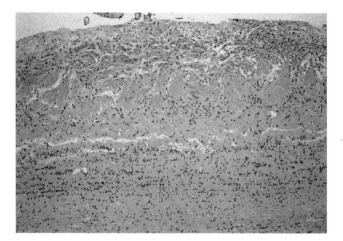

FIGURE 2-101. Olfactory bulb. The olfactory bulb has a distinctive multilayered architecture, beginning with an outer layer of entering olfactory nerve axons, followed by the glomerular layer, external plexiform layer, mitral cell layer, and granular cell layer. The glomeruli are spherical synapse-rich structures that are unique to the olfactory bulb and aid recognition of this structure when encountered in introperative diagnostic frozen sections.

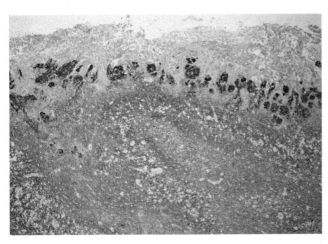

FIGURE 2-102. Olfactory bulb. Because of their high content of synaptic contacts, the olfactory bulb glomeruli are exceptionally well visualized by immunostaining for synaptophysin.

synapse with the dendrites of the mitral cells (Fig. 2-102). The distinctive nested architecture of the glomeruli constitutes a histologic feature that is unique to this component of the nervous system. As would be expected from their dense concentration of synapses, glomeruli are strongly positive for synaptophysin. In the surgical pathology arena, diagnostic intraoperative frozen section interpretation is frequently requested by head and neck surgeons during resection of nasal sinus tumors such as esthesioneuroblastoma; it is therefore wise for all surgical pathologists to become familiar with the normal architecture of this unique structure! The leptomeninges that cover the olfactory bulbs are particularly rich in arachnoid cell nests, which are the cells of origin of olfactory groove meningiomas.

An additional structure of interest that resides in the neighborhood of the olfactory tracts is the terminal nerve plexus (*nervus terminalis, cranial nerve zero*) (Fig. 2-103). This cranial nerve, although the last to be discovered, has

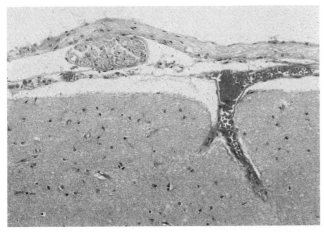

FIGURE 2-103. Cranial nerve zero. The terminal nerve (cranial nerve zero, nervus terminalis) is present in humans as small nerve fascicles in the subarachnoid space overlying the gyri recti between the olfactory tracts. The Schwann cells of cranial nerve zero constitute one potential origin for the subfrontal schwannomas that occasionally arise in this region.

TABLE 2-30. POTENTIAL SCHWANN CELL SOURCES OF ORIGIN FOR SUBFRONTAL SCHWANNOMA

Meningeal branches of the trigeminal nerve
Intracranial segment of the anterior ethmoid nerves
Nervus terminalis (cranial nerve zero)

TABLE 2-31. TUMORS OF THE SUBFRONTAL/OLFACTORY REGION

Olfactory groove meningioma
Subfrontal schwannoma

TABLE 2-32. CONSTITUENTS OF THE HUMAN FILUM TERMINALE

Collagen
Blood vessels
Nerve fascicles
Ependymal remnant[a] (central canal)
(±Adipose tissue)

[a] Source of myxopapillary ependymoma.

TABLE 2-33. TWO UNIQUE NEOPLASMS OF THE FILUM TERMINALE

Myxopapillary ependymoma
Paraganglioma of the filum

an attachment to the brain that is more rostrally located than that of the olfactory nerves and tracts (hence the designation "zero," as the olfactory nerves had previously been designated CN 1). In adult humans, these paired nerves lie in the leptomeninges that cover the gyri recti and each is composed of a microscopic plexus of nerve fascicles of varying calibers. Of the two principal neoplasms that arise in this anatomic neighborhood, olfactory groove meningioma and subfrontal schwannoma, the *Schwann cells of the terminal nerves may account for the origin of at least some of the subfrontal schwannomas* (Table 2-30 and Table 2-31).

The Conus Medullaris and Filum Terminale

The filum consists of the terminal continuation of the spinal cord distal to the conus medullaris (Fig. 2-104). The junction of the filum and conus contains a small remnant of the terminal ventricle (of Kraus). The filum itself is largely composed of collagen from the pia mater, blood vessels, and scattered errant nerve fascicles from the cauda equina (Table 2-32). Of particular clinical significance, however, is the *normal persistence of an ependymal remnant of the central canal throughout the entire length of the filum terminale: this is the cell population of origin of myxopapillary ependymomas* of the filum terminale and conus medullaris. The distinctive morphologic features of this distinctive ependymal neoplasm derive from the intimate association of ependyma with dense connective tissue that occurs only in the filum. Another tumor that is virtually restricted to this neuroanatomic structure is paraganglioma of the filum terminale (Table 2-33). Because normal paraganglia have not been described at this location, the cell of origin of filum paragangliomas is currently unknown.

The Cerebellopontine Angle

Although not a regional organ, the CPA is a richly diverse, anatomically unique and clinically important locale within the CNS with which every clinician, clinical neuroscientist, and student of the nervous system should be fa-

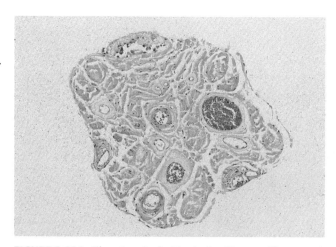

FIGURE 2-104. Filum terminale. The bulk of human filum terminale, seen here in cross section, is composed primarily of collagen with interspersed blood vessels and a few small peripheral nerve fascicles. Importantly, an ependymal remnant of the central canal is present throughout the full length of the filum and constitutes the origin for myxopapillary ependymomas of the filum terminale.

miliar. A large number of different cellular constituents form the CPA cistern and its borders (Table 2-34). A key concept is that the many different types of tumors that can arise in the CPA correspond to the native cellular constituents of the cistern and bordering regions of the CNS (to which list mass lesions arising from developmental rests, such as epidermoid cysts, must also be added). Thus, knowledge of the different cell types normally found in the CPA greatly facilitates formulation of the broad differential diagnosis for mass lesions arising at this site.

BIBLIOGRAPHY

Fuller GN, Burger PC. Central nervous system. In: Sternberg SS, ed. *Histology for pathologists,* 2nd ed. New York: Raven Press, 1997.

TABLE 2-34. CONSTITUENTS OF THE CEREBELLO-PONTINE ANGLE (CPA)

Meningothelial cells of the arachnoid
Leptomeningeal melanocytes
Cranial nerves 7–10
Ependyma of the lateral recess
Choroid plexus of the lateral recess
Blood vessels
CNS parenchyma of the cerebellum and brainstem

3

NEUROCHEMICAL PRINCIPLES

PERSPECTIVE

1. The varied cellular constituents of the nervous system have functional differences just as they have structural and biochemical differences. Neurons are the primary information processing cells, astrocytes maintain structural and biochemical integrity, oligodendrocytes maintain myelin, the ependyma maintain the ventricular lining, and microglia provide defense.
2. Neurons are the primary signaling cellular constituents of the nervous system, and they achieve this task locally by integrating graded excitatory and inhibitory potentials leading to output in the form of the action potential.
3. The graded and self-propagating action potentials depend on the membrane properties of neurons.
4. Much of the signaling activity of the nervous system occurs at synapses where local membrane electrical activity can be briefly modulated or longer duration intracytoplasmic signaling can be effected.
5. The precise nature of synaptic effects is controlled by the specific neurotransmitters and neurotransmitter receptors involved at the particular synapse.
6. Functional systems of neurons may share neurotransmitters and receptors, and diseases can in some cases be classified primarily along neurotransmitter lines.

OBJECTIVES

1. Understand the major functions of the cellular constituents of the nervous system.
2. Be able to distinguish and explain the molecular foundations of the resting potential, graded potentials, and the action potential.
3. Learn the two major classes of neurotransmitter receptors and the functional characteristics of each.
4. Understand the biochemistry, function, distribution, and pharmacology of the major neurotransmitters in relation to normal function, disease, and therapeutics.

NEURONS

The neuron is the central cell of the CNS, permitting those essential operations of spatial and temporal integration, memory, transmission, and plasticity (Figs. 3-1 and 3-2). There are about 10 billion neurons in the adult brain.

These cells have a size range from 5 to 70 μm, but the classical image is the motor neuron with a large nucleus with vesicular chromatin decorated with a prominent nucleolus. The cytoplasm has conspicuous Nissl substance (rough endoplasmic reticulum) and microtubules. Extending from the cell body (soma) are neuronal processes, including dendrites, that, along with the soma, constitute the major receptive fields of neurons (Fig. 3-3). Axo-dendritic and axo-somatic release of neurotransmitters results in graded potentials that are either excitatory (excitatory postsynaptic potentials [EPSPs]) or inhibitory (inhibitory postsynaptic potentials [IPSPs]). In general, excitatory synapses are distributed distally in the dendritic receptive field, while inhibitory synapses exist in the proximal dendritic field or on the cell body. The graded potentials wrought by the interplay of EPSPs and IPSPs are distributed over the surface membrane of the neuron, and it is clear that the proximal receipt of the inhibitory synapses permits modulation by attenuation of incoming excitatory synapses.

The axon is the transmission element of neurons terminating in the synapse (Fig. 3-4). Most neurons have a single axon in contrast to numerous dendrites, and the axon is capable of sustaining an action potential while dendrites perform their work using graded potentials. The junction of the axon with the cell body is the axon hillock where action potentials are initiated; in a sense, the axon hillock is the target of the complex geometric information processing occurring on the cell body and dendritic arborization. Axons can innervate structures in the immediate vicinity of their cell bodies, or they may project great distances throughout the central and peripheral nervous system. In the large projection-class neurons, the axonal volume may exceed by many-fold the volume of the cell body, but the soma is the site of all protein synthesis required to maintain the axon. Proteins synthesized in the cytoplasm as well as organelles such as mitochondria and low molecular weight substances such as neurotransmitter precursors are transported down the axon by an energy-dependent process called "axonal transport" (Fig. 3-5). Axonal transport is, in fact, bidirectional as can be demonstrated dramatically by placing a ligature around the axon, which results in damming up of transported material on both sides of the blockade. In clinical practice, papilledema is the result of retinal ganglion cell axonal swelling at the lamina cribrosa resulting from impaired anterograde axonal transport due to raised intracranial pressure.

There are differing rates of axonal transport, not unlike trucks traveling along freeways at differing speeds (Fig. 3-6). Slow axonal transport creeps along at 0.5–4.0 mm/day, and the cargo consists of structural proteins in-

Axonal Transport

Fast Transport 200-400 mm/day

Neurotransmitter Vesicle Glycoproteins & Enzymes

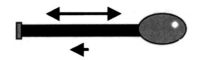

Slow Transport 0.5 - 4 mm/day

Cytoskeletal Proteins

FIGURE 3-6. Aspects of fast and slow axonal transport.

Cells of the Nervous System

Neurons - Information Processors

Glia - "Glue" - Maintainers

Microglia - Defenders

Endothelium - Barrier

FIGURE 3-1. The major classes of cells in the brain parenchyma.

Neurons

Soma 5 μm - 70 μm

Vesicular nucleus with large nucleolus

Rough endoplasmic reticulum (Nissl substance)

Axons and dendrites

FIGURE 3-2. Characteristics of neurons.

Dendrites

Receptive fields of neurons

Excitatory distally

Inhibitory proximally

Graded potentials

FIGURE 3-3. Characteristics of neuronal dendrites.

Axon

Transmission element of neurons

Self-regenerating action potential

Axonal transport

Up to 1 meter long

FIGURE 3-4. The axon is the signal output element of the neuron.

Axonal Transport

Energy dependent

Bidirectional

Variable rate

FIGURE 3-5. Features of axonal transport.

cluding tubulin, neurofilaments, actin, and myosin as well as soluble enzymes required for synaptic energy metabolism. Slow transport is predominantly active only in anterograde direction. Intermediate or saltatory transport cruises along at 15–50 mm/day, and the primary component consists of mitochondria bobbing and weaving bidirectionally along the axoplasm. Fast transport hurls along at 200–400 mm/day in both directions, carrying membrane components such as glycoproteins and glycolipid as well as neurotransmitter synthetic enzymes. Retrograde axonal transport serves to recycle structural and metabolic components, but also is critical for conveying signal molecules from the synaptic outposts back to the soma so that adjustments in metabolic support can be made.

The axon is also the Achilles' heel of the neuron since it serves as the entry route of a number of pathogens and toxins and, due to its large volume, presents a very large target with relatively tenuous supply lines (Fig. 3-7). Rabies virus hops on the motor neurons from the inoculation site in skeletal muscle where initial viral replication occurs, and is obligingly transported into the CNS where it spreads transsynaptically, replicates in the soma, and then is diabolically transported down motor, autonomic, and sensory axons. Herpes zoster virus resides in latency in sensory ganglia, but may, from time to time, be transported by axonal transport to the periphery to produce dermatomal cutaneous eruptions. Similarly, herpes simplex may produce focal encephalitis in areas receiving olfactory input by traveling by axonal transport along the olfactory nerves. In the ancient evolutionary battle between creatures with nervous systems and microbes, the prokaryotes have numerous victories, including the exploitation by *Clostridia tetani* of axonal transport to send tetanus toxin into the nervous system, where it impairs release of inhibitory neurotransmitters (GABA and glycine) from interneurons.

Much of the metabolic activity of the neuronal soma is devoted to axonal maintenance, and if the soma sickens, then the axon withers. Since this form of axonal vulnerability is first felt by the most distal axon and only later by more proximal segments, the process is called a "dying back" axonopathy. Not surprisingly, if this occurs in the peripheral nervous system, the patient experiences acral (fingers and toes) paresthesiae and weakness with loss of distal deep tendon reflexes. The axon itself, however, is the target of a large number of neurotoxic substances that result in a primary axonopathy with clinically identical manifestations. Of course, the primary axonal damage may impair the soma's ability to support intact axon beyond the site of injury, resulting in a superimposed dying back axonopathy.

There is a stereotypic neuronal reaction to axonal injury with perikaryon alterations, including dissolution of the Nissl substance, a process called "chromatolysis" (Fig. 3-8). The redistribution and volume expansion of rough endoplasmic reticulum is preparatory for the reparative protein synthesis. Similar changes may be seen in pellagra. The enlargement of the cytoplasmic volume is associated with migration of the nucleus to an eccentric location, leading to a ballooned neuron with an eerily placed nuclear "eye." Axonal changes distal to a transection site consist of dissolution of the axon—a process called "Wallerian degeneration." Debris from this disintegration is cleared by infiltrating macrophages. The Schwann cells remain as faithful sentinels awaiting the arrival of the slowly regrowing axon still attached to the nuturing soma. The Schwann cells arrange themselves to form hollow tubes or tunnels guiding the regrowing axons to their targets. If the soma is unable to sustain the regrowth of the axon, the Schwann cells give up hope and trigger apoptosis in the process of secondary demyelination. The resulting loss of myelin is easily discerned using a variety of histochemical stains that can be used to map tract degeneration in neurodegenerative

---

Axonal Transport

Deliver samples to soma

Recycle transport vesicles

Entry route for rabies and herpes viruses and tetanus toxin

FIGURE 3-7. Axonal transport's normal functions can be subverted by pathogens.

Reaction to Axonal Transection

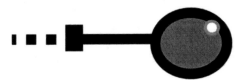

Wallerian Degeneration

Chromatolysis RER Dispersed Nucleus Displaced

FIGURE 3-8. Central chromatolysis is the neuronal somatic response to axonal injury.

Action Potential Conduction Velocity

Fat fibers are fast

Fat = large diameter

Fat = myelinated

FIGURE 3-9. Action conduction velocity is determined by axonal thickness and myelination.

---

disorders or functional connections when these are transected in neuroanatomical studies (Fig. 3-9).

NEUROGLIA

The normal astrocyte is visible only by its round to oval nucleus devoid of a conspicuous nucleolus because its cytoplasm exists as delicate strands blending imperceptibly with the surrounding neuropil (Figs. 3-10 through 3-13). Reactive astrocytes possess eosinophilic cytoplasm rich in glial fibrillary acidic protein and devoid of Nissl substance, nuclei smaller than neurons and without the prominent nucleolus, and multiple delicate processes that touch vessels, neurons, and the pia. The biochemical functions of astrocytes consist of regulation of water and ions in extracellular space, control of metabolic traffic across the blood–brain barrier to and from the blood, serving as metabolic sinks for noxious metabolites, and effecting synaptic modulation of neurotransmitters. Cellular actions of astrocytes include maintenance of structural integrity of CNS tissue, reaction to injury (gliosis), and guiding migration of neurons during development.

Oligodendroglia possess small hyperchromatic nuclei and sharply defined cell margins with clear cytoplasm (Fig. 3-14). The major function of oligodendroglia is production of CNS myelin that ensheaths axons, permitting saltatory conduction of action potentials. Oligodendroglia are relatively recent arrivals on the evolutionary scene and occur only in vertebrates. The invertebrate cephalopods (squid and octopus) have very complex nervous systems and elaborate visual systems, but without central myelin these creatures could attain rapid action potential conduction velocities only by increasing the diameters of their axons. This imposed a fundamental limitation on the degree of brain component miniaturization that these invertebrates could attain. Their loss was our (the vertebrates) gain, for we had access to the giant squid axon that had physical dimensions large enough that measurement of membrane potentials was feasible. Thus, we learned much about fundamental neurophysiology from our brethren in what has been called the second major pinnacle in brain evolution.

Ependyma contain sausage-shaped small nuclei, eosinophilic cytoplasm that is ciliated on one surface (basal body = blepharoplast) (Fig. 3-15). These cells line ventricles and spinal canal, and regulate metabolic traffic between the minute channels of the extracellular space of the neuropil and the vast oceans of the ventricles. The extracellular space actually comprises as much as 15% of

---

Glia

- **Astrocytes**
- **Oligodendroglia**
- **Ependyma**

FIGURE 3-10. The macroglia or true glia are composed of the astrocytes, oligodendroglia and ependyma.

Astrocyte Histology

Eosinophilic cytoplasm (GFAP)

Small nucleus c/o large nucleolus

Delicate cytoplasmic processes

Inconspicuous rough ER

FIGURE 3-11. Astrocyte histology.

Astrocyte Physiology

Outnumber neurons 10:1

Regulation of extracellular milieu

Regulation of BBB metabolic traffic

Metabolic sink of noxious products

Synaptic modulation

FIGURE 3-12. Astrocyte physiology.

Astrocyte Physiology

Structural integrity of CNS tissue

Reaction to injury--gliosis

Guidance of neurons during development

FIGURE 3-13. Astrocyte physiology continued.

Oligodendroglia Histology

Small hyperchromatic nuclei

Clear cytoplasm

Limited number of cellular processes

Myelinate multiple axons

FIGURE 3-14. Oligodendroglial microscopic appearance.

Ependyma Histology

Round to oval nuclei

Cilia and tight junctions

Line ventricles and central canal of spinal cord

Basis of brain: CSF barrier

FIGURE 3-15. Ependyma structure and function.

Microglia

React to injury forming macrophages

Mostly derived from blood monocytes

FIGURE 3-16. Microglia are not true glia but are derived from blood stream monocytes.

Endothelium

The endothelial cells with tight junctions are the structural basis of the blood brain barrier

Molecules penetrate the brain if lipid soluble or transported by endothelium

FIGURE 3-17. The endothelium of the brain capillaries constitutes the blood–brain barrier.

the volume of the neuropil, and is the site of neurotransmitter and metabolite diffusion. Increasing attention is being directed at the movement of molecules through the space and the possibility of long range and relatively diffuse actions of neurotransmitters released into the extracellular space. This type of signaling is known as volume transmission and may have a major role in setting large-scale neuronal excitability or inhibition.

Microglia are reactive cellular elements mostly derived from circulating monocytes (Fig. 3-16). There are resident quiescent monocyte series cells, the microglia, that become activated at the first hint of need. The activated microglial nucleus is elongate and slightly irregular, and is frequently decorated at both ends by tufts of cytoplasm. Activated monocytes coming in from the bloodstream and activated microglia may assume the form of macrophages—giant, sometimes multinucleated, cells filled with ingested debris of victims of their fearsome proteolytic, acidic, oxidizing chemical defense systems. Innocent bystanders such as neurons may, however, suffer from these toxins released from activated macrophages and microglia. Attention is being increasingly directed at the host immune reaction as being exacerbating rather than soothing.

The blood–brain barrier is made from the endothelial cell and its tight junctions (Fig. 3-17). The endothelial cell of brain vessels differs from its systemic counterpart in that it is devoid of cytoplasmic fenestrations, is relatively poor in vesicles for pinocytosis, and is very rich in mitochondria. Furthermore, the endothelial cells cling to one another using tight junctions that completely preclude passage of material between them. Substances can gain entry into the nervous system only by passing through the endothelial cell, either by diffusion through the lipid-laden membranes of the cell or through membrane-bound transporters. Lipid-soluble compounds such as ethanol and benzodiazepine simply diffuse into the brain, illustrating the pharmacologically crucial principle that drug entry into the CNS is largely determined by the drug's lipid solubility or oil/water partition coefficient. Lipophobic drugs simply will not penetrate the blood–brain barrier and must be directly instilled into the cerebrospinal fluid. Other compounds, notably glucose and amino acids, cross the endothelial cell barrier via protein transporters. These transporters may be passive and simply result in facilitated diffusion or they may be active and graciously powered by the endothelial cell mitochondria. Signaling molecules released from astrocytes induce this special blood–brain barrier endothelial cell phenotype. The astrocytes gently place their foot processes circumferentially around capillaries and induce this remarkable phenotype. The pericapillary array of astrocyte foot processes may also play a role in metabolic trafficking, but it does not contribute directly to the physical basis of the blood–brain barrier. The blood–brain barrier permits the brain to conduct its complex metabolic computations insulated from the fluctuations of ions and metabolites. Furthermore, the uncontrolled entry of amino acids that function directly as neurotransmitters is prevented.

MEMBRANES, RECEPTORS, AND NEUROTRANSMITTERS

Membrane Properties of Neurons

Biological membranes consist of lipid bilayers with proteins floating within them. Hydrophobic portions of the proteins extend into the lipid and traverse the membrane, forming ion channels and pumps. Protein segments extending out of the membrane serve as receptor sites. Segments extending into the cytoplasm may effect changes within the cell in response to binding of receptors on the surface.

Electrical Activity of Membranes: Membrane Potential

Sodium, potassium, and chloride are differentially distributed across the cell membrane with sodium being high in the extracellular space, and potassium and chloride being high in the intracellular space. This ion separation is established by expenditure of metabolic energy driving ion pumps in the membrane. The ions tend to leak through the membrane down their concentration gradients; the concentration gradient is counterbalanced by an electrical potential (Fig. 3-18). The voltage across the membrane is determined by the ion with the greatest permeability.

The membrane resting potential is maintained at -70 mV and is dependent on potassium permeability, hence the resting potential is near the potassium equilibrium potential (Fig. 3-19). Potassium channels come in a variety of physiological and pharmacological forms. The channel responsible for the resting potential is voltage independent and is called a "leak channel."

Action Potential

The action potential is a self-regenerating wave of depolarization that spreads bidirectionally from its site of origin, although physiologically this potential arises at the axon hillock and is transmitted orthodromically (Fig. 3-20). Action potential propagation increases with increasing axon diameter, and conduction velocity is increased dramatically with myelination permitting saltatory conduction. At the peak of the action potential the membrane potential is $+40$ mV and is dependent on sodium permeability, which in is turn determined by activity of the voltage gated sodium channel. Membrane sodium permeability increases as membrane potential decreases from its -70 mV resting state toward zero. When the potential reaches -55 mV, the Na channels open catastrophically.

The sodium channel major protein has six membrane spanning domains based on hydrophobicity plots. (Once the amino acid sequence of a protein is known from its cDNA, the sequence is examined for runs of hydrophobic amino acid residues that tend to reside within the lipid membrane. If sequences of about 23 hydrophobic amino acids are found, these portions of the protein are favorable for membrane spanning.) The fourth membrane spanning region, S4, also is rich in basic residues from arginine and lysine, and it is thought that these positively charged residues make up the "voltage sensor" of the sodium channel—changes in the membrane potential alter the positions of these residues leading to changes in the conformation of the channel and subsequent sodium conductance changes. Most voltage-gated channels have the six transmembrane spanning configuration.

A transient increase in sodium permeability is the molecular foundation of the action potential (Fig. 3-21). The increase in Na permeability causes this ion to be dominant and establishes the membrane potential at $+40$ mV. The increase in Na permeability is transient. Potassium channels open as sodium channels close and accelerate the return to the negative resting potential. The potassium channels that open here are voltage dependent, in contrast to the leak channels that account for the resting potential. These are also known as Hodgkin–Huxley channels or delayed potassium channels. This classic potassium channel is inactivated by tetraethyl ammonium chloride (TEA). The closure of the Na channels reestablishes K as the membrane potential determining ion, and the resting potential is restored. There is another voltage-dependent K channel known as the fast K channel that rapidly opens in response to membrane depolarization and hence tends to blunt depolarization and to potentiate hyperpolarization. This six-membrane span-

Neuronal Membrane Potentials

- **Membrane potential**
- **Resting potential**
- **Action potential**

FIGURE 3-18. Neuronal membrane potentials determine the functional state of the neuron.

Resting Potential

- **-50 to -70 millivolts**
- **Dependent on unequal ion distribution across membrane**
- **Potassium permeability establishes resting potential**

FIGURE 3-19. The resting potential of the neuron, like many cells, is established by the potassium equilibrium potential.

Action Potential

- **+ 40 millivolts**
- **Transient increase in sodium permeability**
- **Voltage gated sodium channel dependent**

FIGURE 3-20. The action potential is a transient but self-regenerating depolarization of the neuronal membrane.

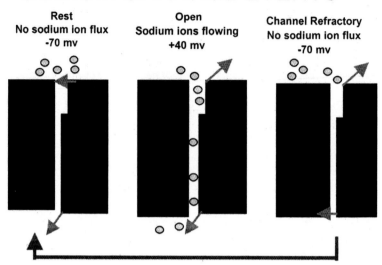

SODIUM CHANNEL EVENTS

FIGURE 3-21. Sodium channel events during the action potential.

ning segment channel will bias an axon toward non-firing. The fast K channel is antagonized by 4-aminopyridine (4AP) which increases the probability with a given depolarization that an action potential will be generated; this activity is the rationale of the experimental use of 4AP in demyelination because the drug should facilitate passage of action potentials along an axon in a demyelinated region by biasing the axon to depolarization. In addition to leak K, slow K, and fast K channels, there are serotonin-dependent K and calcium-dependent K channels, but these play no role in the action potential.

Sodium Channel Toxins

Sodium channel toxins have been derived from a variety of species and have been very useful in illuminating the mechanisms of the sodium channel (Fig. 3-22). Toxins against an evolutionarily ancient and vital protein like the sodium channel are excellent hunting tools for predatory life forms; and many who employ these attack the sodium channel simultaneously at several sites. Rarely (and usually inadvertently) humans may become the targets of such an attack. Therapeutically, local anesthetics may work by blocking the action of the sodium channel.

Na Channel Blockers

The sodium channel blockers bind the outer axonal surface of the channel and prevent maximal Na flux (Fig. 3-23). Tetrodotoxin occurs in the liver and ovaries of puffer fish and results in several deaths annually in Japan despite special licensing of chefs who prepare this delicacy. Sodium conductivity is blocked, but potassium conductance and synaptic transmission are unaffected. Saxitoxin is derived from the dinoflagellate *Gonyaulax catenella* that is consumed by shellfish. The shellfish may in turn be eaten by humans who experience sodium channel blockade manifested as acral paresthesiae, but which may progress to flaccid paralysis.

Sodium Channel Toxins

- **Channel blockers**
- **Channel openers**
- **Channel closure blockers**

FIGURE 3-22. Sodium channel toxins occurring in nature have taught us much about the molecular physiology of the sodium channel.

SODIUM CHANNEL BLOCKERS

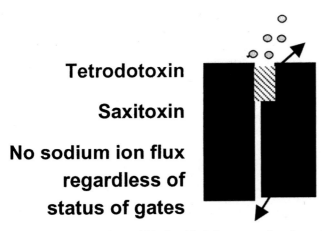

Tetrodotoxin

Saxitoxin

No sodium ion flux regardless of status of gates

FIGURE 3-23. Sodium channel blocker bind the external surface of the channel preventing sodium ion entry.

Na Channel Openers

Batrachotoxin (arrow poison), grayanotoxin and veratridine are alkaloid neurotoxins that pry open the sodium channel and increase the resting membrane conductivity of sodium thereby reducing the resting potential toward zero (Fig. 3-24). Channel blockers block this effect.

Na Channel Closure Blockers

Scorpion and sea anemone toxin block the closure of sodium channels after normal activation, resulting in persistent depolarization (Fig. 3-25). Sodium channel mutations have been discovered in hyperkalemic periodic paralysis and paramyotonia congenita (Fig. 3-26). These mutations occur widely

SODIUM CHANNEL OPENERS

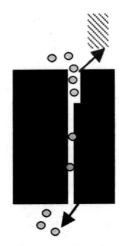

Batrachotoxin

Grayanotoxin

Veratridine

Sodium ions flux continuously

FIGURE 3-24. Sodium channel openers permit continuous sodium ion fluxing.

SODIUM CHANNEL CLOSURE BLOCKERS

Scorpion toxin

Sea anemone toxin

Gates held open; continuous sodium flux

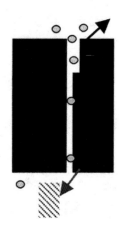

FIGURE 3-25. The sodium channel closure blockers prevent inactivation of the channel.

throughout the sodium channel sequence. In these disorders there is persistent Na conductance implying a failure of channel inactivation.

The specifics of channel operation have to a large extent been clarified using patch clamp measurements in which the activity of a single or very few individual channels can be measured. Molecular genetic techniques are now permitting protein structure–function correlations to be made. Recurrent structural motifs have emerged in channels and receptors, and increasingly we are thinking of these proteins in terms of superfamilies of proteins having structural and functional similarities, and differing only in the details of specific ligands.

SODIUM CHANNEL MUTANTS

Hyperkalemic periodic paralysis
Failure of muscle sodium channel to inactivate at high K concentrations
Periodic paralyses and paramyotonia congentia

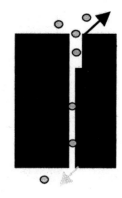

FIGURE 3-26. Increased numbers of mutations of the sodium channels are being described in relationship to the periodic paralyses and paramyotonias.

Receptor Classes

Ionophoric
- Gated channel
- Fast
- TM4 (4 transmembrane domains)
- EPSP or IPSP

Metabotropic
- G Protein-coupled
- Protracted
- TM7 (7 transmembrane domains)
- Cyclase
- Phospholipase
- Ion channels

FIGURE 3-28. Receptors can be either ionophoric, allowing ion fluxes, or metabotropic, functioning via second messengers.

General Features of Neurotransmitters

Neurotransmitters are endogenous compounds that interact with receptors to alter the functional state of the recipient neuron. There are many ways to classify neurotransmitters—according to chemical structure, by physiological effect, according to distribution in the brain, and so forth (Figs. 3-27 and 3-28). Our admittedly somewhat unorthodox approach is to first divide the neurotransmitters into three classes according to their relative abundance in the nervous system—high concentration, mid-range concentration, and low concentration. While this may appear Procrustean at first, we think that this approach is at least as useful as others and has embedded in it some of the history of neurotransmitter research.

High Concentration Neurotransmitters

These are compounds occurring in "industrial" quantities in the brain - μmoles/gram ranges (Fig. 3-29). Included are the amino acid neurotransmitters glutamate, aspartate, GABA, and glycine. Due to their high concentrations and prominent roles in intermediary metabolism, these compounds were not initially considered to be reasonable neurotransmitter candidates. Only when highly selective receptors for these substances were unambiguously demonstrated was it realized that they could indeed be used for cell-to-cell signaling. These compounds proved that neurotransmitters need not be unique special purpose molecules made only for signaling, but that the combination of any appropriate molecule with the right receptor in the correct location were the necessary ingredients for neural signaling. We now realize that these compounds and their receptors are the most abundant neurotransmitter sites in the nervous system, and that they are common targets of both pathological processes and pharmacological interventions.

Intermediate Concentration Neurotransmitters

This group includes the "classical" neurotransmitters that occur in the nanomole/gram concentration range (Fig. 3-30). These include acetylcholine, dopamine (DA), norepinephrine (NE), serotonin (5-HT), and histamine. The neuropharmacology of this group is the best worked out of the three classes of neurotransmitters. Early exploration of these neurotransmitters relied largely on bioassays, but subsequent work has pushed the envelope of molecular biology and pharmacology. These neurotransmitters lent credence to the concept that signaling molecules were quirky small molecules.

Two Types of Gated Channels

Voltage gated
Na, K, Ca

Ligand gated
Neurotransmitter receptors

FIGURE 3-27. Channels can be either voltage or ligand gated.

High Neurotransmitter Levels
- Excitatory amino acids
- GABA
- Glycine

FIGURE 3-29. Neurotransmitters occurring in extremely high concentrations in the brain.

Intermediate Neurotransmitter Levels
- Acetylcholine
- Dopamine
- Norepinephrine
- Serotonin
- Histamine

FIGURE 3-30. The neurotransmitters having intermediate concentrations in the brain constitute the classically described neurotransmitters.

Low Neurotransmitter Levels

- Peptides
- Nitric Oxide
- Carbon Monoxide

FIGURE 3-31. The low concentration neurotransmitters constitute the most novel class of neurotransmitters yet described.

Synaptic Events

Transmitter synthesis in synaptic terminal

Storage in vesicles following Na gradient-dependent uptake

Action potential invades terminal opening voltage-gated calcium channels

Vesicles dock with presynaptic active zone and release NT

FIGURE 3-32. Presynaptic events include neurotransmitter synthesis and storage prior to arrival of a wave of depolarization that triggers release of the transmitter into the synaptic cleft.

Vesicular Storage

Neurotransmitter made in cytosol

Proton gradient-dependent uptake into synaptic vesicles

Transmembrane transporter proteins have structural homologies

FIGURE 3-33. Vesicular storage of neurotransmitter is one of the primary means of preserving an adequate supply of transmitter. Interference with vesicular storage depletes the neurotransmitter.

Synaptic Events

Transmitter diffuses across synaptic cleft

NT activates post-synaptic receptor

NT inactivated by reuptake or enzymatic inactivation

FIGURE 3-34. Postsynaptic events include diffusion across the synaptic cleft, interaction with the receptor and inactivation of the neurotransmitter.

Low Concentration Neurotransmitters

This astonishingly large group of newcomers to the neurotransmitter game includes the neuropeptides and gaseous neurotransmitters that occur in concentration ranges of femtomoles or picomoles/gram (Fig. 3-31). These compounds were discovered only recently due to methodological advances. In essence, any peptide used anywhere else in the body for messenger purposes has been found in the CNS presumably serving neurotransmitter or neuromodulatory functions. Neuropeptides have been found to coexist in neurons using classical or amino acid neurotransmitters.

In addition to neuropeptides, in the late 1980's the mind boggling revelation that nitric oxide (NO) may serve as a neurotransmitter and neuromodulator occurred. NO is a short-lived highly reactive lipophilic molecule generated by nitric oxide synthetase from arginine. This molecule can diffuse rapidly from its intracellular site of synthesis to adjacent cells where it leads to cyclic GMP elevation. It appears that selected neurons may be the site of synthesis and astrocytes may be the target. Interestingly, NO or one of its congeners is the endothelial-derived relaxation factor, which mediates cell to cell communication between vessel endothelium and smooth muscle and may be important in vasospasm. Carbon monoxide (CO) is now regarded as a strong contender for membership in the gaseous neurotransmitter category.

Synaptic Events

All of the neurotransmitters in the three concentration classes exert most of their effects at the synapse with the important exception of the gaseous neurotransmitters. In addition, many of the neurotransmitters play roles in volume transmission where the postsynaptic events are identical to those we are about to describe but where the presynaptic events are not spatially as tightly linked. In classical synaptic transmission, however, there are events that occur in the signaling presynaptic cells and a different set of activities in the receiving or postsynaptic cell (Fig. 3-32). The presynaptic cell must first synthesize neurotransmitter, and for this purpose synthetic enzymes or peptidergic neurotransmitter precursors are transported to the synaptic terminal from the cell body by axonal transport. Local synaptic mitochondria provide energy and some intermediates for synthesis of neurotransmitters. The newly synthesized transmitters are then stored in presynaptic vesicles that undergo quantal exocytosis upon arrival of an action potential into the nerve terminal (Fig. 3-33). Depolarization by the arriving action potential leads to influx of calcium with calcium-coupled translocation of vesicles to active zones resulting in expulsion of the contents of vesicles into synaptic cleft (Fig. 3-34). Even in the absence of an incoming action potential, there is continuous quantal release of neurotransmitter from individual vesicles. The postsynaptic electrical correlate of this quantal release is miniature end-plate potentials (MEPPs). The neurotransmitter released into the synaptic cleft diffuses across that space and binds to postsynaptic receptors triggering postsynaptic physiological events.

The two major mechanisms of receptor action are alteration of ionic conductance and activation of second messengers (Fig. 3-35). Alteration of ionic conductances, also known as ionotropic action, is direct coupled receptor transduction that mediates rapid point-to-point signaling in the nervous system (Fig. 3-36). These fast-acting receptors are sometimes called "class I receptors." Classic examples include excitatory neurotransmitters that increase sodium conductance resulting in membrane depolarization and inhibitory neurotransmitters that increase chloride conductance leading to hyperpolarization. Many of the receptors exhibiting ionotropic action comprise a superfamily of proteins sharing structural similarities. Nicotinic acetylcholine, 5-HT, GABA, glycine, glutamate, kainate and NMDA receptors belong to this superfamily. The ionophore receptors are composed of subunits with four transmembrane domains; the subunits are assembled into tetramers or pentamers.

The second major means of neural signaling, generation of second messengers, also known as metabotropic action, is indirectly coupled receptor transduction and tends to mediate more prolonged effects of synaptic transmission on the postsynaptic cell (Fig. 3-37). The receptors mediating this action are sometimes referred to as "class II receptors." G-protein (guanyl nucleotide-binding protein) coupled transmission mediates transmission for a variety of neurotransmitters, including several peptides, muscarinic acetylcholine receptors, and some of the catecholamine receptors just to name a few. Binding of the ligand to the receptor alters the conformation of an adjacent G protein floating in the cell membrane (Fig. 3-38). The activated G protein may then open an ion channel or activate an enzyme such as a cyclase or hydrolase to effect the generation of second messenger molecules within the cell (Figs. 3-39). G-protein–coupled receptors are composed of a single unit with seven transmembrane domains. Downstream signaling events may include processes as diverse as protein phosphorylation, phosphoinositide hydrolysis, protein carboxyl methylation, phospholipid methylation, and eicosanoid formation (Fig 3-40).

Reuptake or inactivation of neurotransmitter is essential to terminate its action (Fig. 3-41). Failure to inactivate the neurotransmitter leads to continuous postsynaptic activation or inhibition, and functionally is equivalent to shutting down the synapse. Reuptake is the major means of inactivation of most neurotransmitters, although most also have parallel enzymatic inactivation systems. The protein pumps responsible for reuptake share many structural features and comprise a new protein superfamily.

The events occurring at the synapse allow for precise and rigorous criteria for neurotransmitter substances (Fig. 3-42). In order for a putative neurotransmitter to be regarded as a true neurotransmitter, the compound must be present in the nerve terminal, released when the action potential reaches the terminal, application of the putative neurotransmitter postsynaptically must have the same effect as activation of the neuron physiologically, and there must be an inactivation mechanism to terminate the activity of the neurotransmitter.

Specific Neurotransmitter Systems

We will now discuss the major neurotransmitter systems. It is helpful to organize your thinking about neurotransmitters in a systematic fashion rather than regarding this information as isolated biochemical factoids. Consider the synthesis, inactivation, anatomical distribution, the variety of neurotransmitter receptors and their mechanisms, presynaptic and postsynaptic toxins and pharmaceuticals, and disease states associated with the neurotransmitter.

Cholinergic System

Acetylcholine (ACh) undergoes synthesis by choline condensation with acetyl-CoA in a reaction catalyzed by choline acetyl transferase (CAT) (Fig. 3-43). The neurotransmitter synthesizing enzyme CAT is a good immunohistochemical marker for identifying nerve terminals as cholinergic, and can also be biochemically assayed to determine the distribution of cholinergic endings as well as their alterations in disease. This general principle of using enzymes responsible for neurotransmitter synthesis to localize synaptic terminals employing individual neurotransmitters has been used widely to map the neurochemical anatomy of the nervous system. Acetylcholine is inactivated by

---

Two Major Neurotransmitter Mechanisms

- Alteration of ionic conductance fast point to point signaling

- Secondary messenger generation protracted alterations in function

FIGURE 3-35. Neurotransmitters may act rapidly by increasing ionic fluxes or by slower secondary messenger cascades.

Ligand-Gated Channels

Transmitter specificity

Saturability

Reversible action

Functional reconstitution in vitro

FIGURE 3-36. Ligand-gated channel characteristics.

Secondary Messengers

Ligands binding to receptor activate G proteins

G proteins diffuse membrane to interact with effector proteins

G proteins may activate or inhibit effectors

FIGURE 3-37. Secondary messengers have a myriad of effectors.

Secondary Messengers

G proteins may activate or inhibit effector proteins

Effector proteins may include enzymes or ion channels

FIGURE 3-38. Secondary messenger mechanisms involve intracellular processes.

G Protein Cellular Effects

Membrane potential: Channel activation or inhibition

Gene expression: Transcriptional regulation

Metabolism: Enzyme activation or inhibition

Cell shape: Cytoskeletal changes

FIGURE 3-39. The major secondary messenger pathways involve G-proteins that act on downstream messengers.

G Protein Effectors

Adenyl cyclase

Phospholipase

cGMP phosphodiesterase

Potassium and calcium channels

FIGURE 3-40. The complexity of secondary messenger pathways leads to great functional flexibility.

Neurotransmitter Reuptake

Primary means of inactivation of most neurotransmitters

High-affinity sodium gradient-dependent transporter proteins have structural homologies

Neurotransmitter transporters are major targets of neuroactive drugs

FIGURE 3-41. Neurotransmitter reuptake is the most common mechanism of physiological inactivation.

Neurotransmitter Criteria

Present at terminal

Released by action potential

Post-synaptic application mimics physiological action

Inactivation mechanism

FIGURE 3-42. The functional characteristics of synaptic transmission establish the minimal criteria for a substance to be identified as a neurotransmitter.

hydrolysis catalyzed by acetylcholine esterase which releases choline that is promptly taken up by a high-affinity sodium-dependent transporter on the presynaptic neuron.

Cholinergic neurons are found in the medial forebrain complex, as striatal interneurons, in the motor nuclei of peripheral nerves, parabrachial complex, and the reticular formation (Fig. 3-44). They also constitute major elements of the autonomic nervous system as preganglionic neurons of sympathetic ganglia, postganglionic parasympathetic neurons, and sudomotor sympathetic neurons (note that all other postganglionic sympathetic neurons are adrenergic).

Classically, cholinergic receptors are divided into nicotinic and muscarinic, and this scheme remains very useful and valid. It is now recognized, however, that there are multiple subtypes of receptors in these two categories, and that a class of central or neuronal nicotinic receptors exists.

The classical nicotinic receptor exerts its effects by increased sodium conductance with depolarization occurring rapidly and the major pharmacological receptor agonist is nicotine.

Cholinergic nicotinic neurons include the anterior horn cells where the nicotinic receptors reside on the skeletal muscle of the neuromuscular junction, and in the autonomic nervous system where the preganglionic neurons are cholinergic. Central system neurons may possess nicotinic or muscarinic receptors; the central nicotinic receptors are just beginning to be explored.

Neuromuscular junction is a major locus of nicotinic cholinergic disease as well as pharmacology and serves as a useful model of other neurotransmitter-related conditions.

There are multiple general mechanisms that may interfere with synaptic function, including failure to release neurotransmitter, inappropriate and uncontrolled release, receptor blockade or inactivation, and impairment of neurotransmitter degradation. Release blockade of acetylcholine occurs with exposure to botulinum toxin, in the Eaton Lambert syndrome (myasthenic syndrome), in tick paralysis and with beta-neurotoxins of sea snakes (Fig. 3-45). Botulinum, tick paralysis and sea snake toxins acting at the neuromuscular junction can result in severe flaccid paralysis sufficient to lead to respiratory embarrassment and death. Botulinum toxin has been used to great medical advantage using local injections at motor nerve termini to reduce involuntary movements in a variety of movement disorders including torsion dystonia, hemifacial spasm and many others. The occurrence of flaccid paralysis should trigger a careful search of the patient for an inciting tick since removal of the parasite is followed by almost miraculously swift recovery. The Eaton Lambert syndrome is a more chronic condition in which there is impaired calcium mediated vesicular exocytosis; therefore, fewer quanta of acetylcholine are released at the neuromuscular junction in response to action potentials coming down the motor neurons. The patients complain of weakness but with repeated effort or repetitive motor nerve stimulation, they accumulate sufficient non-degraded acetylcholine in the synaptic cleft that more normal neuromuscular transmission occurs. This contrasts with myasthenia gravis (a postsynaptic receptor defect) in which repeated activity or repetitive stimulation leads to fatiguing and a decremental motor response.

Release augmentation of acetylcholine is the mechanism of action of latrotoxin (Black widow spider venom toxin) (Fig. 3-46). The toxin results in painful muscle spasms near the envenomation site due to hyperactivity of skeletal muscles. This may be followed by paralysis especially in small individuals or pets.

Nicotinic receptor inactivation is the mechanism for myasthenia gravis as well as nondepolarizing receptor blockade by curare, alpha-neurotoxins of sea snakes (the damn snakes get the neuromuscular junction coming and going!), cinchona alkaloids, procainamide, and aminoglycoside antibiotics (Fig. 3-47). Myasthenia gravis is by far the most common of these conditions and is characterized by weakness and fatigue particularly with repetitive actions. Electrophysiologically, decrementing muscle activation is seen with repetitive stimulation. Myasthenia gravis results from autoimmune destruction or blockade of the acetylcholine receptors. It should be noted that pharmaceuticals or toxins that act by blocking acetylcholine receptor at the neuromuscular junction will worsen myasthenia gravis via physiological synergism. Depolarizing receptor inactivation can occur with drugs such as succinylcholine that are widely used during general anesthesia to attain complete skeletal muscle relaxation.

Agents that block inactivation of acetylcholine can result in overactivation of both nicotinic and muscarinic receptors and therefore lack the exquisite selectivity seen with receptor targeted agents (Fig. 3-48). Reversible inhibitors of acetylcholine esterase include neostigmine, pyridostigmine, and physostigmine. These agents will augment cholinergic synaptic activity and can be helpful in the diagnoses and treatment of cholinergic receptor blockade conditions such as myasthenia gravis. Physostigmine crosses the blood–brain barrier and interacts with muscarinic ACh receptor as well as nicotinic and is useful in the treatment of CNS effects of atropine intoxication.

Irreversible inhibitors of acetylcholine esterase include organophosphates and carbamates that are extremely useful and potent pesticides. If applied against humans they are called "nerve gas." Receptors can be regenerated using pralidoxime (2-PAM). The organophosphates are emerging as instruments of terrorism in urban areas; hence, physicians must unfortunately become familiar with the emergency treatment of these agents.

The muscarinic acetylcholine receptor exerts its effects by second messengers rather than ion conductance alteration; hence, its actions tend to be more protracted. These receptors are found widely in the CNS and in the autonomic nervous system in postganglionic parasympathetic and sudomotor sympathetic terminals. The receptor agonist after which these receptors are named is muscarine, the active agent in mushrooms of genus Amanita. The physiological effects include parasympathetic hyperactivity manifested by sweating, salivation, miosis, GI hypermotility, airway constriction and secretion. Central effects include vertigo, weakness, confusion, and coma. Muscarinic receptor agonists used in medical practice include pilocarpine, arecoline (doesn't cross the blood–brain barrier and is less apt to cause central effects), methacholine, and carbachol.

The classical muscarinic receptor antagonist is atropine, a powerful pharmaceutical that has central and peripheral effects. It results in mydriasis, decreased salivation, decreased sweating, increased heart rate, decrease airway secretion, and decreased GI motility. Central effects include confusion, restlessness, memory loss, hallucinations, and delirium. Intoxicated individuals are said to be, "Dry as a stone, red as a beet, and mad as a hatter!" Atropine is useful in cholinesterase intoxication by blocking the overactivity induced by accumulation of acetylcholine. Another muscarinic inhibitor, scopolamine, was once used to blunt memories of patients undergoing medical procedures. The effects of the muscarinic inhibitors scopolamine and atropine on memory support the cholinergic hypothesis of Alzheimer's disease (AD) and led to therapeutic development of central cholinesterase inhibitors for the treatment of this disease.

Another anticholinergic agent, Artane, is used to treat Parkinson's disease by antagonizing striatal muscarinic cholinergic neurons.

As mentioned above, AD at a neurochemical level can be regarded as a cortical acetylcholine depletion condition. The neocortex in AD patients is

---

Acetylcholine

Acetyl-CoA and choline catalyzed by choline acetyl transferase

Inactivation by hydrolysis acetylcholine esterase

FIGURE 3-43. Acetylcholine synthesis.

Cholinergic Neurons

Medial forebrain complex

Striatal interneurons

Motor neurons

Reticular formation

Sympathetic preganglionic and sudomotor

Parasympathetic postganglionic

FIGURE 3-44. Cholinergic neurons are widely distributed in the central and peripheral nervous systems.

Acetylcholine Release Blockade

Botulinum toxin

Eaton Lambert myasthenic syndrome

Tick paralysis

ß - toxins from sea snakes

FIGURE 3-45. Acetylcholine release blockade results in weakness.

Acetylcholine Release Augmentation

Latrotoxin

(Black Widow spider toxin)

FIGURE 3-46. Acetylcholine release augmentation.

Acetylcholine Receptor Blockade or Inactivation

Curare

Alpha-neurotoxins of sea snakes

Drugs (succinylcholine, aminoglycosides, quinine, procainamide)

Myasthenia gravis

FIGURE 3-47. Acetylcholine receptor inactivation.

Acetylcholine Esterase Inactivation

Organophosphates

Carbamates

FIGURE 3-48. Acetylcholine esterase inactivation.

relatively deficient in choline acetyl transferase (CAT) that is a marker of cholinergic nerve endings. The degree of depletion correlates with degree of clinical impairment as well as number of plaques. The use of centrally acting anticholinesterase agents (tacrine and donepezil, FDA approved; metrifonate, physostigmine, and rivastigmine in the pipeline) may bolster faltering acetylcholine reserves in the cortex and reduce the clinical manifestations of AD. Note that cortical acetylcholine may activate central nicotinic receptors as well as muscarinic receptors. The basal forebrain complex (anterior perforated substance, nucleus basalis of Meynert, and nucleus of the diagonal band of Broca) accounts of the majority of neocortical acetylcholine. Depletion of cells in this region is seen in AD and correlates with cortical CAT decreases.

The basal forebrain complex projects widely throughout the cortex and serves as a useful model in thinking about other traditional neurotransmitter systems. In particular, there are close analogies with the biogenic amine system in which a variety of chemically similar neurotransmitters generated by relatively small ancient deeply situated nuclei project widely throughout the brain. The cholinergic and biogenic amine systems appear to establish the activity "set point" of the cortex and basal ganglia rather than being heavily involved in fast point to point neural transmission. Disturbances of these widely projecting systems lead to widespread and pervasive alterations of memory, mood, cognition and movement; and appear to be important in conditions such as AD, schizophrenia, manic depressive disorder, and Parkinson's disease, just to name a view.

Biogenic Amine Systems

The biogenic amines are a set of classical neurotransmitters synthesized from amino acid precursors. They are among the most extensively studied neurotransmitters, and the initial breakthrough that allowed their microanatomical localization was based on the fact that these compounds fluoresce in the presence of formaldehyde vapor. The neurotransmitters in this group include DA, NE, and 5-HT. DA is located in three major systems in the brain: the mesolimbic system, nigrostriatal system and tuberoinfundibular system (Fig. 3-49). The mesolimbic dopaminergic system may play a role in schizophrenia, with relative excess of DA activity being present in that disease. The therapeutic efficacy of neuroleptics is related to DA receptor binding affinity and therefore blockade of DA receptors (D2) in this system. Undesirable side effects include binding and blockade of striatonigral DA receptors, leading to extrapyramidal symptoms, and blockade of the tuberoinfundibular system, leading to hyperprolactinemia.

In the nigrostriatal system, DA deficiency underlies Parkinson syndromes. Treatment of these syndromes with DA receptor agonists can lead to excessive mesolimbic activity with hallucinations and agitated confusion, mimicking schizophrenia. Conversely, of course, treatment of psychiatric disease with DA receptor blocking agents leads to secondary Parkinsonism and other movement disorders. Secondary Parkinsonism can result from medical use of DA antagonist agents such as neuroleptics, phenothiazine antiemetics, alphamethyl-DOPA and metoclopramide. Neurotoxic depletion of DA in the striatonigral system occurs with exposure to MPTP or manganese.

The tuberoinfundibular system runs from the arcuate nucleus to the median eminence. DA secreted by this system is prolactin inhibitory factor (PIF); therefore, DA normally inhibits prolactin release from the pituitary. DA agonists such as bromocriptine can be used to involute prolactinomas as well as in the treatment of Parkinsonism. Neuroleptics that block DA's effect lead to hy-

---

Dopamine Neurons

Mesolimbic system

Striatonigral neurons

Tuberoinfundibular system

FIGURE 3-49. Anatomic distribution of dopamine neurons.

perprolactinemia with gynecomastia, galactorrhea, menstrual irregularities, loss of libido, and impotence.

The biogenic amine NE is found in heavy concentrations in the locus ceruleus and raphe nuclei of the brainstem, from which widely projecting axons arise (Fig. 3-50). Similarly, 5-HT–secreting neurons reside in the raphe nuclei of the brainstem. The amine hypothesis of affective disorders holds that affective disorders result from relative deficiency (depression) of biogenic amine action or relative excess (mania). Support comes from the observations that biogenic amine storage depletors lead to depression, whereas reuptake inhibitors ameliorate depression. Additionally, drugs such as cocaine and amphetamine that result in massive biogenic amine activity induce manic states. The relative roles of NE and 5-HT in affective disorders remains unclear, and there may be interindividual and syndromic variability. Contrast the affective disorders with schizophrenia which is thought to represent mesolimbic dopaminergic hyperactivity with a possible role for 5-HT.

Biochemical Aspects of Catecholamines

Tyrosine is the amino acid precursor of catecholamines, DA, and NE, and this precursor gains entry into the brain via a stereoselective aromatic amino acid transporter on the endothelial cells of brain capillaries. Competition for this amino acid transport carrier across the blood–brain barrier might inhibit entry of tyrosine into the CNS and this may be relevant in some aminoacidopathies as well as acquired metabolic disorders. Once safely inside the brain, tyrosine is taken up at the synaptic endings of dopaminergic and noradrenergic neurons where it encounters a series of enzymes that sequentially remove the amino acid's hydroxyl group (tyrosine hydroxylase) producing dihydroxyphenylalanine (DOPA), which is then decarboxylated (DOPA decarboxylase) to produce DA (Fig. 3-51). DA can then be hydroxylated to produce NE. In the peripheral autonomic system and the medulla of the adrenal gland, NE is methylated to produce epinephrine.

Tyrosine hydroxylase is the first and rate-limiting step. The tyrosine hydroxylation reaction can be inhibited by a variety of compounds but this is of very limited clinical utility. For example, alpha-methyl-*p*-tyrosine has been used to treat inoperable pheochromocytoma so as to reduce production of catecholamines. DOPA can itself cross blood–brain barrier using the aromatic amino acid transporter, and this has been used to great therapeutic advantage in Parkinson's disease to help replenish central DA levels by providing the precursor levodopa (DOPA). The neurotransmitter itself, DA, cannot be used because of severe peripheral vascular side effects and it is not transported into the brain. DOPA is decarboxylated to DA in CNS by DOPA decarboxylase, which is a B_6-dependent enzyme. It is really an aromatic amino acid decarboxylase and as such exists both in the CNS and the periphery. Peripheral aromatic amino acid decarboxylase destroys therapeutically administered levodopa. Decarboxylase inhibitors such as carbidopa permit therapeutic efficacy with lower doses of levodopa, thereby reducing peripheral side effects. Before decarboxylase inhibitors became available, patients on levodopa had to avoid vitamin B_6 as pyridoxine is a cofactor for the decarboxylation reaction. Potent inhibitors of the CNS decarboxylase exist but are not very effective in reducing tissue levels of neurotransmitters. The decarboxylases are not selective, therefore other compounds, "false neurotransmitters," may compete for their action which then results in pharmacologically inactive compounds.

There are a remarkable number of naturally occurring compounds as well as purposefully created pharmaceuticals that act on the catecholamines. The loci of action include synthesis and vesicular storage, release into the synaptic

---

Norepinephrine

Raphe nuclei of brainstem

Locus coeruleus

Maintenance of consciousness and affect

FIGURE 3-50. Anatomic distribution and function of norepinephrine.

Dopamine Synthesis

Tyrosine is precursor amino acid

Tyrosine hydroxylase is first and rate limiting reaction

Tyrosine hydroxylation leads to dihydroxyphenylalanine (DOPA)

DOPA decarboxylated to dopamine

FIGURE 3-51. Dopamine synthesis begins with tyrosine.

cleft, the receptors, and finally inactivation that in the case of the biogenic amines is done largely by reuptake.

The Rauwolfia alkaloids (reserpine) and tetrabenazine are classical biogenic amine depletors that inhibit vesicular storage, thereby accelerating cytoplasmic presynaptic degradation of the catecholamines immediately after synthesis. These compounds are therefore antagonists of biogenic amine actions.

In contrast, agents that augment release or inhibit reuptake of NE and DA increase the actions of these neurotransmitters. Amphetamine augments release of NE and DA, but most of its effect probably comes from reuptake inhibition. While enzymatic degradation is important in catecholamine metabolism, the major route of physiological inactivation is high affinity reuptake of these neurotransmitters (Fig. 3-52). This contrasts with the degradative inactivation of acetylcholine, and provides a new set of molecular targets for therapeutics and pathogens.

Inhibition of enzymatic degradation by monoamine oxidase (MAO) serves to augment biogenic amine action by inhibiting degradation. Pargyline and iproniazid are such MAO inhibitory drugs. Monoamine oxidase exists in two functionally distinct types: type A, which deaminates NE and 5-HT, and type B, which deaminates phenylethylamine and benzylamine.

Type A MAO produces the primary breakdown product of NE in the CNS, MHPG, which, when measured in CSF, gives some indication of NE status. Type B MAO in part deaminates 5-HT; however, much attention has recently focused on the role of MAO type B in converting MPTP into toxic products that induce destruction of dopaminergic neurons. The MPTP Parkinsonism syndrome can be aborted in experimental animals by pretreatment with the MAO type B inhibitor deprenyl. Deprenyl may slow the progression of idiopathic Parkinson's disease.

The other major route of enzymatic degradation of the catecholamines is Catechol-*O*-methyltransferase (COMT). COMT exists both in the periphery and in the CNS. Tolcapone is an inhibitor of peripheral COMT that may reduce fluctuations and prolong efficacy of levodopa.

Physiological inactivation of catecholamine synaptic action is primarily through reuptake by sodium gradient–dependent high-affinity transporter proteins belonging to a superfamily of such transporters having broad physio-

CATECHOLAMINE METABOLISM

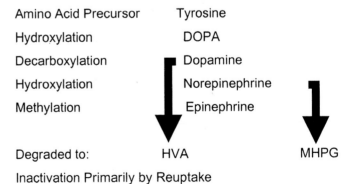

Amino Acid Precursor	Tyrosine
Hydroxylation	DOPA
Decarboxylation	Dopamine
Hydroxylation	Norepinephrine
Methylation	Epinephrine
Degraded to:	HVA MHPG

Inactivation Primarily by Reuptake

FIGURE 3-52. Catecholamine metabolism leads to breakdown products that can be measured in the cerebrospinal fluid.

logical importance. Any pharmaceutical that inhibits reuptake augments the activity of the neurotransmitter by increasing its synaptic residence time and concentration. NE-targeted tricyclic antidepressants such as desipramine prevent reuptake, and the recreational pharmaceuticals cocaine and amphetamine exert their "energizing" effects by preventing NE reuptake. DA synaptic levels are increased by amphetamine and benztropine, which are DA reuptake inhibitors.

There are numerous different catecholamine receptors, and even receptor subtypes. The unifying theme is that these receptors are mostly type 2 slow receptors—mostly adenyl cylase stimulators or inhibitors. The major NE and epinephrine (E) receptors include NE subtypes a, b, and c involved in peripheral vascular regulation, E subtypes a, b, and c involved in sympathetic actions peripheral mostly, and β receptors (β1) in the heart and cortex where NE and E are equally effective, as well as (β2) in lung and cerebellum where epinephrine is much more potent than NE.

There are at least five DA receptors (D1–D5) broken into two families. DA family 1 consists of D1 and D5, which lead to stimulation of adenyl cyclase when bound with DA; bromocriptine is an antagonist and neuroleptics are weak antagonists of this family. DA family 2 consists of D2, D3, D4, which lead to inhibition of adenyl cyclase when bound to DA; bromocriptine is an agonist and neuroleptics are strong antagonists of members of this family.

The final biogenic amine to be considered is 5-HT. This neurotransmitter is synthesized by neurons residing in the raphe nuclei of the brainstem projecting widely to the cortex and limbic structures (Fig. 3-53 and 3-54). 5-HT is involved in sleep regulation and vigilance, and pharmacological destruction of serotonergic neurons leads to insomnia in experimental animals. Such insomnia is lethal in a relatively short period of time. 5-HT exerts broad "mellowing" effects on affect, aggression, and vigilance.

Of intense interest are the activities of 5-HT in vascular regulation where it inhibits release of substance P, neurokinin A, and calcitonin gene-related protein (CGRP) on cerebral and dural vasculature. Release of these compounds is important in the Moskowitz sterile neuroinflammation hypothesis of migraine, which posits that vasculature efferent innervation by the trigeminal nerve, exhibits hyperactivity leading to release of substance P, neurokinin A, and CGRP, which in turn vasodilate vessels, increase platelet aggregation, and degranulation of mast cells releasing histamine, provoking a sterile "neuroinflammatory" response leading to the pain of migraine. Inhibition of this cascade by 5-HT agonists provides dramatic and effective therapy for migraine (Fig. 3-55).

Synthesis of 5-HT parallels that of DA and NE except that an indole skeleton is provided by the amino acid tryptophan rather than catechol skeleton provided by tyrosine.

Serotonin Metabolism

Precursor	**Tryptophan**
Hydroxylation	**5 - Hydroxy-tryptophan**
Decarboxylation	**5 - Hydroxy-tryptamine**
Degraded to	**5 - HIAA**
Inactivation primarily by reuptake	

FIGURE 3-53. Serotonin synthesis and breakdown.

Serotonin

Raphe nuclei of brainstem

Project widely

Sleep regulation and vigilance

Other broad "mellowing" effects

Inhibits release of sub P, neurokinin A, and calcitonin gene related protein (CGRP) on cerebral and dural vasculature - Moskowitz sterile neuroinflammation hypothesis of migraine

FIGURE 3-54. Serotonin neurochemistry and distribution.

Serotonin

Sumatriptan is a potent serotonin 5HT1D receptor agonist. This results in inhibition of release of sub P, neurokinin A, and CGRP, which reduces the sterile neuroinflammatory reaction leading to migraine.

FIGURE 3-55. Serotonin plays a major role in migraine.

Tryptophan is starting substrate that is transported across the blood–brain barrier by the neutral amino acid transport system. Tryptophan is dehydroxylated by tryptophan hydroxylase to 5-hydroxy-tryptophan which is then decarboxylated by aromatic amino acid decarboxylase to 5-hydroxytryptamine (5-HT). 5-HT is degraded to (5-hydroxyindole acetic acid) 5-HIAA via MAO, but as with the catecholamines, physiological inactivation is primarily through reuptake.

The neuropharmacology of 5-HT overlaps the catecholamines in many areas. There are seven 5-HT receptor subtypes and within the subtypes are sub-subtypes: 5-HT1, 2, 4, 5, 6, and 7 are G protein–coupled receptors, while only 5-HT subtype 3 is an ionophore receptor. A few very specific aspects of 5-HT are discussed here, but the diversity of 5-HT receptors and the broad range of functions of these receptors lead to an astonishing cornucopia of neuropharmacological actions for agonists and antagonists. Augmentation of 5-HT by dietary tryptophan has been used (with limited success) in the treatment of intractable myoclonus. The powerful hallucinogen LSD is a nonselective 5-HT agonist leading some to believe that the hallucinations of schizophrenia and other psychotic states may arise from serotonergic dysfunction. Sumatriptan is a potent 5-HT1D receptor agonist. This results in inhibition of release of substance P, neurokinin A and CGRP, which reduces the sterile neuroinflammatory reaction leading to migraine. Ergots also act on 5-HT receptors but are less specific and therefore have more side effects. Please note that neither sumatriptan nor ergots can cross the blood–brain barrier, but the cranial and dural vessels that mediate migraine reside outside of the pharmacological blood–brain barrier. The recently developed novel anxiolytics buspirone and gepirone are also 5-HT1A receptor agonists. 5-HT agonists have been implicated in conditions as divergent as headache, anxiety, and myoclonus as well as Hippie Day hallucinations and New Age mellowness!

Methysergide and cyproheptadine are classical 5-HT receptor antagonists, and rather paradoxically, these two agents have effectiveness in some forms of migraine. Methysergide (blocks 5-HT2A/2C) is a cogenitor of LSD but lacks the hallucinogenic features of that recreational drug, and is used in cluster headache as well as for diarrhea and malabsorption in the carcinoid syndrome. The atypical antipsychotic medication clozapine is a 5-HT2A/2C receptor antagonist in contrast to most antipsychotics that are predominantly DA antagonists. The 5-HT selectivity of this drug reportedly leads to fewer extrapyramidal side effects, making it the drug of choice in the management of hallucinations in Parkinson's disease. Risperidone is an antipsychotic agent that has both 5-HT (5-HT2A/2C) and DA (D2) blocking effects.

5-HT's actions are terminated physiologically by high affinity reuptake pumps rather than by degradation. The tricyclic antidepressants work by inhibiting this reuptake, thereby increasing synaptic presence of the neurotransmitter. The tricyclics work for all of the biogenic amines (DA, NE, and 5-HT), but they exhibit some selectivity. The tricyclic antidepressants imipramine and amitriptyline are active for all of the amines while fluoxetine (Prozac) and sertraline (Zoloft) are reuptake inhibitors that are relatively selective for 5-HT. The tricyclic antidepressant, clomipramine, is also relatively selective for 5-HT and is of use in the management of obsessive-compulsive disorder (OCD).

Amino Acid Neurotransmitters

The amino acid neurotransmitters are the most abundant neurotransmitters in the brain, but they were not initially regarded as plausible neurotransmitter candidates because of their ubiquitous roles in intermediary metabolism and protein synthesis (Fig. 3-56). The miserly economy of evolution has co-opted these small molecules for cell-to-cell signaling by providing very selective receptors precisely distributed and spatially isolated from the more mundane functions of the amino acids.

Aspartate and glutamate are the excitatory amino acids that produce cation channel opening and hence depolarization. These amino acids are widely distributed and occur in very high concentrations. Several classes of receptors have been identified with each having specific agonists and anatomical distribution. Much interest is focused on the role of these neurotransmitters in neuronal injury—the excitotoxic hypothesis—and in convulsive disorders. If the excitotoxic mechanism is more generalized and operates across protracted time periods, then neurodegenerative disorders such as amyotrophic lateral sclerosis may result from failure to inactivate these toxic neurotransmitters, excessive receptor sensitivity to them or exposure to exogenous excitotoxins. The potential role of exogenous excitotoxins in chronic neurological disorders is highlighted by neurolathyrism induced by l-beta-*N*-oxalyl-alpha,beta-diaminopropionic acid from Lathyrus sativus, and the amyotrophic lateral sclerosis/Parkinson/dementia complex of Guam induced by beta-*N*-methylamino-L-alanine from Cycad seed.

Receptors for the excitatory amino acids include ionotropic and metabotropic classes with bewildering variety (Fig. 3-57). Several of these, however, serve as good models for the entire group.

The *N*-methyl-D-aspartate (NMDA) receptor is a very complex cation channel that is gated by concurrent multiple ligand binding and voltage sensing (Fig. 3-58). Physiologically, this channel is activated by binding with glutamate or aspartate, but this step while necessary is not sufficient to open the channel. In a fascinating twist of evolution, the major inhibitory amino acid of the spinal cord, glycine serves as an obligatory co-agonist by acting at a different site on the receptor. Even simultaneous binding of glutamate and glycine to the receptor is insufficient to cause it to open. Action of the receptor is also voltage dependent because a magnesium cation (Mg) occupies the channel at resting potential, blocking conductance even if the ligand sites are bound with agonist. If the membrane is depolarized, however, the Mg is displaced from the channel, and cations including Ca, Na, and K flow through the channel (Ca being the most important). In summary, the NMDA recep-

---

Amino Acid Neurotransmitters

Excitatory – glutamate & aspartate

Inhibitory – GABA & glycine

FIGURE 3-56. Amino acid neurotransmitters.

Excitatory Amino Acid Neurotransmitters

Ligand-gated channels
- **NMDA**
- **Kainate**
- **Quisqualate A**

Second messenger linked
- **Quisqualate B**

FIGURE 3-57. Classes of excitatory amino acid receptors.

NMDA RECEPTOR LIGAND + VOLTAGE GATING

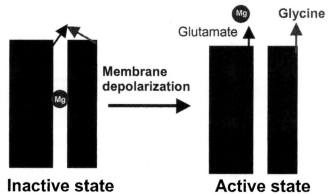

FIGURE 3-58. Mechanism of action of the NMDA receptor.

tor fluxes cations only if two separate ligand sites are occupied by two different ligands whilst the membrane is already depolarized. This is one carefully controlled channel! Such tight control is essential because one of the major cations allowed into the cell by this channel is calcium—a versatile cellular signaling molecule at low concentrations but at high concentrations it becomes a cellular assassin, activating proteases and quenching mitochondria at high cytoplasmic concentrations.

Like the old strategic missile protocols of the Cold War where two individuals turning two different keys simultaneously could launch nuclear weapons only under specific levels of defense readiness, the NMDA receptor is subject to multilevel concurrent regulation lest intracellular Armageddon be unleashed.

NMDA receptors are widely distributed throughout the neocortex, hippocampus (particularly CA1), and anterior horn motor neurons. Activation occurs physiologically only after the membrane bearing the receptor has already been depolarized by some other stimulus; hence, the NMDA activation prolongs or augments the initial depolarization. Such augmentation may "strengthen" the synapse or make it more likely to fire with the next incoming depolarization. The physiological consequence is long-term potentiation which may be good for building memories and learning, but may be bad if it leads to pathological firing in convulsive disorders. During cellular energy failure induced by ischemia, there is collapse of membrane potentials (depolarization) and uncontrolled synaptic and transmembrane release of excitatory amino acids into the extracellular space. NMDA receptors are exposed to high concentrations of their ligands while residing in a depolarized membrane and will open, allowing calcium to enter the already miserable cell (Fig. 3-59). Intracellular proteins are destroyed by calcium-activated proteases and mitochondrial proton potentials responsible for ATP generation are abolished by calcium sequestration in the matrix.

In view of the important potential role of excitotoxicity, a large number of NMDA receptor antagonists have been developed and several of these compounds have reached use in clinical trials. The classical NMDA antagonists are the noncompetitive receptor blockers MK801, ketamine, CGS19755, and CPP, as well as the competitive blocker AP5-7. In addition to receptor blockers, there are compounds such as eliprodil that down-modulate the NMDA polyamine site.

Convulsions have as their underlying pathophysiological substrate long term potentiation mediated in part at least by glutamate receptors. Several of the more recently introduced antiepileptic drugs exert most or some of their action at the glutamate receptor. Felbamate acts at the NMDA and AMPA receptors to block the glycine co-agonist site. Lamotrigine blocks release of glutamate.

Neurodegenerative diseases may also have contributions from excitotoxicity. In particular, the motor neurons of the cranial nerve motor nuclei and anterior horns of the spinal cord are major recipients of glutaminergic synaptic endings. The recently introduced drug riluzole blocks the presynaptic sodium channel that effects excitation-release coupling for glutamate. This drug modestly slows the progression of bulbar amyotrophic lateral sclerosis and has fueled continued interest in glutamate antagonist drugs in this condition. Glutamate is inactivated at the synapse by reuptake, and defects in the amino acid transporters that carry out this function may result in raised synaptic concentrations of glutamate with subsequent disease development. There is evidence accumulating that excitatory amino acid transporter defects may be found in amyotrophic lateral sclerosis. Clearly if this is verified, development of drugs that augment synaptic transport of excitatory amino acids will be an important area of investigation.

Excitotoxicity

Inappropriate activation of the NMDA receptor

Membrane depolarization

Influx of calcium

Activation of hydrolytic enzymes and quenching of mitochondria

FIGURE 3-59. Excitotoxicity is one of the major mechanisms of neuronal death in a variety of neurological diseases.

Another major excitatory amino acid receptor is the AMPA receptor that is also known as the quisqualate receptor since its first described agonists were quisqualate and AMPA. This receptor has several antagonists such as NBQX (quinoxalinediones).

The final class of excitatory amino acid ionotropic receptors to be considered here are the kainate receptors that can be activated by the complex organic acids kainate and domoate. No specific clinically useful antagonists have been developed for this receptor which is common in the neurons of the limbic system and CA3 hippocampus. Due to the hippocampal localization, these receptors have been implicated in the pathogenesis of seizure disorders. There have been several instances of domoate neurotoxicity due to ingestion of contaminated shellfish. This remarkable syndrome is characterized by seizures and memory disturbance.

There are a number of metabotropic glutamate receptors and like other second messenger receptors, activation of many of these results in adenyl cyclase inhibition mediating long term action. Antibodies raised to metabotropic glutamate receptors leads to a epileptic syndrome in rabbits closely resembling Rasmussen's epilepsy—a rare progressive asymmetrical seizure syndrome that sometimes requires hemispherectomy for control. Some patients with this condition have autoantibodies to metabotropic glutamate receptors and have been successfully treated with plasmapheresis. The burgeoning number of both ionotropic and metabotropic glutamate receptors make these receptors promising targets for disease processes and therapeutic intervention.

Inhibitory Amino Acids

GABA (gamma-amino butyric acid) and glycine are the two major inhibitory amino acids in the CNS. GABA-ergic systems occur throughout the nervous system but predominate in the brain and brainstem, and may play a major role in the suppression of neuronal hyperexcitability that may have clinical expression as diverse as seizures or anxiety (Fig. 3-60). Some of the most effective anxiolytics and anticonvulsants exert effects on GABA neurons. In addition, the anti-spasticity drug baclofen acts on GABA-B receptors. Also, relative deficiency of GABA in Huntington's disease has been implicated in the clinical manifestations of that disease.

GABA-A receptors are ionotropic and operate by causing increased chloride (Cl) conductance leading to hyperpolarization of the neuronal cell membrane. There are at least five binding sites including the GABA site, barbiturate locus, benzodiazepine site, picrotoxin site, and the steroid binding site. Augmentation of receptor function occurs in response to binding by the benzodiazepams and barbiturates, and this underlies these drugs' antiseizure and anxiolytic actions. A variety of anti-seizure drugs act on the GABA-A receptor either directly or by modifying GABA metabolism (Fig. 3-61). The very

---

GABA-A Receptor

Increased chloride conductance

Hyperpolarization

Site of action of benzodiazepines, barbiturates, and valproate

Antagonists: Picrotoxin and bicuculline

FIGURE 3-60. GABA-A receptor properties.

GABA Metabolism

Precursor   **Glutamic acid**

Decarboxylation   **GABA**

Degraded to   **Succinic acid**

     Alpha-ketoglutarate

Inactivation primarily by reuptake and resynthesis

FIGURE 3-61. GABA-B receptor properties.

widely used drug sodium valproate enhances GABA synthesis and decreases its degradation while simultaneously blocking depolarizing cation channels. Muscimol is a direct agonist as is ethanol. Progabide is a GABA pro-drug that activates the GABA-A receptor. The neuroactive steroids including alphax-alone are agonists of this receptor. Gabapentin is not a direct agonist despite its name, but it does antagonize picrotoxin- and bicuculine-induced seizures by down-modulating the picrotoxin site that normally inactivates the channel. Vigabatrin (gamma-vinyl-GABA) blocks GABA aminotransferase thereby reducing GABA breakdown augmenting receptor function.

The GABA antagonists picrotoxin and bicuculine are classical potent convulsant neurotoxins. These compounds bind the GABA-A receptor at specific regulatory sites and decrease its activity moving the membrane potential away from a hyperpolarized state to a more depolarized and hence more excitable state.

The GABA-B receptor is activated by G protein-linked cation channel inhibitors (Fig. 3-62). Cation channel inhibition biases the membrane away from depolarization toward hyperpolarization. The major clinical agonist is baclofen which is used to decrease spasticity.

Glycine is the other major inhibitory amino acid neurotransmitter in the CNS (Fig. 3-63). Glycine, like GABA, stabilizes the membrane potential by increasing chloride conductance. The anatomical distribution is different, however, with glycine favoring the spinal cord whereas GABA is seen more in higher centers above the foramen magnum. Spinal cord and to a lesser extent brainstem inhibitory interneurons are glycinergic. The glycine receptor is non-competitively blocked by strychnine that has no effect on GABA receptors. Tetanus toxin works in part by inhibiting release of glycine and GABA. These two neurotoxins lead to uncontrolled neuronal activation due to loss of normal amino acid inhibition with resultant tetanic contraction, increased tone and seizures. The synthetic precursor of glycine is serine, and its action is terminated by reuptake. It is important to remember that glycine has a role in NMDA receptor control by acting as an obligatory co-agonist.

Peptides and Gases

The very low concentration neurotransmitters, including the neuropeptides and gaseous neurotransmitters nitric oxide and carbon monoxide, are the most recently described cellular signaling molecules described in the nervous system. The neuropeptides are among the most numerous recently discovered neurotransmitters. The first of these—the enkephalins—were found during a search for endogenous opiate receptor agonists. Subsequently, most peptide messengers found elsewhere in the body have been found in the brain. Synthesis is complex and, in some cases, involves differential mRNA splicing. Degradation involves endogenous peptidases of several varieties. The literature on these substances is vast and growing, and undoubtedly these compounds play a major role in nervous system functioning.

The general features of peptidergic neurotransmitters includes synthesis occurring in the cell body in the form of larger precursor proteins that are transported down the axon to the synapse; therefore, synaptic replenishment depends on cellular protein synthesis and axonal transport. Peptides may coexist in the synaptic terminal with other neurotransmitters where peptides tend to occupy large dense core vesicles and classical neurotransmitters occupy small vesicles. Peptide may modulate postsynaptic responsiveness to classical neurotransmitters, and exert protracted postsynaptic effects by acting on second messenger receptors. Postsynaptic action is terminated by extracellular proteases and by diffusion. The fact that these transmitters may diffuse widely in the extracellular space exerting far-flung effects makes them major participants in volume transmission.

GABA-B Receptor

G protein linked action

Slow sustained activity

FIGURE 3-62. GABA metabolism shows the fabulous yin and yang of the brain—the amino acid precursor for the major inhibitory neurotransmitter is the most abundant excitatory amino acid glutamate.

Glycine

Increased chloride conductance

Hyperpolarization

Major inhibitory neurotransmitter in the spinal cord

Antagonist: Strychnine

FIGURE 3-63. Glycine is the major inhibitory amino acid below the foramen magnum.

Nitric Oxide Synthesis

l-Arginine + NADPH + O₂

Citrulline + NADP⁺ + NO

The reaction is catalyzed by nitric oxide synthetase (NOS) which was known classically as NADPH diaphorase. The enzyme requires flavin mononucleotide, flavin adenine dinucleotide, iron-protoporhyrin IX, and tetrahydrobiopterin as co-factors.

FIGURE 3-65. Nitric oxide synthesis.

The gaseous signaling molecule, nitric oxide (NO), is critical in vasomotor control, inflammation, and neuronal communication (Fig. 3-64). NO is produced by tissue specific isoforms (neuronal, endothelial, and macrophage) of nitric oxide synthetase (NOS) from arginine, and rapidly and radially diffuses to adjacent target cells where it interacts with iron centers stimulating cGMP synthesis (Fig. 3-65). NO from neurons does not serve as a fast point to point signaling molecule but rather sets the functional state of adjacent cells, and in that respect resembles the classical biogenic amine neurotransmitters. NO has a short half-life and is oxidized to nitrate and nitrite. Peroxidation products of NO may be produced in a variety of pathophysiological states including head trauma and stroke, and lead to damage of nucleic acids, proteins and lipids (Fig. 3-66). NO released from endothelial cells acts on vascular smooth muscle cells where it induces relaxation and hence vasodilatation. NO-mediated vasoregulation may be central to CNS vascular autoregulation. NO released from inflammatory cells occurs in extraordinarily high concentrations and kills target cells and innocent bystander cells by binding iron centers in the electron transport chain used in energy generation. Due to this compound's toxicity, neurons that synthesis it have protective enzymes to mitigate damage. Chronic excess NO may play a role in neurodegeneration while acute elevations may contribute to damage in ischemia and trauma. NO synthesis is augmented by NMDA receptor activation by glutamate; therefore, NO may synergize excitotoxicity.

Carbon monoxide (CO) is the most recently defined neurotransmitter and its function and potential role in neuropathophysiology is just now being defined. This compound is proof that discovery of new neurotransmitters is an ongoing process and no matter how improbable a putative neurotransmitter appears at first glance, an open and inquisitive mind is essential for the clinical neuroscientist.

Nitric Oxide

- NO used in cell-to-cell signaling interacts with iron containing guanylate cyclase in the target cell leading to increased cyclic GMP
- NO used in host defense binds with iron-sulfur center containing enzymes in the mitochondria to impair energy production and DNA synthesis
- Oxidation intermediates of NO degradation are themselves toxic

FIGURE 3-64. Nitric oxide is the most recently described neurotransmitter and is a gas!

CNS Nitric Oxide Metabolism

- NO is diffusible and highly reactive
- Synthesized by neuronal nitric oxide synthetase (NOS) in NADPH-diaphorase neurons
- Diffuses into adjacent cells
- Activates guanylate cyclase
- Inactivated by oxidation
- Inappropriate NO activation may enhance excitotoxicity and free-radical damage

FIGURE 3-66. The dark side of nitric oxide–inappropriate activation may enhance excitotoxicity and free radical damage.

4

NEUROGENETICS

PERSPECTIVE

1. The nervous system is the most complex biological structure known, and this complexity is reflected by the fact that at least one-third of the entire genome is involved in genes expressed in the nervous system.
2. Classical Mendelian genetics involves autosomal recessive, X-linked, and autosomal dominant disorders. In autosomal recessive disorders, both copies of an allele are defective; hence, there is a loss of function of the protein coded by this allele. In X-linked disorders, the allele on the X chromosome is defective and there is no corresponding allele on the puny Y chromosome, so once again there is a loss of function. Autosomal dominant disorders have only recently begun to give up their secrets, and here the mutation on one allele leads to altered function of the protein product leading to a "gain of function," which is a polite way to say a gain of toxicity.
3. Mitochondrial genetic disorders are maternally inherited because we receive all of our mitochondria with their minute but highly important endogenous genomes from our mothers. Energy-dependent organs such as the brain and skeletal muscles are primary targets in the mitochondrial disorders.
4. In addition to classifying genetic disorders according to mode of inheritance, gene defect, and protein product, it is helpful in a clinical setting to work backwards from phenotype to genotype.

OBJECTIVES

1. Understand the basics of molecular genetics and how study of the genetics of the nervous system and its diseases has expanded the frontiers of genetics.
2. Distinguish among the mechanisms of the classical Mendelian disorders.
3. Understand the consequences of trinucleotide repeat amplification.
4. Learn the nature and mode of transmission of the mitochondrial genetic disorders.

About one-third of all genetic diseases find expression in disorders of the nervous system broadly defined to include the CNS, peripheral nerve, and skeletal muscle. Study of neurogenetic diseases has had a profound impact on both neurology and medical genetics. In recent years, the molecular pathogenesis of a number of "sporadic" as well as genetic diseases has been clarified using genetic techniques. The careful study of rare genetic pedigrees expressing the same phenotype as common sporadic diseases has provided major insights into Alzheimer's disease, Parkinson's disease, and amyotrophic lateral sclerosis to name just a few. Hereditary diseases are also yielding their secrets leading to a greater understanding of these conditions, and permitting development of molecular biology-based diagnostic assays and potential therapeutics. Finally, and possibly most important, the study of neurologic genetic diseases has resulted in the discovery of entirely new mechanisms of disease. Trinucleotide repeat amplification in myotonic dystrophy, fragile X mental retardation, Huntington's disease, spinocerebellar ataxias, etc. was a fundamental breakthrough in genetics. Clinical mitochondrial genetics has largely been the result of study of neurologic diseases. Gene duplication (PMP22 in Charcot Marie Tooth disease) and deletion in the same gene in tomaculous neuropathy has provided insights into unequal crossover in the genesis of disease. Finally, the study of prion disorders—both sporadic and familial—is revolutionizing concepts of cellular information transfer and challenges the central dogma of molecular biology.

BASIC MOLECULAR BIOLOGY

Genetic information flow:

"Central Dogma of Molecular Biology": DNA → RNA → protein

"Modification of Central Dogma Forced by Retroviruses": RNA → DNA → RNA → protein

"Modification of Central Dogma Forced by Prions": protein → protein

All prokaryotes and eucaryotes transmit genetic information from generation to generation via deoxynucleic acid (DNA). In eucaryotes, the DNA resides in the nucleus in association with proteins to form the chromosomes. Two lengths of complementary nucleotides (Adenosine/Thymidine and Cytosine/Guanine) interacting via hydrogen bonds form the double helix of DNA. DNA replication occurs when the double-stranded DNA unravels to form single stranded DNA that can be acted upon by DNA polymerase to form two new molecules identical to the originating molecule. Ribonucleic acid (RNA) can similarly be manufactured because the nucleotides of RNA also form complementation pairs (Uracil/Thymidine and Cytosine/Guanine).

In addition to permitting maintenance of genetic fidelity between generations, the other major function of DNA is to specify the sequence of amino acids in proteins synthesized within the cell. A given protein is the final expression of a given gene. In eucaryotes, genes consist of exons (sequences of DNA which find expression in protein amino acid sequence) and introns (intervening sequences between exons which are not expressed in the final protein amino acid sequence). Genes also possess regulatory sequences involved in controlling gene expression.

TRANSCRIPTION

DNA is transcribed into heteronuclear ribonucleic acid (hnRNA), which contains both introns and exons. The hnRNA is edited so that introns are excised and adjacent exons are fused (spliced) together to give a final RNA product—messenger RNA (mRNA). Different mRNAs can be spawned from a single gene by alternative splicing of the hnRNA. RNA synthesis and editing occurs in the nucleus, and mRNA is transported from the nucleus into the cytoplasm where translation occurs. Defective slicing underlies the mouse mutation of central myelin (jimpy) and abnormal tau isoform expression in frontotemporal dementia. Ribosomal and transfer RNA are also generated in the nucleus, and are transported to cytoplasm for their essential roles in translation (protein synthesis).

TRANSLATION

Messenger RNA is translated into protein on the cytoplasmic ribosomes. Transfer RNA (tRNA) complexed with amino acids bind to mRNA on the ribosome with complementation of three nucleotides on the mRNA specifying which tRNA will bind. The linear sequence of nucleotides on mRNA is translated into the primary sequence of the synthesized protein. The primary structure of the protein is simply the sequence of amino acids comprising the protein. These strands of amino acids then fold to form the secondary structure of the protein. The functional characteristics of the protein are generally determined by the secondary structure of the protein.

ASSAYS USED IN MOLECULAR BIOLOGY

The major methods of assaying DNA and RNA depend on hybridization of the sequence of interest with a probe consisting of a complementary strand of DNA or RNA bearing a signaling isotope or chromophobe. Such hybridization is usually conducted on nylon membranes with nucleic acids bound to them in an array corresponding to the nucleic acids separated by molecular weight. Individual genes can be studied using DNA hybridization, while RNA hybridization is used to study levels of gene expression and alternative splicing. Measurement of protein is done using antibody probes. These assays are named Southern blots for DNA, Northern blots for RNA, and Western blots for proteins. Technological advances in gene analysis are proceeding very rapidly, and the emergence of microarray chips on which hybridization of thousands of gene loci can be carried out simultaneously promises to revolutionize molecular genetics and clinical medicine.

Polymerase chain reaction (PCR) permits the selective exponential amplification of nucleic acid sequences of interest. Primers at either end of the sequence of interest are used to confer selectively, then multiple cycles of nucleic acid synthesis are carried out. Only nucleic acid residing between the primers will be amplified to produce sufficient material so that further analysis can be conducted including Southern blotting or direct sequencing. PCR permits the study of nucleic acid from very small samples, allows selective study of nucleic acid of interest, and permits detection of genetic material that does not belong to the host (i.e., infectious agent nucleic acid).

CLASSES OF MUTATIONS

Defects in genes can arise from a variety of structural defects in the linear array of nucleotides altering the message or in subsequent processing. Initially there was a focus on exonic mutations but more is being learned about the role of intronic sequences in the expression of the information contained in the genes, novel classes of mutation are being uncovered.

Single DNA base change → Missense →   Abnormal protein

Nonsense →   No or truncated protein

	Premature stop →	No or truncated protein
mRNA processing →	Splicing mutation →	Abnormal protein
Codon →	Frameshift →	Abnormal protein
Insertion or	Codon insertion →	Abnormal protein
Deletion	Codon deletion →	Abnormal protein
Gene fusion →	Fusion mRNA →	Chimera protein
Triplet repeat →	Polyglutamate runs →	Abnormal protein
Amplification	Abnormal methylation	
Mitochondrial →	Deletions →	No protein
	tRNA deletions →	Many proteins not made

HUMAN KARYOTYPE

The human genetic material resides on the chromosomes comprised of 22 pairs of autosomal chromosomes and one pair of sex chromosomes. Normal somatic cells possess this precise 46 chromosome complement and are said to be diploid (2N), while normal germ cells (ovum and spermatozoa) possess one-half this number—23 individual chromosomes not in pairs—and are haploid (N). During the cell cycle when an individual cell is synthesizing a duplicate of its genetic material, the chromosome number grows from 46 to 92 (tetraploid, 4N) just before mitosis. In tumors, individual cells may possess chromosome numbers that are not haploid, diploid, or tetraploid, and such cells are said to be aneuploid. It is also possible during germ cell development (meiosis) for chromosomes to be maldistributed, leading to too few or too many in the progeny. The most common karyotype abnormalities resulting from this are trisomy disorders where an extra full or partial chromosome is present.

Autosome chromosomes	22 pairs
Sex chromosomes	XX (female): beyond embryogenesis random X-inactivation occurs
	XY (male)

KARYOTYPE ABNORMALITIES

Trisomy 21: Down's syndrome
14/21 Translocation
Trisomy 13
Trisomy 18
Fragile X

PATTERNS OF INHERITANCE OF GENETIC DISEASES

Genes are paired structures with each copy of the gene (allele) residing on one of the paired autosomes or sex chromosomes. The puny Y-chromosome does not bear all of the alleles that reside on the X-chromosome; therefore, a male has a lower safety margin for mutations on the sex chromosomes—this is manifested by the X-linked recessive disorders, which are manifested almost exclusively in males.

Autosomal Dominant

One damaged allele is sufficient to produce disease. Fifty percent of offspring of an affected individual will have the defective allele and will therefore have the disease. The degree of expression (penetrance) of the defect is variable according to the specific disease. Huntington's disease has 100% penetrance—all individuals bearing the defective gene are affected. Neurofibromatosis type 1 has variable penetrance—some individuals are severely affected, while others have a mild phenotype.

A number of autosomal dominant disorders of great neurological significance result from trinucleotide repeat amplification. Part of normal genetic polymorphism includes the possession of repeating trinucleotide sequences. Some of these repeats may be amplified during germ cell development or during development, and such amplification leads to disease. Transgenerational trinucleotide repeat amplification accounts for the occurrence of anticipation—the onset of hereditary disease of greater severity at a younger age in progeny.

Autosomal Recessive

Both alleles must be damaged in order for the disease to be manifest. Possession of a single normal allele is sufficient to compensate for the defect of the matching allele. Many of the classic inborn errors of metabolism are autosomal recessive. Twenty-five percent of the offspring of two carriers are affected. The affected individual receives one defective allele from the father and one from the mother. Carriers usually are asymptomatic but may have levels of the protein coded for by the defective gene occurring at levels between normals and affected individuals.

X-Linked Recessive

Alleles on the sex chromosomes are abnormal in these disorders. The Y-chromosome does not contain a full complement of alleles to match the X-chromosome. If the male offspring receives a defective unmatched allele from his carrier mother, he will be affected. Fifty percent of the male offspring will receive the defective X-chromosome, and 50% will receive the mother's normal X-chromosome; therefore, 50% of male progeny will be affected. The female offspring of the same mother will be normal or, at worst, be carriers.

TABLE 4-1. NEUROGENETIC DISEASES WITH EXPANDED TRINUCLEOTIDE REPEATS

Disease	Gene	Repeat	Normal Length	Disease Length
Type 1: repeats not translated into protein				
Fragile X syndrome				
FRAX-A	*FMR-1*	CGG	6–54	200 to >1,000
FRAX-E	*FMR-2*	CCG	6–25	200 to >1,000
Myotonic dystrophy	*myotonin*	CTG	5–37	200 to >1,000
Friedreich's ataxia	*frataxin*	GAA	8–22	120 to >1,000
Type 2: repeats translated into protein				
Kennedy's disease	*androgen receptor*	CAG	11–33	40–66
Huntington's disease	*huntingtin*	CAG	10–34	37–121
SCA1	*ataxin-1*	CAG	19–36	42–81
DRPLA	*atrophin-1*	CAG	7–34	49–83
Machado-Joseph disease (SCA3)	*MJD1 Ataxin-3*	CAG	13–36	68–79
SCA2	*ataxin-2*	CAG	15–29	35–59
SCA6	*ataxin-6*	CAG	4–16	21–27

TABLE 4-2. NEUROGENETIC DISEASES BY CLINICAL MANIFESTATION

Disease	Protein	Chromosome
Dementia		
Familial Alzheimer's disease	Amyloid protein precursor	21
	Presenilin-1	14
	Presenilin-2	1
Familial frontotemporal dementia	Tau	17
Familial Prion disorders Creutzfeldt–Jakob Fatal familial insomnia GSS	Prion protein	20
Movement disorders		
Huntington's disease	Huntingtin	4
Familial Parkinson's disease	α-Synuclein	4
Torsion dystonia	Dystonin	9
Ataxia		
Friedreich ataxia	Frataxin	9
DRPLA		12
Spinocerebellar ataxia 1	Ataxin-1	6
Spinocerebellar ataxia 2	Ataxin-2	12
Spinocerebellar ataxia 3/MJD	Ataxin-3	14
Spinocerebellar ataxia 4	Ataxin-4	16
Spinocerebellar ataxia 5	Ataxin-5	11
Spinocerebellar ataxia 6	Ataxin-6	19
Spinocerebellar ataxia 7	Ataxin-7	3
Episodic ataxia 1	Potassium channel	12
Episodic ataxia 2	Gated P/Q type calcium channel	19
Familial hemiplegic migraine	Gated P/Q type calcium channel	19
Motor neuron disease		
Wernig-Hoffman disease	SMN, NAIP, BTFII	5
Familial ALS	Superoxide dismutase	21
Kennedy's disease	Androgen receptor	X
Neuropathy		
CMT	PMP22	17
Tomaculous neuropathy	PMP22	17
Myopathy		
Dystrophinopathies Duchenne's Becker's	Dystrophin	X
Myotonic dystrophy	Myotonin	19
Hyperkalemic periodic paralysis	Sodium channel	17
Paramyotonia congenita		
Hypokalemic periodic paralysis	Calcium channel	1
Malignant hyperthermia	Ryanodine receptor	19
Epilepsy		
Progressive myoclonic epilepsy	Cystatin B (protease inhibitor)	21
Mental Retardation:		
Fragile X MR (FXMR)[a]	FMR1	X
Stroke		
Cerebral autosomal dominant arteriopathy with subcorical infarcts and leukoencephalopathy (CADASIL)[b]	Notch 3	19
Familial cavernous malformation	(CCM1)	9

(continued)

TABLE 4-2. (*continued*)

Disease	Protein	Chromosome
Phakomatoses		
Neurofibromatosis 1 (NF1)	Neurofibromin	17
Neurofibromatosis 2 (NF2)	Merlin	22
von Hippel–Lindau	VHL (elongation factor)	3
Tuberous sclerosis	TSC1	9
	TSC2 (tuberin)	16

GSS, Gerstmann–Sträussler–Scheinker disease; DRPLA, dentatorubropallidoluysial atrophy; MJD, Machado–Joseph disease; ALS, amyotrophic lateral sclerosis; CMT, Charcot–Marie–Tooth disease.
[a] FXMR now appears to result in defective dendritic maturation and maintenance.
[b] CADASIL, episodic ataxia 2, and familial hemiplegic migraine all map to 19. CADASIL results from a defect of notch 3, while EA2 and FHM appear to be different phenotypes resulting from damage to the same allele coding for the voltage-gated P/Q type calcium channel.

Mitochondrial

The mitochondria within our cells are genetically semi-autonomous due to the presence of 10–12 circular genomes within each mitochondria coding for an independent protein synthetic apparatus that makes components of the electron transport chain. At fertilization, the ovum contributes all of the mitochondria and the sperm contributes none. Mitochondrial inheritance is exclusively maternal. Furthermore, during early development, the mitochondria do not segregate randomly; therefore, there is some mitochondrial genetic variability from tissue to tissue (heteroplasmy). Mitochondrial genetic disorders lead to impaired oxidative energy metabolism and are therefore expressed predominantly in tissues with high bioenergetic activity, including brain, skeletal and cardiac muscle, and kidney.

The accompanying tables (Tables 4-1 and 4-2) list hereditary disorders classified by clinical category. The diseases are chosen because they are common, or the genetic mechanisms of disease shed light on the basic pathogenesis of the disease, or the genetic defects are particularly illustrative of novel genetic principles. This list is by no means comprehensive, and the details of the disease phenotypes are described in other parts of this book. It is impossible for print to keep up with the torrent of newly elucidated neurogenetic disorder; therefore, use of the Internet is particularly essential in this area. Two web sites that are very useful are www.ncbi.nlm.nih.gov/Omim (National Center for Biotechnology Information Online Mendelian Inheritance in Man) and www.genetests.org (University of Washington compendium of available genetic tests and testing sites).

5

NEUROANATOMY ESSENTIALS

PERSPECTIVE

1. Clinical localization is the first essential step in generating a differential diagnosis for a patient with neurological disease.
2. By knowing where a lesion is, you have a pretty good idea what the lesion is.
3. Coupling the time course of the illness with the clinical localization to render a differential diagnosis is the essence of neurology.
4. The pathologist and radiologist also generate differential diagnoses based on clinical, radiological and gross localization of the lesion.
5. Neuroradiology is gross neuropathology in black and white.

OBJECTIVES

1. Understand the major levels of the nervous system and the signs and symptoms produced by lesions at these different levels.
2. Be able to distinguish between a lesion of the peripheral and central nervous system.
3. Learn how to determine if a lesion is at the spinal level, in the posterior fossa, in the basal ganglia or in the cerebral hemisphere.
4. Understand how to distinguish in extradural, intradural extramedullary, and intramedullary spinal cord process, and the implications of this distinction.
5. Explain the difference in signs and symptoms of an intra-axial brainstem, fourth ventricular, cerebellar, or extra-axial posterior fossa lesion.
6. Be able to localize within the basal ganglia according to the type of movement disorder observed.
7. Understand the anatomical basis and localizing significant of visual field abnormalities.
8. Know the major motor, sensory, and cognitive consequences of lesions of the frontal, parietal, occipital, temporal, and limbic lobes.

The basic reason for studying neuroanatomy (other than the intrinsic beauty of the nervous system) is to permit effective localization of lesions based on clinical findings from the neurological history and examination. With localization come focused differential diagnosis and rational deployment of neuroimaging or electrophysiological testing. Conversely, the neuroradiologist or the pathologist examining either an image of the brain or the brain itself may deduce likely clinical manifestations of any lesions seen (Fig. 5-1). Ideally, the localization and differential diagnosis of the clinician is precisely congruent with the findings on direct examination of the brain.

Radiology is Gross Pathology in Black and White

If you know gross pathology, you know radiology. If you know radiology, you know gross pathology.

FIGURE 5-1. Knowledge of gross pathology immediately translates into knowledge of neuroradiology.

The analysis of neurological signs and symptoms is often misconstrued by the novice as an archaic and almost magical process, but in reality, neurological differential diagnosis consists of applying a few relatively simple neuroanatomical principles in an organized and disciplined fashion. The first objective is to determine if the disease process localizes to the central versus the peripheral nervous system. If the disease involves the peripheral nervous system, then the root, plexus, peripheral nerve, neuromuscular junction, or muscle must be distinguished as the potential locus. If the process involves the CNS, one ascertains if the disease is in the spinal cord, posterior fossa, or supratentorial compartment. Determination of the level of the nervous system involved is essential to refining the differential diagnosis. One must always be mindful, however, that disease may be multifocal and so involve multiple levels, or may involve functional systems that span several levels.

In the CNS, the first step is to determine if the lesion is above or below the foramen magnum. Lesions below the foramen magnum, by definition, produce signs and symptoms of spinal cord disease—a myelopathy. The spinal cord is the primary conduit through which motor instructions leave and sensory data travels to the brain. Disorders of the spinal cord can disrupt these processes with catastrophic consequences for the patient.

SPINAL CORD LEVEL

> **Key Concept:** Damage to the spinal cord interferes with motor function below the spinal segment injured while sparing motor function above the segmental level of injury.

Damage to the cervical spinal cord will result in weakness (paresis) or complete loss of motor function (plegia) in the arms and the legs. Since four extremities are rendered weak, the resulting motor condition is known as quadriparesis or quadriplegia. Damage to the thoracic or lumbar spinal cord will result in weakness of the lower extremities only which is called paraparesis if some strength remains or paraplegia if the limbs are completely paralyzed. Immediately after the insult, the intact spinal cord below an area of damage is unable to function. Muscle tone and reflexes are absent, and voluntary movement is impossible. After days to weeks, the intact but isolated spinal cord below a level of damage begins to exhibit autonomous activity manifested by the return reflexes and tone. The reflexes are hyperactive and the overactive muscle stretch reflex may lead to repetitive cyclical coordinated muscle contractions (extensors then flexors then extensors . . .). This repetitive activity is called clonus. The tone is also increased in the extremities, and may attain sufficient force to allow weight bearing. The increase in tone and reflexes is called spasticity, which can be exploited in rehabilitation but may also pose problems because the extremities may become fixed in position. Increased reflexes and tone, and the release of primitive reflexes such as the Babinski reflex, indicate damage to the upper motor neurons which project from the motor cortex to the motor neurons of the brainstem and spinal cord. Weakness with hyperreflexia, spasticity and release of primitive reflexes is known as upper motor neuron weakness. In contrast, if the lower motor neurons (anterior horn cell motor neurons in the spinal cord and motor cranial nerve nuclei in the brainstem) are damaged, reflexes are lost or diminished, tone decreases, and no primitive reflexes appear. The skeletal muscle innervated by the lower motor neuron undergoes neurogenic atrophy. Hence, weakness with hyporeflexia, decreased tone, and muscle atrophy is lower motor neuron weakness. Both upper and lower motor neuron weakness can be seen in spinal cord disorders.

> **Key Concept:** Damage to the spinal cord interferes with sensory function below the spinal segment injured while sparing sensory function above the segmental level of damage.

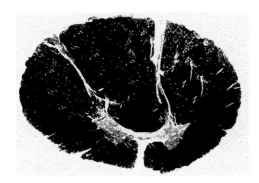

FIGURE 5-2. A cross section of the spinal cord with a myelin stain shows the normal myelin as dark and the H-shaped gray matter as light. In diseases in which myelin is lost secondary to axonal degeneration, the functional systems involved can be highlighted with a myelin stain. Myelin will, of course, also be lost in primary demyelinating disease, but here functional systems are not followed.

Damage to the cervical spinal cord will result in diminished sensation (hypesthesia) or complete loss of sensation (anesthesia) in all four extremities and the trunk. Damage to the thoracic or lumbar cord leads to sensory loss of the lower extremities and lower trunk.

When a spinal cord lesion is suspected, a *sensory level* (area of transition from normal to diminished sensation), is crucial in localizing the site of the lesion.

Definition: A patient with upper motor neuron signs and a sensory level is myelopathic. These signs result from a spinal cord disease process or myelopathy.

Key Concept: Partial damage to the spinal cord at a given level may involve selected motor and sensory tracts to a lesser or greater degree depending on the precise anatomy of the lesion (Figs. 5-2 and 5-3).

Classic examples of anatomy illustrating conditions are:

A. Spinal cord hemisection syndrome (Brown–Sequard syndrome) in which the cord on one side is sectioned to the midline. This syndrome is quite rare in real life, although occasional knife-yielding homicidal maniacs do manage to do this. The damaged structures include:
   1. Dorsal columns (f. gracile and cuneate [leg and arm]) results in ipsilateral loss of fine touch.
   2. Lateral corticospinal tracts leading to ipsilateral upper motor neuron below the level of damage.
   3. Lateral spinothalamic tract with loss of contralateral pain and thermal sensation one or two segments below the level of damage.
   4. Anterior horn damage at the level of injury leads to segmental lower motor neuron weakness.
B. Anterior spinal artery infarct—this results in damage to the anterior two-thirds of the cord, sparing the dorsal columns and dorsal horns (Fig. 5-4).

Classic Spinal Cord Syndromes

- **Brown-Sequard syndrome: hemisection--Charles Edouaard Brown-Sequard (1817-1894)**
- **Anterior spinal cord syndrome**
- **Central cord syndrome**
- **Complete transection**

FIGURE 5-3. There are several classical spinal cord syndromes that are clinically and anatomically distinct.

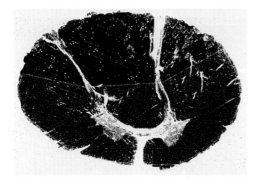

FIGURE 5-4. The anterior spinal cord syndromes disrupts the anterior 2/3 of the spinal cord leading to weakness and loss of pain and thermal sense below the level of the lesion. The posterior columns are spared so the patient can feel fine touch and the position of the paralyzed limbs. This condition may complicate vascular surgery on the aorta or result from atherosclerosis or vasculitis of the anterior spinal artery.

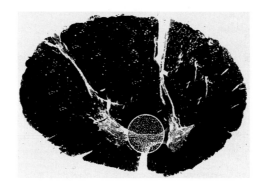

FIGURE 5-5. The central cord syndrome results from an intramedullary neoplasm or syringx. The second order pain and thermal sense axons are interrupted as they cross leading to segmental (cape or shaw distribution) loss of sense of pain and temperature.

This syndrome is seen with atherosclerosis and other vascular diseases of the aorta and its branches, and results in damage to the following:

1. Lateral corticospinal tracts on both sides leading to spastic paraplegia or quadriplegia depending on the segmental level of damage.
2. Lateral spinothalamic tracts bilaterally leading to loss of thermal and pain sensation below the level of damage.
3. Anterior horns at the level of damage leading to flaccid paralysis at that segment.

    The dorsal columns are spared permitting preservation of fine touch and proprioception below the level of damage.

C. Syringomyelia is the occurrence of a cyst within the center of the spinal cord most commonly at the cervical level (Fig. 5-5).

1. Anterior commissure conveying the decussating lateral spinothalamic axons. This leads to bilateral loss of pain and thermal sense at the segmental level just below the lesion. The zone of sensory loss forms a band around the trunk and follows a shawl distribution over the shoulders and arms when the syringx is in the cervical cord.
2. The anterior horn cells may also be involved leading to lower motor neurons signs in segments involved (the arms and hands for a cervical lesion).

> **Key Concept:** Some diseases selectively involve specific tracts or gray matter of the spinal cord to give characteristic sets of signs of symptoms that may be strongly suggestive of the diagnosis (Fig. 5-6).

Vitamin B_{12} deficiency leads to selective damage of the dorsal columns (loss of fine touch and position sense) and lateral corticospinal tracts (upper motor neuron weakness). Tabes dorsalis resulting from tertiary syphilis selectively damages the dorsal columns leading to loss of fine touch and position sense. Motor neuron disease (amyotrophic lateral sclerosis) leads to selective loss of upper and lower motor neurons without sensory involvement. Poliomyelitis leads to relatively selective loss of anterior horn cells leading to flaccid lower motor neuron weakness (Fig. 5-7 through 5-9).

> **Key Concept:** When considering masses involving the spinal cord, it is important to ascertain whether the mass resides within one of three spaces—the extradural spinal space, the intradural extramedullary space, or within the intramedullary space (this is, within the spinal cord itself) (Fig. 5-10).

    The extradural space is the fat and blood vessel-filled space surrounding the thecal sac (Fig. 5-11). The spinal cord and its surrounding cerebrospinal

---

Selective Damage of Tracts or Neuronal Populations

- Vitamin B_{12} deficiency
- Tabes dorsalis
- Motor neuron disease
- Poliomyelitis

FIGURE 5-6. Certain diseases damage selected neuronal populations leading to selective tract degeneration that can be recognized on myelin stained sections of the spinal cord.

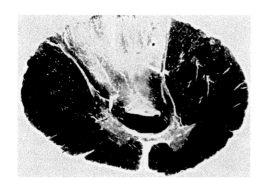

FIGURE 5-7. Tabes dorsalis from neurosyphilis leads to degeneration of the dorsal columns with clinically profound loss of joint position sense and fine touch.

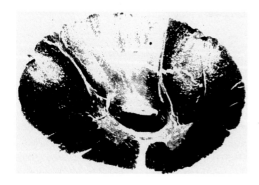

FIGURE 5-8. Vitamin B_{12} deficiency leads to combined (motor and sensory) system degeneration with loss of the ascending dorsal columns and descending corticospinal tracts. A similar picture can be seen in nitrous oxide abuse, vitamin E deficiency, and early Friedreich's ataxia.

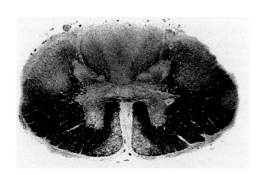

FIGURE 5-9. Friedreich's ataxia leads to loss of dorsal columns, lateral corticospinal tracts, and anterior and posterior spinocerebellar tracts.

Spinal Cord Spaces

- **Extradural space - 1**
- **Intradural extramedullary - 2**
- **Intramedullary - 3**

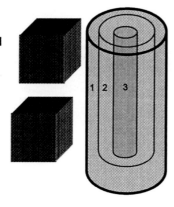

FIGURE 5-10. In the evaluation of spinal cord masses, it is appropriate to determine in which of the three major myelographic spaces the mass resides.

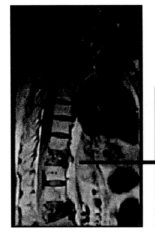
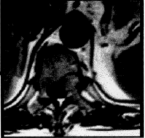

FIGURE 5-12. Sagittal and axial spinal MRI showing metastatic tumor destroying several vertebral bodies with compromise of the spinal canal.

Spinal Epidural Masses

- **Neoplasms: usually metastatic to spine**
- **Abscess**
- **Herniated intervertebral disc**

> **Local pain**
> **Radicular pain**
> **Myelopathy**

FIGURE 5-11. Epidural masses are usually metastatic, abscess, or herniated intervertebral disc.

Intradural Extramedullary Masses

- **Neoplasms: arise from nerve roots and meninges**
  - **Schwannoma**
  - **Neurofibroma**
  - **Meningioma**

> **Radicular pain**
> **Myelopathy**

FIGURE 5-13. Intradural extramedullary spinal cord masses are usually neoplasms arising from the nerve roots and their coverings.

fluid (CSF) and dural sac reside within the epidural space, and the nerve roots emerging from the spinal cord traverse the epidural space.

Space-taking lesions in the epidural space include:

1. Neoplasm: most commonly these are tumors metastatic to the vertebral body and these tumors then extend into the epidural space (Fig. 5-12).
2. Abscess: localized collections of purulent material (pus).
3. Herniated intervertebral disc: especially in the cervical and lumbar regions, fragments of the intervertebral disc may protrude into the epidural space.

Note that masses in the epidural space may compress the spinal cord leading to a myelopathic picture, or they may compress individual nerve roots emerging from the spinal cord. Compression of a nerve root leads to pain and loss of sensation in the dermatome served by that root, weakness in the muscles innervated by that root, and loss of reflexes in the distribution of the nerve root. Compression of a nerve root with these signs and symptoms is called a "radiculopathy."

The intradural extramedullary space is the CSF-filled space between the dural sac surrounding the spinal cord and the spinal cord itself (Fig. 5-13). The nerve roots reside in this space. The most common masses in this space

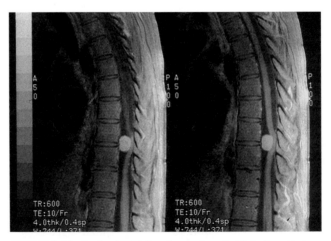

FIGURE 5-14. Sagittal MRI showing a discrete high signal intensity meningioma at T8.

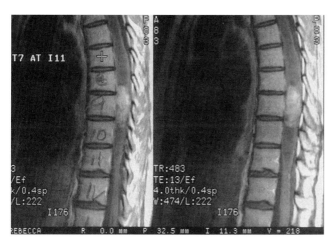

FIGURE 5-16. Sagittal MRI showing an intramedullary ependymoma expanding the spinal cord in the mid-thoracic region.

are tumors arising from the nerve roots themselves and the dura surrounding the roots (Fig. 5-14). Such tumors may produce radicular as well as myelopathic symptoms.

The *intramedullary space* is the spinal cord proper (Fig. 5-15). The common masses arising within the spinal cord are tumors which we will for now refer to as gliomas which arise from astrocytes, oligodendroglia or ependyma (Fig. 5-16). The syringomyelia we mentioned earlier is also an intramedullary mass.

INFRATENTORIAL LEVEL: BRAINSTEM, FOURTH VENTRICLE, AND CEREBELLUM

The brainstem is an area particularly well suited to application of the discipline of clinical localization (Figs. 5-17 and 5-18). You should attempt to determine where a lesion is in a rostral-caudal axis (midbrain, pons, medulla) and on which side (right or left) the lesion is located. Once you have ascertained these features, then attempt to determine whether the lesion is in near the midline or is more lateral.

Intramedullary Masses

- **Neoplasms: arise from cells indigenous to the CNS**
  - **Astrocytoma**
  - **Ependymoma**
  - **Oligodendroglioma**

  Myelopathy

FIGURE 5-15. Intramedullary neoplasms arise from the denizens of the neuropil and are usually gliomas. Occasionally a hemangioblastoma, metastasis, granuloma, abscess, or hematoma will be seen. Syringomyelia may also occupy space within the cord.

Posterior Fossa Structures

- **Brainstem - Long tract + cranial nerves**

- **Fourth Ventricle - CSF obstruction**

- **Cerebellum - Ataxia**

FIGURE 5-18. The location of a lesion in the posterior fossa determines the likely clinical manifestations.

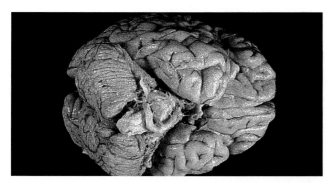

FIGURE 5-17. The whole brain seen from below shows the brainstem, cerebellum, cranial nerves and vasculature in addition to the basal aspects of the frontal and temporal lobes.

"Crossed Signs" = Brainstem

- Ipsilateral cranial nerve
- Contralateral arm/leg motor and sensory

FIGURE 5-19. Clinical syndromes involving an ipsilateral cranial nerve and contralateral long tract findings are seen in with brainstem lesions.

Localize Rostral Caudal Using Cranial Nerves

Localize in Medial to Lateral Plane Using Tracts

FIGURE 5-20. The level of the brainstem involved is determined by which cranial nerve is involved. The lateral to medial distribution of the lesion at a given level depends on the tract involvement.

Localize Rostral Caudal Using Cranial Nerves

- Midbrain: 3 & 4
- Pons: 5, 6, 7
- Pontomedullary: 8
- Medullary: 9, 10, 11, 12
- Pontomedullary Cervical: Spinal nucleus/tract 5

FIGURE 5-21. Distribution of cranial nerve nuclei within the brainstem.

Key Concept: The prime characteristic of brainstem lesions is "crossed" sensory and motor signs. Cranial nerve nuclear and nerve signs are ipsilateral to a brainstem lesion while ascending sensory tracts have decussated, and descending motor pathways will decussate leading to contralateral signs on the body (arms, trunk, legs) (Fig. 5-19).

Key Concept: You should localize lesions in a rostral caudal axis (that is midbrain, pons, or medulla) based on which cranial nerve nuclei are involved (Figs. 5-20 and 5-21).

Key Concept: You should localize lesions in the medial to lateral plane using tract (corticospinal, spinothalamic, medial lemniscus, and autonomic) involvement primarily.

Key Concept: Remember that the fourth ventricle and cerebellum reside dorsal to the brainstem. Lesions of the cerebellum produce ataxia, dysmetria and inability to perform rapid alternating movements ipsilateral to the cerebellar hemisphere involved. Disruption of the cerebellar inflow and outflow tracts in the brainstem will produce ataxia and dysmetria which is either ipsilateral or contralateral depending on whether the involved tracts have decussated yet.

Key Concept: Mass lesions in the fourth ventricle may encroach on the brainstem or the cerebellum to produce symptoms and signs referable to these structures, but early on, ventricular masses tend to produce signs and symptoms of CSF flow obstruction—headache, nausea, vomiting, head enlargement in children and infants before the skull sutures fuse, and papilledema.

The following are some of the more common brainstem syndromes illustrating these localization principles.

LESIONS OF THE MEDULLA

The medulla is the first structure encountered in the ascent from the spinal level to the infratentorial level of the neuraxis (Figs. 5-22 and 5-23). This transition is marked by the decussation of the descending corticospinal tracts com-

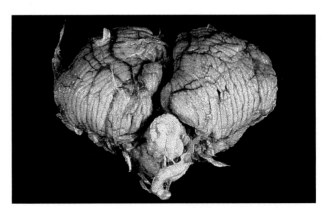

FIGURE 5-22. The medulla is surrounded by the spinal cord below, the pons above and the cerebellar tonsils behind.

Medulla

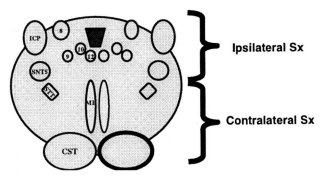

FIGURE 5-23. Internal structure of the medulla including corticospinal tracts (CST), medial lemniscus (ML), inferior cerebellar peduncle (ICP) and cranial nerve nuclei.

prising the ventrally disposed medullary pyramids at the cervicomedullary junction.

The ascending proprioceptive and fine touch system has its relay nuclei, the nucleu gracilus for lower extremity and trunk, and the nucleus cuneatus for upper extremity, neck, and upper trunk, also at the cervicomedullary junction. The second order neurons from these nuclei decussate to form the medial lemniscus that ascends through the brainstem to eventually innervate the ventral posterior lateral (VPL) nucleus of the thalamus. In the medulla, the medial lemniscus is arranged as a vertical (ventral to dorsal) strip of fibers in the midline with the upper extremity fibers being most dorsal and the lower extremity fibers being most ventral; i.e., the sensory homunculus in the medulla is "standing straight up." The medial lemniscus rotates to the horizontal in the pons and by the time it reaches the midbrain has rotated further so that the fibers from the lower extremity are now more dorsal than those of the upper extremity. Imagine a reveler on Bourdon Street in New Orleans. Early in the evening, the individual is standing vertically against a lamppost enjoying the libations and this is analogous to the position of the medial lemniscus in the medulla. By mid-evening, the partygoer slides down the lamp post and lays on the street analogous to the increasingly horizontal disposition of the medial lemniscus is the pons. Finally, the besotted reveler is pulled from the street by his ankles by the local constabulary analogous to the "feet up" orientation of the medial lemniscus in the midbrain.

The ascending thermal and pain fibers of the spinothalamic system decussated at the spinal level and also end on the VPL. The spinal tract and nucleus of the trigeminal reside in the dorsolateral medulla and subserve ipsilateral facial pain and thermal sensibility, and the second order neurons decussate in the trigeminothalamic fibers to ascend throughout the brainstem to the ventromedial posterior (VPM) nucleus of the thalamus. In the medulla, these fibers reside in the dorsolateral area, and they grow more and more integral as they travel through the brainstem.

Important cerebellar circuitry resides in the medulla in the form of the inferior cerebellar penducle carrying information about the ipsilateral proprioception as well as input from the inferior olive to the dentate nucleus.

The cranial nerve nuclei of the medulla are the spinal nucleus and tract of the trigeminal nerve, the nuclei of the glossopharyngeal and vagal nerves, and the motor neurons of the hypoglossal nucleus mediating tongue motility. All of these nuclei innervate ipsilateral face, tongue, and pharynx. The parasympathetic autonomic functions of the vagus also originate in the nucleus ambiguous of the medulla, and immediately adjacent in the dorsolateral medulla are descending sympathetic fibers from the hypothalamus.

A. *Medial medullary syndrome (anterior spinal artery syndrome)* (Fig. 5-24). Affected structures and resultant deficits include:
1. Corticospinal tract (medullary pyramid). Lesions here result in contralateral spastic hemiparesis.
2. Medial lemniscus. Lesions here result in contralateral loss of tactile and vibration sensation from the trunk and extremities.
3. Hypoglossal nucleus or intra-axial root fibers CNXII. Lesions here result in ipsilateral flaccid hemiparalysis of the tongue. When protruded, the tongue points to the side of the lesion (i.e., to the weak side).

B. Lateral medullary syndrome *[posterior inferior cerebellar artery (PICA) syndrome; Wallenberg syndrome]* is characterized by dissociated ("crossed") sensory loss (Fig. 5-25). This is the most common brainstem stroke and results more commonly from occlusion of the ipsilateral vertebral artery which gives rise to the PICA rather than the PICA itself. Affected structures and resultant deficits include:
1. Vestibular nuclei. Lesions here result in nystagmus, nausea, vomiting, and vertigo.
2. Inferior cerebellar peduncle. Lesions here result in ipsilateral cerebellar signs [e.g., ataxia, dysmetria, dysdiadochokinesia].
3. Nucleus ambiguus of CN IX, CN X, and CN XI. Lesions here result in ipsilateral laryngeal, pharyngeal, and palatal hemiparalysis [i.e., loss of gag reflex (efferent limb), dysarthria, dysphagia, and dysphonia)].
4. Glossopharyngeal nerve roots. Lesions here result in loss of the gag reflex (afferent limb).
5. Vagal nerve roots.
6. Spinothalamic tracts (spinal lemniscus). Lesions of these tracts result in contralateral loss of pain and temperature sensation from the trunk and extremities.

Medulla: Medial Medullary Syndrome

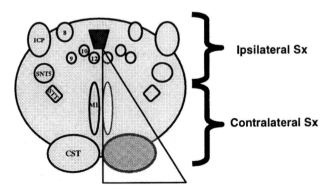

FIGURE 5-24. Structures impacted by a medial medullary lesion.

Medulla: Lateral Medullary Syndrome

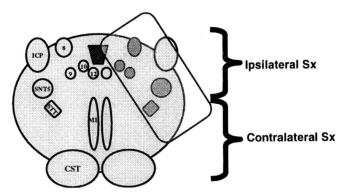

FIGURE 5-25. Structures impacted by a lateral medullary lesion that is most commonly an infarct resulting from vertebral artery occlusion compromising flow to the posterior inferior cerebellar artery (PICA) territory.

7. Spinal trigeminal nucleus and tract. A lesion here results in ipsilateral loss of pain and temperature sensation from the face (facial hemianesthesia).

8. Descending sympathetic tract. Lesions here result in ipsilateral Horner's syndrome (ptosis, miosis, hemianhidrosis, and apparent enophthalmos).

LESIONS OF THE PONS

The pons is a protuberant expansion of the midbrain having an uncanny and unflattering resemblance to the "beer belly" of many middle aged individuals (Figs. 5-26 through 5-28). The belly of the pons is composed of horizontally oriented fibers which will enter the cerebellum as that structure's primary cortical input system, the middle cerebellar peduncle. Interspersed are vertically disposed descending corticobulbar and corticospinal fibers which will decussate prior to innervation of their lower motor neuron targets in the brainstem and spinal cord. Key among these supranuclear projections are fibers which

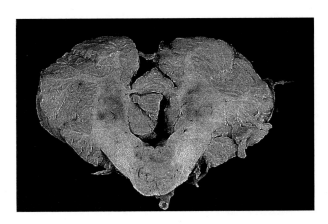

FIGURE 5-26. The pons is bordered below by the medulla, above by the midbrain, posteriorly by the 4th ventricle and cerebellum, and anteriorly by the clivus.

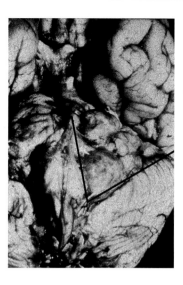

FIGURE 5-27. The confluence of the pons, medulla and cerebellum is the cerebellopontine angle—a site of a variety of tumors, the most common of which is the schwannoma of the eight cranial nerve.

end in the paramedian pontine reticular formation (PPRF) immediately adjacent to the sixth nerve nucleus. The PPRF integrates horizontal conjugate gaze commands from the cortical frontal eye fields, smooth pursuit systems, and the vestibular and proprioceptive systems. The yoked conjugate eye control system of the oculomotor, trochlear, and abducens nuclei tied together by the medial longitudinal fasciculus (MLF) receives vertical gaze and papillary control commands in the midbrain and horizontal gaze commands as well as data about the position of the head and neck in the pons. From an evolutionary standpoint, this system allows a creature to visually acquire a target and maintain fixation even in the face of head and body movements as the target is approached. The Darwinian imperatives executed continuously by the CNS are the so-called 4F's of behavior—feeding, fighting, fleeing, and finding a mate—and for these critical missions a steady gaze is essential!

In addition, the pons contains the nuclei most responsible for facial sensation and action—cranial nerves 5 and 7. The chief sensory nucleus of 5 me-

Pons

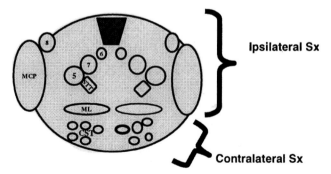

FIGURE 5-28. Internal structure of the pons with the middle cerebellar peduncle (MCP), the now horizontally disposed medial lemniscus (ML) and the cranial nerve nuclei. Note that the ascending sensory systems are beginning to converge.

diates fine touch from the face and so is essential for nuzzling, exploring and other pleasant facial sensory activities. The spinal nucleus and tract of 5 mediating pain and thermal sense from the face, begin in the pons but descend through the purgatory of the medulla and upper cervical spinal cord. The mesencephalic nucleus of 5 mediating jaw prioproception and the jaw jerk reflex ascends into mesencephalon where it forms an eye catching string of neurons. These sensory components of the trigeminal nerve are complemented by the motor nucleus of 5 that is responsible primarily for the ferocious mastication of the predator. The seventh cranial nerve mediates minor aspects of sensation, but is largely responsible for the subtle and at times coarse emotional signaling associated with facial expressions. As such, the seventh nerve motor nucleus receives complex cortical and limbic inputs permitting the coy smile, the fearsome scowl and the supercilious raised brow essential for the successful execution of the Darwinian imperatives. The facial musculature of the lower face receives predominantly input from the contralateral cortex via crossed corticobulbar fibers whereas the brow receives bilateral innervation. Hence, a supranuclear (central) seventh nerve palsy will result in the lower two-thirds of the contralateral face being weak with sparing of the brow, while a peripheral or nuclear palsy will result in weakness of the entire face ipsilateral to the lesion.

The lower pons and upper medulla play host to the vestibular and cochlear nuclei which receive auditory and head position data from the vestibular and cochlear systems in the temporal bone. Nuclear, cranial nerve, or sensory apparatus damage can lead to ipsilateral hearing loss or tinnitus if the cochlear system is involved. The semicircular canal and the utricle of the vestibular sensory system are differential activated by head positional changes, hence, if the head changes position in the horizontal plane, one semicircular canal is activated while the corresponding contralateral semicircular canal becomes less active. This translates directly into differential activity of the vestibular nuclei which is analyzed by multiple CNS systems. If a lesion results in diminished or increased (vestibulitis) activity, this leads to the CNS being misinformed by the vestibular system about the position of the head in space. The visual system and proprioceptive system will be providing data of high fidelity and the mismatch between the malfunctioning vestibular input and these systems will be subjectively experienced as vertigo. The evolutionarily primitive and nonsuppressible vestibular input to the conjugate gaze control system will lead to involuntary slow conjugate horizontal gaze deviation to the side of the less active vestibular system. Once the horizontal gaze deviation has reached its maximal excursion, the frontal eye field will issue a rapid corrective command for the eyes to move back to the midline. The slow horizontal deviation followed by the rapid corrective movement back to the midline is called "nystagmus." The rapid correct excursion is more conspicuous to the observer and the direction of the nystagmus is designated as the direction of the nystagmus. Hence, the eye's slowly deviate toward the less active ("dead") vestibular system, but the rapid corrective movement is away from the inactive vestibular system. Conversely, if one vestibular system is inappropriately active, the eyes will slowly deviate away from the lesioned side but the rapid corrective movement will be toward the hyperactive side.

A. *Medial inferior pontine syndrome results from occlusion of the paramedian branches of the basilar artery (Fig. 5-29). Affected structures and resultant deficits include:*
   1. Corticospinal tract. Lesions here result in contralateral spastic hemiparesis.

Pons: Medial Inferior Syndrome

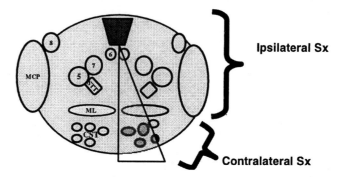

FIGURE 5-29. Structures impacted by a medial pontine lesion.

2. Medial lemniscus. Lesions here result in contralateral loss of tactile sensation from the trunk and extremities.
3. Abducent nerve roots. Lesions here result in ipsilateral lateral rectus paralysis.

B. *Lateral inferior pontine syndrome [anterior inferior cerebellar artery (AICA) syndrome]* (Fig. 5-30). Affected structures and resultant deficits include:
1. Facial nucleus and intra-axial nerve fibers. Lesions here result in:
   a. Ipsilateral facial nerve paralysis.
   b. Ipsilateral loss of taste from the anterior two-thirds of the tongue.
   c. Ipsilateral loss of lacrimation and reduced salivation.
   d. Loss of corneal and stapedial reflexes (efferent limbs).
2. Cochlear nuclei and intra-axial nerve fibers. Lesions here result in unilateral deafness.
3. Vestibular nuclei and intra-axial nerve fibers. Lesions here result in nystagmus, nausea, vomiting, and vertigo.

Pons: Lateral Inferior Syndrome

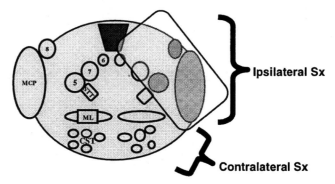

FIGURE 5-30. Structures impacted by a lateral pontine lesion.

4. Spinal trigeminal nucleus and tract. Lesions here result in ipsilateral loss of pain and temperature sensation from the face (facial hemianesthesia).
5. Middle and inferior cerebellar peduncles. Lesions here result in ipsilateral limb and gait ataxia.
6. Spinothalamic tracts (spinal lemniscus). Lesions here result in contralateral loss of pain and temperature sensation from the trunk and extremities.
7. Descending sympathetic tract. Lesions here result in ipsilateral Homer's syndrome.

C. *MLF* syndrome (internuclear ophthalmoplegia) interrupts fibers from the contralateral abducent nucleus that project, via the MLF, to the ipsilateral medial rectus subnucleus of CN III. It results in a medial rectus palsy on attempted lateral conjugate gaze and nystagmus in the abducting eye; convergence remains intact. This syndrome is frequently seen in patients with multiple sclerosis, but may rarely be seen in infarcts or tumors.

LESIONS OF THE MIDBRAIN

The midbrain is the site of vertical gaze control with supranuclear projections from the frontal eye field as well as the occipital smooth pursuit systems converging on the reticular system adjacent to the nuclear complexes of cranial nerves three and four (Figs. 5-31 through 5-33). Pupillary light reflex circuitry also resides in the midbrain where tectal projections from the retinae trigger papillary constriction in response to bright light. Also, circuits in the midbrain mediate the linkage of ocular convergence with papillary constriction. It is not surprising then that midbrain lesions lead to disturbances of vertical gaze, papillary reflexes and convergence.

In addition to the cornucopia of neuro-ophthalmological circuitry, the midbrain hosts the major outflow projections of the cerebellum. Dentate nuclear fibers travel in the superior cerebellar peduncles, decussate in the midbrain and send projections to the red nuclei and eventually the ventrolateral nuclei of the thalamus. Disruption of these dentatorubrothalamic projections lead to furious appendicular tremor reminiscent of the flapping of wings in

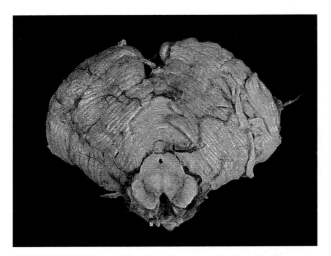

FIGURE 5-31. The midbrain is bordered below by the pons, above by the basal ganglia and internal capsule, and posteriorly by the upper cerebellum and pineal gland.

Midbrain

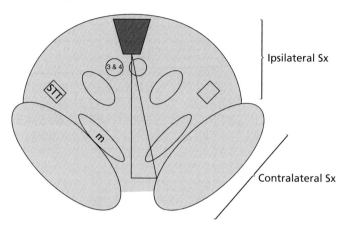

Ipsilateral Sx

Contralateral Sx

FIGURE 5-32. Internal structure of the midbrain. The corticospinal tracts now reside in the cerebral peduncles anteriorly, the ascending sensory pathways form a line (ML medially, spinothalamic laterally) as they converge toward the thalamus. The cranial nerve nuclei of 3 and 4 are in the midline and are closely anatomically and physiologically intercalated.

birds and is called "wing-beating" tremor. The substantia nigra vesicles immediately dorsal to the cerebral peduncles and the dopaminergic neurons of this critical nucleus project to the ipsilateral globus pallidus. Disruption of these projections by either death of the nigral neurons or transection of their axons leads to contralateral hemiparkinsonism. Functionally, the substantia nigra goads the basal ganglionic circuits into action and facilitates eventual corticospinal and corticobulbar pathway activation. Conversely, another denizen of the midbrain and lower diencephalons, the subthalamic nucleus, inhibits the motor output of the basal ganglionic circuitry. Lesions of the subthalamic nucleus remove this steady inhibition leading to contralateral flinging appendicular movements called "hemiballismus."

Midbrain

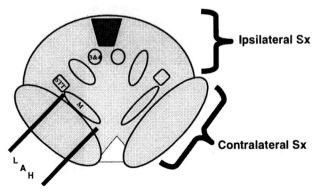

Ipsilateral Sx

Contralateral Sx

FIGURE 5-33. Note the internal structure of the cerebral peduncle with the corticospinal tract functional distribution of leg laterally, arm midway, and head medial.

Dorsal Midbrain Parinaud Syndrome

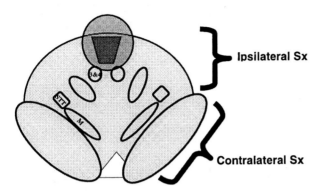

FIGURE 5-34. The Parinaud syndrome results of compression of the midbrain from behind usually by a pineal tumor. The aqueduct may be compressed leading to hydrocephalus, and pressure on the cranial nerve nuclei leading to disturbances of vertical gaze, accommodation and pupillary control.

Finally, the cerebral peduncles are composed of descending corticospinal and corticobulbar fibers residing in the inner three-fifths of the peduncle. These descending motor control axons will decussate in most instances prior to arrival at their targets, hence, peduncle lesions lead to contralateral upper motor neuron type weakness below the level of the midbrain.

A. Dorsal midbrain (Parinaud) syndrome is frequently the result of a tumor of the pineal region (Fig. 5-34). Affected structures and resultant deficits include:
   1. Superior colliculus and pretectal area. Lesions here result in paralysis of upward and downward gaze, pupillary disturbances, and absence of convergence.
   2. Cerebral aqueduct. Compression results in a noncommunicating hydrocephalus.
B. *Paramedian midbrain (Benedikt) syndrome* (Fig. 5-35). Affected structures and resultant deficits include:
   1. Oculomotor nerve roots (intra-axial fibers). Lesions here result in complete ipsilateral oculomotor paralysis; eye abduction and depression are caused by the intact lateral rectus (CN VI) and superior oblique (CN IV). Ptosis (paralysis of the levator palpebrae muscle) and an ipsilateral fixed and dilated pupil (complete internal ophthalmoplegia) also occur.
   2. Dentatothalamic fibers. Lesions here result in contralateral cerebellar ataxia with intention tremor.
   3. Medial lemniscus. Lesions here result in contralateral loss of tactile sensation from the trunk and extremities.
C. *Medial midbrain (Weber) syndrome. Affected structures and resultant deficits include:*
   1. Oculomotor nerve roots (intra-axial fibers). Lesions here result in complete ipsilateral oculomotor paralysis; eye abduction and depression are due to intact lateral rectus (CN VI) and superior oblique (CN IV) muscles. Ptosis and an ipsilateral fixed and dilated pupil also occur.
   2. Corticospinal tracts. Lesions here result in contralateral spastic hemiparesis.

Paramedian Midbrain

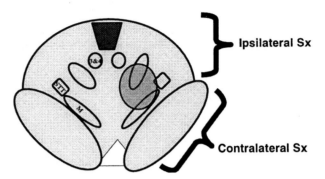

FIGURE 5-35. Structures impacted in the midbrain by a paramedian lesion (usually an infarct) disrupting the superior cerebellar peduncle outflow and red nucleus leading to ataxia as well as ipsilateral disturbances of cranial nerve 3.

3. Corticobulbar fibers. Lesions here result in contralateral weakness of the lower face (CN VII), tongue (CN XII), and palate (CN X). (The upper face division of the facial nucleus receives bilateral corticobulbar input, and is therefore intact). The uvula and pharyngeal wall are pulled toward the normal side (CN X), and the protruded tongue points to the weak side.

The syndromes discussed here have been based on classical vascular intra-axial infarcts historically described in patients with neurosyphilis. Bear in mind that intra-axial tumors, foci of inflammation (brainstem encephalitis) and areas of myelin loss can produce the same syndromes or hybrids of these syndromes as several vascular territories may be transgressed.

THE CEREBELLUM

The cerebellum ("little brain") is classically regarded as an adjunctive motor system which facilitates timing and amplitude of motor acts. It receives command inputs from the premotor frontal cortex via fibers that descend through the cerebral penduncle of the midbrain and decussate in the belly of the pons to form the middle cerebellar peduncle. Proprioceptive data from the extremities and vestibular system data enter the cerebellum via the inferior cerebellar peduncle. All of these data are integrated in the cerebellar cortex and are relayed to the dentate nucleus and fibers from this nucleus leave the cerebellum via the superior cerebellar peduncle. These departing dentatorubrothalamic fibers end in the contralateral red nucleus and ventrolateral (VL) nucleus of the thalamus. The VL is also the thalamic destination of the basal ganglion system outflow, hence convergence of these two major motor systems occurs in this key nucleus. Lesions of the cerebellar hemisphere will produce ipsilateral appendicular ataxia and inability to perform rapid alternating movements while lesions of the cerebellar midline (vermis) produces trunkal ataxia. Lesions of the cerebellar inflow and output fibers of the middle and superior cerebellar peduncles will produce either ipsilateral or contralateral manifestations depending on precisely where in the course of the circuit the lesion occurs. Lesions of the inferior cerebellar peduncle or its contributing fibers produce ipsilateral problems.

The Cerebellar Pontine Angle Syndrome

There is a common extra-axial tumor called the "schwannoma," which arises from Schwann cells myelinating the eighth cranial nerve as it emerges from the brainstem. The eighth nerve is knocked out primarily, but the innocent bystander 7 and 5 may be involved. This tumor is analogous to tumors arising in the extramedullary intradural space of the spinal cord. A tumor at the cerebellar pontine angle (CPA) produces damage to:

1. Cochlear CN VIII leading to unilateral tinnitus (ringing in the ear) and deafness.
2. Vestibular CN VIII leading to nystagmus and vertigo (subjective sense of spinning or tumbling in space).
3. Facial CN VII leading to ipsilateral LMN facial weakness.
4. Trigeminal CN V leading to ipsilateral loss of facial sensation.

These tumors are treatable (curable) by surgical removal although hearing cannot always be preserved. The CPA is a cellularly diverse neighborhood and so may spawn neoplasms including the meningioma, neurofibroma, choroid plexus papilloma, ependymoma, juvenile pilocytic astrocytoma or fibrillary brainstem astrocytoma with exophytic extension, and medulloblastoma. Tumors arising in the adjacent bony surrounds can also intrude here and include the chordoma, chondrosarcoma, osteosarcoma, and endolymphatic sac tumor. As always, with any mass in the nervous system, the unseemly visitation by metastases must be considered.

To summarize, lesions in the posterior fossa may be extra-axial impinging on cranial roots or they may be intra-axial involving either the brainstem, ventricular system or cerebellum. Extra-axial lesions produce ipsilateral cranial neuropathies, brainstem lesions produce crossed ipsilateral cranial nerve plus contralateral tract manifestations, ventricular lesions produce increased intracranial pressure, and cerebellar lesions produce ipsilateral ataxia and disdiadochokinesis or trunkal ataxia.

The Basal Ganglia

The basal ganglia are a collection of nuclei residing deep in the cerebral hemispheres extending into the midbrain including the putamen and caudate nuclei (striatum), globus pallidus interna and externa, subthalamic nucleus and the substantia nigra. These nuclei receive motor command inputs from the premotor areas of the ipsilateral cerebral cortex, process and refine that command information, and initiate and maintain movements via outputs to the ventrolateral nucleus of the thalamus back to the premotor cortex. As indicated previously, the ventrolateral nucleus of the thalamus is a site of convergence of the cerebellar and basal ganglionic circuits—the two great modulators of cortical motoric output. As currently conceived, the motor commands are refined in the basal ganglia with the subthalamic nucleus normally putting the brakes on or inhibiting motor output and the substantia nigra normally being the accelerator or facilitating motor output.

Diseases of the basal ganglia lead to movement disorders—there can be either too little (hypokinetic) or too much (hyperkinetic) movement. These movements are involuntary, but some modulation can sometimes be consciously exerted. The abnormal movements may or may not persist during sleep. In conceptualizing movement disorders, it is also helpful to regard initiation and maintenance of thoughts as "actions" analogous to motor acts, hence basal ganglionic disturbances can result in disturbances of the speed, focus and continuity of mental activities that are analogous to the more visible external kinetic manifestations.

Hypokinesis usually takes the form of rigidity, where there is trouble initiating movement so that the patient has reduced motility. The resting tone of the muscles may be increased so that if you try to move the patient's arm you will encounter continuous involuntary resistance to movement (lead pipe rigidity). Parkinson's disease is the prototype of a hypokinetic movement disorder. It is important to recognize that these individuals may also have difficulty initiating and maintaining mental actions and so may manifest slowness or paucity of thought. In addition, they cannot carry out the normal rapid corrective postural and autonomic responses to movement in a gravitational field and may experience postural instability and hypotension.

In the hyperkinetic disorders, there is involuntary (spontaneous) movement. Huntington's disease is the prototypical disease in this category. The abnormal movements can take several forms and some are listed below:

Dystonia: slow sustained writhing contraction of an extremity or the trunk and neck.

Athetosis: slow writhing contraction of the extremities, similar to dystonia but not as sustained.

Chorea: brief, jerky, "fidgety" movements usually of the extremities.

Hemiballismus: wild, flinging, high amplitude involuntary movement of an extremity. Usually the result of an infarct or other damage in the subthalamic nucleus.

Tremor: repetitive rhythmic oscillatory movement of the extremities or head.

Please recognize that the various forms of movement can occur in an individual patient (a Parkinson's disease patient can be rigid yet have a tremor), and the movements may fuse into one another (a patient with Huntington's disease can have chorea and athetosis which run together as choreoathetosis). Also, imagine, if thought processing is impinged upon by the same chaos as motor processing, the patient may experience a torrent of unwelcome and uncontrolled thoughts that may be clinically manifested by psychosis. Also, the patient may be unable to completely modulate and refine motor and verbal actions with resulting motor tics and explosive speech with potentially politically incorrect or scatological utterances.

In cases of unilateral basal ganglionic lesions, the motor manifestations are in the contralateral face, body and extremities since the basal ganglion ultimately express themselves via the corticospinal and corticobulbar cortical output systems that decussate prior to innervation of the relevant lower motor neurons. Unilateral movement disorders suggest an underlying structural lesion such as a tumor or infarct while bilateral (even if a bit asymmetrical) movement disorders are strongly suggestive of neurodegenerative or neurotoxic disorders.

The Cerebral Hemispheres

The cerebral hemispheres are the most recent evolutionary addition to the CNS. These are grotesquely amplified in humans and permit incredible refinement of our methods of achieving the Darwinian 4F's. Much more sophisticated analysis of visual, auditory and somatosensory information is carried out in the parietal, temporal and occipital lobes with linkage to the distributed emotive and memory circuitry of the limbic system and hippocampus. Motor output involves the frontal lobe motor and premotor areas, and in addition to complex motor output, the human brain is capable of symbolic output in the form of spoken and written language. The vast expanses of cerebral cortex, particularly of the frontal lobes, permits planning, anticipation, cunning, running of simulations prior to initiation of motor acts increasing the complexity, variability and unpredictability of human behavior.

Despite this complexity, however, several simplifying principles can be applied to clinical localization of cerebral hemispheric lesions. First is the fact that the cerebral hemisphere is concerned with the contralateral universe—the left hemisphere controls right-sided motor activities, processes sensory information from the right side of the body and face, and is concerned with the right hemifield of visual space. Second, the frontal lobe is concerned with action—either mental or motor—while the parietal, occipital and temporal lobes are predominantly involved with sensory processing and synthesis. Third, there is asymmetrical distribution of language and emotive functions such that in most humans, the left hemisphere is dominant for language—basically, all right handed persons are left dominant and about half of left-handed persons are left cerebral hemisphere dominant.

The visual pathways provide a beautiful localization system in the supratentorial compartment with specific visual field defects being associated with precise localization from the orbit to the occiput. Visual data from one eye travels ipsilateral to the retina until the optic chiasm, hence lesions of the eye, retinal or optic nerve will lead to monocular visual defects. In the optic chiasm, which resides below the hypothalamus and above the pituitary fossa, fibers concerned with lateral or temporal visual fields of space cross to join the fibers subserving temporal space from the ipsilateral eye. For example, due to the geometric inversion imposed by the optics of the lens, data from the right visual field of space will fall on the left temporal and the right nasal retinae. Fibers from the left temporal retina subserving the right visual field will proceed to the chiasm, will not cross, but will continue in the left optic tract to the left lateral geniculate nucleus and thence to the left occipital cortex via the left optic radiations. Fibers from the right eye's nasal retina subserving the right visual field, proceed to chiasm, cross to the left optic tract and travel with the left temporal retina fibers to the left genigulate nucleus and thence to the left occipital lobe via the left optic radiations. Data from the right visual field carried in the left optic tract innervates separate layers of the left lateral geniculate nucleus, and convergence of data from the left and right retinae does not actually occur until fibers of the left optic radiations converge on the ocular dominance columns of the left occipital lobe.

Lesions of the optic chiasm lead to bitemporal hemianopic visual field defects by interrupting the crossing nasal retinae fibers from both eyes. This location is the only site where a bitemporal hemianopic visual field defect can be produced. Once the fibers have negotiated the optic chiasm, impingement on the optic tracts, optic radiations or occipital lobes will lead to contralateral homonymous hemianopic visual field defects. As the occipital lobes are approached, the visual field defects become increasingly congruous. The retinal fibers are closely packed in the optic tracts, but in the optic radiations, the fibers from the lateral geniculate nucleus are dispersed such that fibers subserving the upper temporal quadrate of visual space, reside in the temporal white matter while those subserving the inferior contralateral temporal field of visual space travel in the parietal white matter. Lesions in the temporal lobe impinging on the optic radiations produce a superior contralateral homonymous quandrantanopsia ("pie in the sky" visual field cut) while parietal lobe lesions led to an inferior contralateral homonymous quadrantanopsia ("pie in the mud" visual field cut). Once the occipital lobes are reached, lesions here are characterized by extreme congruity with macular sparing.

As indicated earlier, language is usually localized to the left cerebral hemisphere. The sensory aspect of language—receipt and analysis of spoken or written material—is processed by the angular gyrus and occipital lobes respectively, while the prefrontal motor area handles the generation of written or spoken language. The major sensory areas and motor areas are connected by the arcuate fasciculus. Abnormalities of language resulting from damage to these areas are called "aphasias" and are classically categorized as receptive, conductive, and expressive aphasia. If damage occurs in the angular gyrus the patient is unable to interpret incoming linguistic data and the reception area is no longer able to monitor output of the more anterior motor speech area (Wernicke's aphasia). As a result, the patient cannot understand language whether it comes from an external source or arises internally; therefore, there is profound defect of comprehension and since speech output is unfettered by quality control monitoring, copious verbal gibberish is generated. Conversely, if the anterior (Broca's) speech generation area is damaged, comprehension is intact but speech is very slow and laborious and may be punctuated by scatological limbic eruptions. Interestingly, individuals with either Broca's or Wernicke's aphasia are incapable of verbal repetition. In some instances, the arcuate fasciculus connecting the receptive and motor speech areas is interrupted leading to conduction aphasia in which comprehension is impaired, speech output is slow and concrete and repetition is impaired. In general, repetition of a syntactically complex structure such as "there are no ifs, ands, or buts about the matter" is the most sensitive indicator of aphasia. Milder forms of these classical forms of aphasia are common with smaller lesions and in some instances the cerebral cortex adjacent to the primary speech reception and generation areas is damaged leading to transcortical aphasia in which repetition is intact but comprehension is impaired (transcortical receptive aphasia) or linguistic output is impaired (transcortical expressive aphasia). Language content disturbances most commonly arise from lesions of the dominant (usually left) cerebral hemisphere, however, the nondominant hemisphere does play a role in language by influencing the cadence and inflection (prosody) of speech which encodes implicit emotive content. Hence a person with a nondominant hemisphere language defect will often have monotonous robotic speech devoid of the normal melodious fluctuations that so often provide the listener with insight into the speaker's emotion state.

Writing is very much like speaking and is executed by the motor speech areas of the dominant hemisphere. Symbolic expression can occur either by activation of the muscles of the larynx or by activation of the muscles of the hands and fingers; a person with an expressive aphasia cannot write anymore than they can speak. Reading requires activity of areas more posterior to the speech receptive area in the parietal occipital region so it is possible to have a selective loss of reading comprehension (alexia) without a loss of speech comprehension. Also it appears that written linguistic output is less dependent on internal monitoring than is speech, because individuals can experience alexia without agraphia (inability to read with preserved ability to write). Such persons can and often do write copious grammatically correct text which they cannot read. This most commonly results from lesions of the dominant occipital lobe and splenium of the corpus callosum isolating the nondominant visual cortex from the dominant lobe.

Disturbances of the parietal lobe lead to difficulties with spatial orientation and construction. The person may become lost in familiar surroundings and if asked to draw objects such as clock faces or box houses will generate primitive renditions. In the most extreme forms of spatial agnosia, the patient

roots are incised and the cord is removed with cauda equina and dorsal root ganglia intact. If entry into the thoracic and abdominal cavities is not permitted, the spinal cord can be removed posteriorly by incising along the spinous processes from occiput to sacrum, reflecting the skin and underlying soft tissues laterally, and cutting through the posterior elements that are removed en bloc to expose the spinal cord. The spinal cord can be formalin fixed along with the brain.

After fixation, the brain is weighed and examined externally for abnormalities. The adult brain weighs 1,200–1,500 g. The cerebral and cerebellar hemispheres are examined for softening by touch, and are inspected for hemorrhage, dusky discoloration, or purulent material. Softening is usually indicative of an infarct and the relationship of the softening to vascular territories should be noted; softening may, however, indicate an underlying neoplastic or inflammatory process. The cerebral hemispheres are gently pried apart and the corpus callosum is visualized and cingulate herniation is sought. The base of the brain is inspected for the presence of uncal herniation—marked asymmetry of the unci with compression of the oculomotor nerve and hemorrhagic necrosis are the definitive elements of uncal herniation. There is normally a parahippocampal sulcus that must not be mistaken for uncal grooving. Cerebellar tonsillar herniation is definite when the tonsils are touching vigorously enough to experience hemorrhagic pressure necrosis; milder degrees of tonsillar herniation may occur but must be interpreted with caution. The arteries of the circle of Willis are inspected for the presence of atherosclerosis manifested as yellow white discoloration predominantly at bifurcations. Severe atherosclerosis may distort rheology sufficiently that the course of arteries may be altered; in particular, the basilar artery may exhibit extreme tortuosity (ectasia) sufficient to result in encroachment on cranial nerves and brainstem. The arteries must also be examined carefully for the presence of saccular aneurysms.

The brainstem and cerebellum are detached from the cerebral hemispheres by a cleanly axial incision through the midbrain at its most rostrally accessible level. When properly done, this incision reveals a perfectly flat midbrain disclosing the substantia nigra, cerebral peduncles and aqueduct of Sylvius. A shallow incision is then made down the length of the right side of the brainstem to allow distinction of the left and right sides of the brainstem microscopic sections. The brainstem and cerebellum can be cut together using through and through axial incisions, or the cerebellum can be detached from the brainstem by cutting through the cerebellar peduncles. The brainstem is cut axially at 3–4-mm intervals, while somewhat thicker sections are permissible for the cerebellum.

The midbrain sections are examined for substantia nigral pigmentation bearing in mind that this nucleus does not fully pigment until age 12 years of age; loss of pigmentation is suggestive of Parkinson's disease that must be confirmed with microscopic sections. The cerebral peduncles should be symmetrical; asymmetry may reflect axonal degeneration due to damage of motor neurons residing in the motor strip. This atrophic process takes months to develop. At the transition between the midbrain and the pons, the locus ceruleus is conspicuous at the corners of the emerging forth ventricle; this noradrenergic nucleus may undergo atrophy in Parkinson's disease. The most conspicuous medullary landmarks are the inferior olivary nuclei and medullary pyramids. Like the cerebral peduncles, the medullary pyramids may undergo atrophy with damage to the upper motor neurons whose axons comprise these structures.

The cerebral hemispheres are left together and the base of the brain facing upward, coronal sections at 1-cm intervals are made from the frontal tips

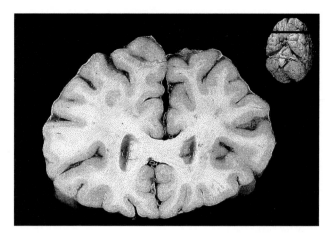

FIGURE 5-36. At brain cutting, one of the standard coronal cuts is made at the level of the temporal tips. This will go through the genu of the corpus callosum and just graze the anterior tips of the frontal horns of the lateral ventricles. If most of the ventricle can be seen, then ventriculomegaly is present.

to the occipital poles. Particular care should be taken to make a cut precisely at the temporal tips as this will assure that the cuts are lined up left and right, and this cut will pass through the genu of the corpus callosum and should just graze the anterior tips of the frontal horns of the ventricles (Fig. 5-36). If capacious ventricles are seen in this cut, then ventriculomegaly is present. A cut targeting the optic chiasm is also useful as the coronal sections will usually reveal the anterior commissure and the underlying basal nucleus of Meynert (Fig. 5-37). The next coronal cut should target the mammillary bodies to assure that these are inspected for hemorrhage and atrophy of Wernicke's encephalopathy. The next coronal cut is directed at the plane defined by two-thirds of the way along an imaginary line from the interpeduncular fossa of the midbrain to the ventricular aqueduct (Fig. 5-38). A properly placed incision in this plane will reward the examiner with a perfect view of the hippocampus at the level of the lateral geniculate body.

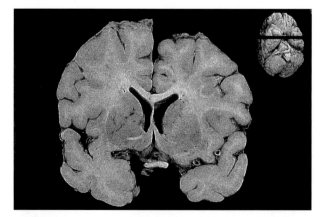

FIGURE 5-37. A coronal cut at the level of the optic chiasm shows the lateral ventricles, head of caudate, putamen, and often the anterior commissure. The gray matter beneath this commissure contains the basal nucleus of Meynert—the major cholinergic nucleus of the cerebral cortex.

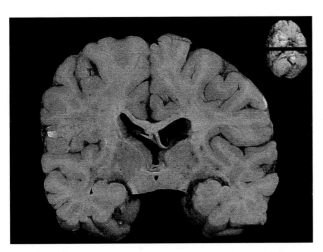

FIGURE 5-38. A coronal cut made about two-thirds of the way along an anterior to posterior line through the midbrain will go through the hippocampus.

The coronal sections are systematically inspected—the cortical ribbon, the white matter, the basal ganglia, the corpus callosum, and the ventricles. Any asymmetries, discoloration, softening, mass effect, or atrophy should be noted. The left and right hemispheres provide reciprocal controls facilitating detection of even subtle abnormalities. The white matter should be glistening white and smooth without any granularity or gray discoloration although punctuation by small individual vascular channels is permitted; sometimes abnormalities of the white matter become apparent as the coronal slices dry slightly.

Selected areas of the brain are cut into "blocks" that are approximately 4 mm thick and 2 × 2 cm square for subsequent processing for microscopic examination. There are honest differences of opinion among neuropathologists about how many blocks constitute an adequate sampling of a routine brain, but most would agree that, at a minimum, the frontal, parietal, occipital, temporal, and cingulate cortex with underlying white matter should be examined along with hippocampus, striatum, midbrain with particular attention to the substantia nigra, pons with special attention to the locus ceruleus, medulla, and cerebellar cortex with underlying white matter and dentate. Cortex, hippocampus, and basal ganglia from both cerebral hemispheres is not absolutely essential although the blocks should have contributions from both. Similarly, the cerebellum can be sampled with a single block. Some would insist that bilateral sampling of the cerebral cortex, hippocampus, basal ganglia, and thalamus is necessary, and this certainly leads to a more thorough examination, but is attended by higher costs.

The slides produced from the brain cutting are usually stained with hematoxylin and eosin, the workhorse stain of diagnostic histopathology. Additional stains can be obtained and a plethora of beautiful staining methods have been part of the tradition of neuropathology. In particular, silver stains to highlight neurofibrillary tangle and plaques have enjoyed immense popularity, however, increasingly, immunohistochemical methods are replacing the older methods because of specificity, sensitivity and increasingly, cost considerations—most hospital histopathology laboratories are adept at immunohistochemistry and often use robotic automation, while silver stains combine the liabilities of dark art and high reagent cost.

ANATOMICAL VARIANTS AND INCIDENTAL AUTOPSY FINDINGS

There are a number of eye-catching anatomical variants and other incidental findings often seen at brain cutting that may cause confusion in the novice. Many of these structures can also be seen on neuroimaging studies and, if misinterpreted as pathological, may lead to diagnostic and therapeutic misadventure. Following are the most salient and commonly encountered incidental (clinically unimportant and asymptomatic), but visually arresting, oddities likely to be encountered at autopsy.

1. Cavum septi pellucidi: The two layers of the septum pellucidum usually fuse to form a single septum by the first few months after birth. However, they may remain separate in adults, enclosing a space termed the cavum septi pellucidi, which is a commonly noted incidental finding on magnetic resonance imaging (MRI) scans. The septi fuse from posterior to anterior; it is most common to find a cavum located anterior, with normal fusion of the posterior septi. A patent cavum posteriorly, beneath the splenium of the corpus callosum, is more rare, and is given a separate name: cavum Vergae.

2. Xanthogranulomas of the choroid plexus: Xanthogranulomas are postulated to form as a reaction to extravasated blood in the choroid plexus, which subsequently lyses and provokes an inflammatory reaction that includes macrophage infiltration. Xanthogranulomas may be unilateral, but bilaterality is also common. Neuroradiologists are familiar with these lesions and usually diagnose them accurately on neuroimaging studies. At autopsy, the gross appearance varies from bright yellow (due to lipid-laden macrophages cells) to dark black-golden brown (due to hemorrhage and hemosiderin deposition) and often suggests tumor metastasis. In this situation it is wise to bear in mind that solitary, isolated metastasis to the choroid plexus although certainly possible, is rare in the absence of other metastatic foci and, in cases of bilateral masses, isolated bilateral metastasis would be very exceptional and xanthogranulomas are far more likely. Histologic examination confirms the diagnosis.

3. Cystic change of the choroid plexus: Another gross morphologic change frequently seen in the choroid plexus at autopsy is cystic change. Large fluid-filled delicate cysts may be present in one or both glomera choroidea (the glomera are the large masses of choroid plexus located in the atria of the lateral ventricles).

4. Arachnoid plaques: Flat white plaques most frequently arise in the spinal leptomeninges, but may also be more rarely seen over the cerebrum or cerebellum as well. There may be only a single small plaque or several dozen blanketing the entire spinal cord. Even in the latter case, they are usually completely asymptomatic. Most plaques consist of hyaline fibrous material histologically, similar to fibrous plaques of the pleura; rare examples may calcify or ossify.

5. Calcified and ossified plaques of the dura: Calcification or ossification of the dura is sometimes seen at autopsy, particularly superiorly along the superior sagittal sinus and in the falx cerebri. In many cases, these hard plaques are easier to feel by palpation of the dura than to be seen. The plaques are asymptomatic.

6. Incidental lipoma: Small incidental lipomas are not infrequently identified at autopsy, attached to the dura or in the leptomeninges. The vicinity of the tuber cinereum and infundibulum at the base of the brain is a common location. Even very small lipomas stand out due to their bright yellow color.

7. Incidental subependymoma of the fourth ventricle: Subependymomas are low grade gliomas that grow exophytically into the lateral or fourth ventricle. If they attain sufficient size, they may obstruct the interventricular foramen of Monro or the outlet foramina of the fourth ventricle and cause obstructive hydrocephalus; however, small subependymomas will be asymptomatic and are often only discovered as an incidental finding at autopsy.

8. Incidental meningioma: Meningiomas are among the most common tumors of the nervous system, so it is not surprising that incidental examples are very frequently seen at autopsy attached to the dura overlying the cerebral convexities or at the skull base.

9. Incidental cystic pineal gland: Small fluid-filled cysts are present in the pineal gland of all normal adults. Rarely, a pineal cyst can attain sufficient size to compress adjacent neural structures and cause symptoms; much more commonly even large cysts of 1 cm in diameter are usually asymptomatic. They are, however, very conspicuous on neuroimaging studies and also at autopsy when the pineal is sectioned.

10. Heavily pigmented leptomeninges of the brainstem: As discussed in Chapter 2, melanocytes are normal constituents of the leptomeninges, particularly around the upper cervical cord and brainstem medulla. In some individuals, the pigmentation can be so heavy as to be conspicuously visible to the naked eye as a dusky brown-black discoloration of the pia covering the medulla. The characteristic anatomic distribution, which can extend from the upper cervical cord as far rostrally as the gyri recti, located between the olfactory bulbs and tracts, provides the key to correct identification.

11. Incidental Rathke cleft cyst: Similar to the pineal gland, the pituitary gland also normally contains microscopic cysts of the pars intermedia. Occasionally these cysts can reach sufficient size to compress the infundibulum, producing "stalk effect" and mild elevation of serum prolactin. Usually, however, they are asymptomatic and discovered incidentally at autopsy.

12. Asymmetric obliteration (fusion) of the tips of the occipital horns of the lateral ventricles: The tips and angles of all of the cerebral ventricles, along with the central canal of the spinal cord, are prone to coalesce and fuse during development, especially the small, slender horns of the occipital lobes. Moreover, the occipital horns are often asymmetrically fused to different extents, as will be obvious on axial or frontal sections taken through them. Histologically, tissue sections from the area of fusion will show nests and rosettes of ependymal cells.

13. Incidental arachnoid cyst: Arachnoid cysts, which are actually intra-arachnoid in anatomic location (located within a split of the arachnoid membrane) are most commonly seen in the rostral Sylvian fissure in association with a posteriorly compressed temporal lobe pole. They may also occur at any site within the CNS in which arachnoid is present.

14. Ecchordosis physaliphora: These benign rests of the embryonic notochord material (with a very impressive name!) are typically seen adherent to the ventral aspect of the brainstem, especially over the pons in close proximity to the basilar artery. One must be very meticulous in closely examining the basal aspect of the brainstem as well as the clivus of the skull base if one hopes to ever see this entity. Ecchordoses are small, lobulated gelatinous gray masses of a few millimeters to a half centimeter or so in size. Microscopically, they are composed of cells with prominently vacuolated cytoplasm termed physaliferous cells, literally "bubble-bearing" cells. The same name is given to their malignant cousins seen in chordomas.

15. Leptomeningeal glial heterotopias: Sometimes small (1–3 mm in diameter) white nodules of soft tissue are noted in the leptomeninges at autopsy, particularly around the ventral aspect of the pons and medulla. Invariably,

these turn out to be either glial (most common) or glioneuronal (less common) herotopias on histologic examination. The single most common site for microscopic leptomeningeal glial heterotopias is in the interpeduncular fossa between the crus cerebri of the midbrain.

SUMMARY OF CLINICAL LOCALIZATION IN THE NERVOUS SYSTEM

Localization Synthesis #1: Weakness
  Arm, leg, face on one side: *Full Hemiparesis*
  Arm and leg on one side, face on the other: *Crossed hemiparesis—Brainstem*
  Leg and arm on one side sparing face: Partial Hemiparesis
  Both legs: *Paraparesis*
  Both arms and legs: *Quadriparesis*
  One arm or one leg: *Monoparesis*

Full Hemiparesis: The lesion is in the cerebral hemisphere or upper brainstem. Are there visual field defects and/or disturbances of higher function?
  Yes—Cerebral hemisphere contralateral to motor deficit.
  No—Lesion is below the cerebral hemisphere but above the decussation of the facial corticobulbar fibers—i.e., high brainstem. Look for other midbrain or high pons signs.

Crossed hemiparesis: The lesion must be in the brainstem in the pons (CN 7) on the same side as the facial weakness. The body weakness should be contralateral to the pontine lesion. For confirmation, double check to be sure that the facial weakness is LMN CN 7 weakness (brow, cheek and chin equally involved). Look for an ipsilateral CN6 deficit.

Partial Hemiparesis: The lesion is probably below the level of the pons since the face is spared. Rarely, very focal lesions may knock-out the descending corticospinal fibers in the internal capsule or cerebral peduncles while sparing the corticobulbar fibers. Also lesions of the cerebral motor cortex may affect arm and leg more than face, or the arm and face more than leg due to the spread-out nature of the motor homunculus. Check for visual field defects and disturbances of higher cortical function to verify cortical and hemispheric involvement. Look for associated cranial nerve and sensory signs to evaluate for medullary involvement. Look for a sensory level for spinal cord (cervical level since the arm and leg are affected).

Paraparesis: Strongly suggestive of spinal cord lesion below the cervical level. Look for a sensory level to ascertain the segmental level of the myelopathy. Confirm the UMN weakness by eliciting hyperreflexia and primitive reflexes (beware that acutely these may be absent). If you do not see UMN findings, but rather detect flaccid paralysis, diminished or absent reflexes, and muscle atrophy in the legs consider a cauda equina lesion leading to LMN weakness of the lower extremities. Rarely paraparesis will result from midline cerebral hemispheric lesions compromising the leg and foot portions of both motor homunculi. Such lesions are associated with UMN weakness, no sensory level, and may have accompanying disturbances of higher function.

Quadriparesis: Strongly suggestive of spinal cord lesion in the cervical region or lower medullary brainstem. Look for a sensory level and lower cranial nerve deficits. You will expect to see hyperreflexia and primitive reflexes bespeaking an UMN lesion. Be aware that if UMN signs are not present, the cervical cord may still be in spinal shock. Also, however, quadriparesis may result from LMN processes at every level from the anterior horn cells, spinal roots and peripheral nerves, neuromuscular junction or even from profound muscle weakness itself. Obviously to produce quadriparesis, multiple levels of anterior roots, nerves, neuromuscular junctions or muscle must be involved.

Monoparesis: Suggests a segmental spinal cord, multiple roots, or plexus. Look for associated spinal level as well as sensory disturbances in the distribution of roots, plexi or individual nerves. Is the weakness really confined to a single nerve in the extremity and only portions of the extremity are weak.

Localization Synthesis #2: Numbness: The approach to the problem of numbness is remarkably similar to the analysis of motor disturbances. First, define as precisely as possible the areas involved, and in the case of sensory disturbances, define which modalities are involved since these are spatially separated in the spinal cord but converge as they ascend through the neuraxis above the foramen magnum.

Full Hemisensory loss/all modalities: Must be above the sensory nuclei of V. Look for hemispheric signs (visual field defects and disturbance of higher function). Rarely, isolated thalamic or internal capsule lesions can lead to isolated (pure) hemisensory loss.

Partial Hemisensory (arms and leg sparing face) loss/all modalities: The spinothalamic tracts and secondary neurons of the nucleus gracilis and cuneatus have converged but not yet met up with the facial sensory fibers. Rare, look for associated high brainstem findings. Sometimes lesions of the cerebral cortex sensory homunculus will lead to partial hemisensory defects—look for associated disturbances in higher cortical function and visual field defects.

Crossed Hemianesthesia: Ipsilateral facial numbness and contralateral body numbness. Must be in the brainstem from mid-pons (sensory nucleus of CN5) all the way down to C2 (spinal nucleus and tract of CN5). The more caudal the lesion, the greater the likelihood that the sensory loss will be dissociated (involves only pain and thermal sense while sparing fine touch).

Sensory Level: Strong evidence for a spinal cord lesion at the level of the transition from normal to abnormal sensory loss. Dissociation of modalities may be seen with partial spinal cord lesions.

Segmental Dissociated Sensory Loss: Loss of pain and thermal sense over several spinal segments with normal pain and thermal sense above and below the level of abnormality. Posterior column function normal throughout. This indicates interruption of the crossing ascending secondary neurons in the anterior spinal commissure. Seen in central spinal cord lesions such as syringomyelia or spinal cord tumors.

Dermatomal Sensory Loss (All modalities): Indicates a radicular lesion. Verify with motor and reflex testing of the offending root. Is the sensory loss dermatomal or does it follow the distribution of a peripheral nerve? Compare and contrast the sensory loss seen in a median neuropathy versus a C6 radiculopathy, an ulnar neuropathy versus a C8 radiculopathy, a superficial cutaneous branch of the peroneal nerve and an L5 radiculopathy.

6

INCREASED INTRACRANIAL PRESSURE

PERSPECTIVE

1. Space-taking lesions of any cause may produce a common set of signs and symptoms by increasing intracranial pressure (ICP) and leading to herniation syndromes.
2. Increased ICP can result in compromised cerebral perfusion and, if the pressure is asymmetrical between dura-defined compartments of the intracranial vault, can lead to herniation.
3. The major herniation syndromes are cingulate, uncal, central, and tonsillar herniation.
4. Ipsilateral cranial nerve III dysfunction from uncal herniation is the most significant clinical localization sign in increased ICP because it is exquisitely localizing and occurs when the process is still potentially reversible.
5. Death occurs in increased ICP due to cerebral perfusion failure, compression of medullary cardiopulmonary control circuits, and brainstem hemorrhages (Duret hemorrhages).
6. Increased ICP can result from inappropriate accumulation of cerebrospinal fluid (CSF)—hydrocephalus.

OBJECTIVES

1. Understand the basic principles of cerebral perfusion and the impact of increased ICP on this process.
2. Know the major features clinically and pathologically of cingulate, uncal and tonsillar herniation.
3. Understand the cause and significance of "false localizing" findings in increased ICP and herniation.
4. Be able to distinguish between communicating and noncommunicating hydrocephalus.

The single most important and unique aspect of the brain's existence from a general pathophysiological viewpoint is that:

THE BRAIN LIVES IN A CLOSED BOX!

The volume of the intracranial contents is made up by the brain, the CSF, and the blood going to and from the brain. Any disease process which takes up space does so at the expense of either brain, CSF, or blood (Fig. 6-1). This is a verbal expression of the Monro-Kelly hypothesis, which states:

$$\text{Intracranial Volume} = \text{Volume}_{CNS} + \text{Volume}_{CSF}$$

$$+ \text{Volume}_{Blood} + \text{Volume}_{Lesion}$$

Such space-occupying lesions may occur in diseases from every major category of disease with the exception of degenerative disorders.

The immediate consequence of trying to fit more volume into the fixed space of the intracranial vault is an increase in ICP. The normal mean ICP is less than 200 mm H_2O or 15 mm Hg for a patient in the lateral decubitus position. The pressure can be measured by lumbar puncture or by placement of an ICP transducer. As ICP increases, the patient experiences headache, confusion, drowsiness, and may develop papilledema. The first line of physiological compensation is reduction in CSF volume; hence, the ventricles are compressed to small slits and sulci are effaced.

If the volume of the lesion takes up more space than the reduction in CSF volume can compensate for, then reduction in the blood volume takes place. This reduction in cerebral blood flow may have immediate adverse consequences since the brain is critically dependent upon an uninterrupted supply of oxygen and nutrients.

BRAIN HERNIATION SYNDROMES

If the lesion expands further, then the only structure remaining to "give" is the brain itself. The intracranial compartment is subdivided by dural boundaries—the tentorium cerebelli divides the vault into the supra- and infratentorial compartments, and the falx divides the supratentorial compartment into two equal right and left compartments. Depending on the location of the space-occupying lesion, the brain may be forced out of one compartment into another—such shifts are called "brain herniations" (Figs. 6-2 and 6-3).

Cingulate Herniation

If one hemisphere is forced under the falx, the cingulate lobe is the first portion of that hemisphere to be displaced. Such herniations are called "subfalcine" or "cingulate" herniations. An individual experiencing such a herniation becomes confused and drowsy. The anterior cerebral artery is also displaced beneath the falx, and infarction within this vessel's territory may occur, leading to contralateral lower extremity weakness and urinary incontinence. The displacement of this vessel may be seen angiographically, and shifting of the other normally midline structures may be seen by CT and MRI.

Intracranial Volume

- **Brain**
- **Blood**
- **Cerebrospinal fluid**
- **Lesion**

FIGURE 6-1. The intracranial volume.

Herniation Syndromes

- **Cingulate (falcine)**
- **Uncal**
- **Cerebellar tonsillar herniation**
- **Upward herniation**
- **External herniation (cerebri fungoides)**

FIGURE 6-2. The major herniation syndromes.

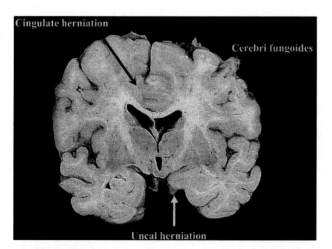

FIGURE 6-3. Composite image showing midline shift—cingulate herniation, downward displacement—uncal herniation, and protrusion from the cranial cavity—cerebri fungoides.

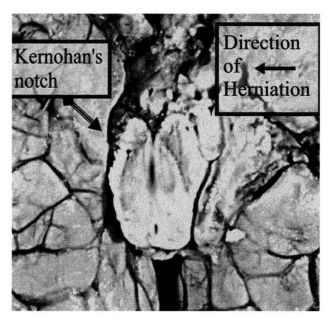

FIGURE 6-4. Uncal herniation shifting the midbrain across the midline compressing the contralateral cerebral peduncle against the tentorium leading to Kernohan's notch.

Uncal Herniation

If one hemisphere is forced from the supratentorial compartment toward the infratentorial compartment, the medial temporal lobe (the uncus) is the first portion of the hemisphere displaced; therefore, this is an uncal or transtentorial herniation. The ipsilateral oculomotor nerve (cranial nerve III) is crushed by the displaced temporal lobe leading to ipsilateral pupillary dilatation and paresis of all the extra-ocular muscles except the lateral rectus (cranial nerve VI) and the superior oblique (cranial nerve IV). The unopposed action of the lateral rectus leads to the eye "looking" laterally.

As medial displacement continues, the midbrain is shifted away from the displaced hemisphere with the contralateral cerebral peduncle being driven into the unyielding tentorium. This crushing injury of the cerebral peduncle is known as Kernohan's notch and results in hemiparesis on the same side of the body as the offending mass (Fig. 6-4). Since a hemispheric mass will normally produce hemiparesis on the opposite side of the body, this paradoxical finding of ipsilateral hemiparesis may be clinically confusing and is called a "false-localizing" sign.

The downward and medial displacement of the hemisphere through the tentorial opening may also result in compression of one or both posterior cerebral arteries as they make their ways from the infratentorial compartment to the now crowded supratentorial compartment. Such compression may impair blood flow to the occipital lobes sufficiently to result in infarction with attendant visual field disturbances bearing no obvious relationship to the inciting mass. This occipital lobe infarction and its attendant signs is also "false-localizing."

While the uncal herniation syndrome is very ominous, it is reversible with removal of the offending mass and it compels rapid definitive neurosurgical intervention. Temporary measures aimed at reducing ICP include mannitol administration to literally osmotically shrink the brain, and hyperventilation to reduce PCO_2, inducing cerebral vasospasm thereby reducing cerebral blood volume and therefore pressure. These measures may gain the patient sufficient time for neurosurgical treatment.

Here is a summary of false localizing (non-localizing) signs:

1. Hemiparesis ipsilateral to lesion resulting from Kernohan's notch.
2. Homonymous hemianopsia due to PCA compression—occipital lobe infarction (if both occipital lobes infarct, cortical blindness ensues).
3. Cranial nerve 6 palsies.
4. Papilledema.

Central Herniation

If both hemispheres herniate transtentorially, the central herniation syndrome is said to be present. Both pupils dilate; flaccidity and coma ensue.

Cerebellar Tonsillar Herniation

If the infratentorial compartment becomes crowded either from migrating supratentorial contents or from a mass arising in the infratentorial compartment, the brainstem and cerebellum may seek egress through the foramen magnum. The cerebellar tonsils and medulla are forced together at this opening with lethal compression of vital medullary centers. This bleak situation is called "tonsillar herniation." Mild tonsillar grooving is frequently seen at brain cutting and probably does not reflect significant antemortem increased ICP. Many neuropathologists require that the cerebellar tonsils are touching and preferably necrotic and hemorrhagic before rendering a definitive diagnosis of tonsillar herniation (Fig. 6-5).

As if things weren't bad enough, immediately before and following tonsillar herniation, the downward displacement of the brainstem may literally wrench vessels from their parenchymal beds within the midbrain and pons leading to multiple linear hemorrhages known as Duret hemorrhages or secondary hemorrhages of herniation (Fig. 6-6). These hemorrhages may coalesce, becoming difficult to distinguish from hypertensive pontine hemorrhage, although extensive midbrain involvement speaks strongly against the latter entity.

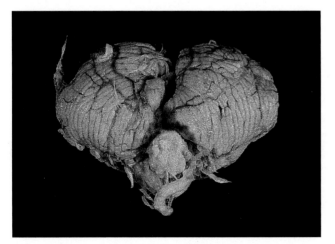

FIGURE 6-5. Cerebellar tonsillar herniation with dark hemorrhagic discoloration and necrosis. The tonsils touch in the midline and compress the medulla.

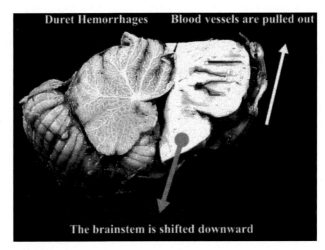

FIGURE 6-6. Downward shift of the brainstem leading to Duret hemorrhages.

Fungus Cerebri

If a traumatic or surgical defect is present in the skull, brain under increased pressure may spew like oatmeal from the opening. This process is known as fungus cerebri.

CEREBRAL EDEMA

Another pathophysiological process that may contribute to increased ICP is the development of cerebral edema. Cerebral edema may complicate any process which gives rise to increased pressure, and can set up a self-perpetuating cycle in which increasing edema begets increasing pressure which in turn begets more edema.

Cerebral edema is at a fundamental level an absolute increase in brain water content. The amount of water in brain tissue is tightly controlled by the rate of production of CSF, the rate of egress of CSF from the cranial vault, and the flux of water across the blood–brain barrier. The blood–brain barrier compartmentalizes the brain from the circulation so that only lipid-soluble molecules or molecules which can access specialized transport systems can enter the brain. The structural basis of the blood–brain barrier is the endothelial cell with its tight junctions lining the cerebral vessels. Water can enter the brain uncontrollably if the barrier is disrupted or if osmotic forces across the barrier are sufficient to drive water into the cerebral tissues. Three major forms of cerebral edema may occur:

1. Cytotoxic edema: Water is driven across an intact blood brain barrier by osmotic forces arising either because of failure of cells within the brain to maintain osmotic homeostasis or because of systemic water overload. In either case, water is driven down its concentration gradient into the cerebral tissues until equilibrium occurs.

2. Vasogenic edema: The blood–brain barrier disintegrates permitting uncontrolled entry of water into the tissues. This is the commonest cause of edema, and is seen with neoplasms, abscesses, meningitis, hemorrhage, contusions, and lead poisoning. A combination of cytotoxic and vasogenic edema is common in infarcts. The above processes may disrupt the barrier properties of the endothelium, or the vessels formed in neoplasms may be defective from

their inception. Vasogenic edema often responds dramatically to the administration of corticosteroids that restore barrier integrity even in tumors.

3. Interstitial edema: While cytotoxic and vasogenic edema involve water fluxes across the endothelium, interstitial edema involves overproduction or failure of egress of CSF so that the fluid seeps across the ependymal lining of the ventricles to accumulate within the white matter.

HYDROCEPHALUS

Related to interstitial edema is hydrocephalus, which is accumulation of CSF within the ventricles resulting in dilatation of these structures (Fig. 6-7). Certainly, when the ventricular distension is sufficiently advanced, fluid will leak trans-ependymally into the white matter, causing interstitial edema. Accumulation of CSF can arise from one of two processes:

1. Overproduction of CSF: This is very rare, occurring only in the context of tumors of the choroid plexus.

2. Failure of CSF egress from the cranial vault: This is the commonest mechanism. If the blockage occurs within the ventricular system itself, ventricles proximal to the block will dilate, whereas those situated downstream from the block will be spared. This form of hydrocephalus is obstructive, or noncommunicating, hydrocephalus (Fig. 6-8). The most common site of block is at the ventricular system's narrowest strait—the aqueduct of Sylvius connecting the third and fourth ventricles.

If the block exists after the CSF has left the ventricular system and is traveling over the cerebral convexities to the arachnoid granulations, which usher the fluid into the venous sinuses, then all of the ventricles dilate and the process is referred to as communicating hydrocephalus, meaning that the ventricles are in unobstructed fluidic communication. Communicating hydrocephalus may complicate subarachnoid hemorrhage or inflammation resulting in arachnoid scarring, or may result from thrombosis of the dural sinuses themselves.

The clinical features of hydrocephalus depend on the age of the patient. In infancy and childhood before the cranial sutures have fused, the head enlarges sometimes to grotesque proportions as the ventricles dilate. Since hy-

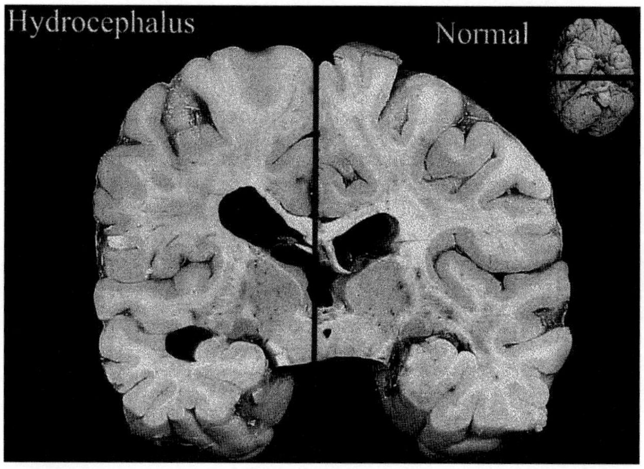

Acute CSF Obstruction

- Colloid cyst of the third ventricle
- Positional "ball-valve" at foramen of Monro
- Intermittent positional obstruction with recurrent headaches may precede catastrophe

FIGURE 6-8. Positional CSF obstruction may rarely result from a colloid cyst of the third ventricle.

FIGURE 6-7. Digital composite image comparing normal ventricular size with the enlarged rounded ventricles hydrocephalus.

Brain Death AAN 1995

Prerequisites
- Clinical or imaging features of CNS catastrophe
- Exclusion of medical conditions that confound assessment
- No drug intoxication or poisoning
- Core temperature above 32 C (90 F)

Findings
- Comatose – no cerebral motor response to pain
- Absent brainstem reflexes
- Apnea – no spontaneous respiratory movements

FIGURE 6-9. The American Academy of Neurology (AAN) 1995 guidelines for the clinical criteria for brain death.

Absence of Brainstem Reflexes

- No pupillary light responses
- No ocular motility
  - No oculocephalic response
  - No oculovestibular response (50 ml cold water each ear)
- No corneal reflex, grimace to painful stimuli
- No jaw jerk reflex
- No gag reflex or cough response to bronchial suctioning

FIGURE 6-10. The brainstem reflexes must be absent. To ascertain this, they must be tested.

Apnea Test

- Not hypothermic or hypotensive
- Deliver 100% oxygen at 6 L/min into trachea
- Disconnect from ventilator, observe for 8 minutes
- No respiratory movements
- pCO_2 greater than 60 mmHg or 40 mmHg above baseline

FIGURE 6-11. The apnea test to assess for spontaneous respirations must also be done rigorously.

Confirmatory Tests

- EEG – isoelectric at maximum sensitivity
- Absence of cerebral blood flow

FIGURE 6-12. Electroencephalography and cerebral blood flow studies performed rigorously are confirmatory.

drocephalus is common in infants and treatable by shunting, measurement of the head circumference is a fundamental part of the pediatric physical examination.

After suture fusion has occurred, hydrocephalus finds its expression not in head enlargement, but in increased ICP with headache, confusion, drowsiness, papilledema, and vomiting. Ventricular enlargement proceeds at the expense of cerebral tissue volume so that in advanced cases only a mantle of several millimeters thickness remains.

Remarkably, such individuals may retain substantial cognitive abilities, although spasticity may cloak the expression of this intelligence.

In older persons, hydrocephalus may develop insidiously, with gradual enlargement of the ventricles being clinically expressed as progressive dementia, gait impairment, and urinary incontinence as the long white matter fibers connecting portions of cortex to one another and lower motility centers are stretched apart by the relentless expansion of the ventricles. This condition is usually accompanied by normal ICP and is therefore called "normal pressure hydrocephalus" and is shunt-responsive in about two-thirds of cases.

All of the above forms of hydrocephalus result from disturbance of CSF dynamics, and should be distinguished from hydrocephalus *ex vacuo*, which is compensatory enlargement of the ventricles in response to loss of CNS tissue from other diseases. This is most commonly seen in the dementing illnesses leading to diffuse cortical atrophy, although focal destruction, such as occurs at the site of an old infarct, leads to focal compensatory ventricular enlargement.

BRAIN DEATH AND PERSISTENT VEGETATIVE STATE

Disturbances leading to increased ICP may result in compromise of cerebral blood flow sufficiently severe to result in the clinical state of brain death. Similarly, lack of oxygen or profound structural disruption wrought by trauma or intraparenchymal hemorrhage may result in irreversible cessation of brain function. The definition of brain death has evolved since first codified in the United States in 1968, but basically requires irreversible loss of consciousness without preservation of reflexes or cardiopulmonary neural control above the level of the foramen magnum (Figs. 6-9 through 6-13). Individuals meeting brain death criteria can be declared dead even in the presence of a heartbeat, and their organs can be harvested with the consent of the next of kin. Care must be taken to avoid rendering the diagnosis of brain death in the face of drug intoxication or hypothermia, where the clinical and physiological criteria of death can be obtained, but clearly irreversibility does not apply. Similarly, neurologically naive individuals may mistake profound neuromuscular blockade or brainstem infarction leading to "locked-in" syndrome for brain death.

The neuropathology of rigidly defined brain death usually takes the form of "respirator brain" where the brain is soft, congested, and autolyzed. No acute tissue reaction is present since no inflammatory cells could be carried into the brain due to the lack of blood flow and the endogenous reactive elements are necrotic. There may, however, be some residual histological alterations reflecting pathological processes preceding brain death. The tissue from such a brain fixes poorly in formalin and usually tissue sections are blandly eosinophilic. Of forensic interest is the occurrence of visually striking gas-filled cavities in the autolytic brain of un-embalmed corpses due to the activity of gas-forming organisms. This results in a brain full of holes, called "Swiss cheese" brain.

An area of considerable contemporary interest is the neuropathology of persistent vegetative state, in which individuals reside in a state of profoundly reduced sentient interaction with their surroundings but have preservation of vital functions sufficient to sustain life. Such an individual may breathe independently, and, if nutrition and good nursing care is given, prolonged corporeal survival may occur. A small fraction of individuals in persistent vegetative state may resume consciousness; therefore, ethical decisions in this venue revolve around resource allocation rather than organ donation. The neuropathology of persistent vegetative state is still being charted, but widespread cerebral cortical or thalamic damage is commonly seen with relative preservation of the brainstem. Thalamic damage, if bilateral, is sufficient to render the individual vegetative by depriving the otherwise functional cerebral cortex of input, activation and synchronization.

Paroxysmal Disorders

- **Patients with epilepsy have a 3X increased chance of sudden death**
- **Respiratory or cardiac dysfunction?**

FIGURE 6-13. Individuals with epilepsy have a higher than expected incidence of sudden death.

7

TUMORS

PERSPECTIVE

1. Cell proliferation, differentiation, and programmed cell death are under genetic control.
2. At the most fundamental level, cancer is a set of disorders characterized by mutations or deletions of genes regulating cell growth, differentiation, and death.
3. Tumor progression results from the sequential acquisition of new mutations or deletions that confer selective advantage.
4. Nervous system tumors, like tumors elsewhere, are named according to the phenotypic similarity of the tumor cells to normal cells and tissues of the developing and mature nervous system.
5. Nervous system tumors produce symptoms by compressing or invading adjacent neural tissue; therefore, focal signs and symptoms are common in patients with these tumors. In addition to focal effects, CNS tumors also produce increased intracranial pressure with its attendant signs and symptoms.

OBJECTIVES

1. Learn the essential details of the major types of nervous system tumors according to histological classification.
2. Become familiar with the appropriate differential diagnosis for CNS mass lesions according to anatomic location.
3. Learn the major clinicopathologic features of primary CNS lymphoma.
4. Understand the embryologic derivation, histologic subtypes, and clinical features of craniopharyngioma.
5. Understand how and why tumors of the pituitary gland can produce endocrine disturbances, neurological findings, or a combination of the two.
6. Learn the major features of meningiomas: characteristics of the cell of origin, gross locations, histopathological features, and grading criteria.
7. Compare and contrast schwannoma and neurofibroma.
8. Learn which tumors commonly metastasize to the nervous system and which do not.

INTRODUCTION

The current (2000) World Health Organization Classification of Tumours of the Nervous System, written by Kleihues and Cavenee, includes the codification of over 100 different neoplasms. Morphologic analysis of hematoxylin and eosin (H&E)–stained tissue sections by light microscopy, aided by electron microscopy, special stains, and immunohistochemistry, continues to serve as the basis for diagnosis, classification and grading of this varied and complex group of tumors. However, the era of molecular classification is rapidly dawning. Cytogenetic analyses and loss of heterozygosity (LOH) studies of the past decade provided crucial leads for the current progress towards more exact molecular genetic characterization, and translation of this exponentially accruing knowledge into better, more clinically useful, and less subjective classification systems for brain tumors will not lag far behind. Among the first examples is the use of LOH for 1p and 19q to predict chemosensitivity of oligodendroglial tumors. In this chapter, the essentials of traditional nervous system tumor morphology will be accompanied by relevant genetic information to the degree known at the time of writing; with the current pace of advances, seemingly by the week, there is no substitute for keeping a close eye on the literature!

> **Key Concept:** Histologic pattern recognition by light microscopic examination currently remains the primary tool used for classification of nervous system tumors; however, molecular genetic alterations are being increasingly used for more precise diagnosis and subclassification.

The wide range of neoplasms that involve the CNS can be organized into four major categories: (1) tumors arising from intrinsic cellular constituents, which can be further subdivided into tumors of neuroectodermal origin unique to the nervous system, such as gliomas and ganglion cell tumors, versus tumors of intrinsic constituents that are also common to other organ systems, such as primary brain sarcomas and primary CNS lymphoma, (2) tumors arising from the cellular constituents of anatomic structures that surround the brain and spinal cord that secondarily involve the nervous system by direct compression and/or invasion, such as meningiomas and bone and cartilaginous tumors of the skull and vertebral column, (3) tumors that arise from developmental rests of tissues not normally found within the nervous system, such as germ cell tumors, and (4) tumors that metastasize from systemic organs to the nervous system via the blood stream, of which the most common are lung carcinoma, breast carcinoma, renal cell carcinoma, melanoma, and gastrointestinal carcinomas. In addition, tumors of the peripheral nervous system (PNS) and tumors of the pituitary gland, which is a unique composite organ that is half CNS (neurohypophysis) and half foregut derivative (adenohypophysis), will also be presented in this chapter.

TUMORS DERIVED FROM NEUROECTODERM

Early in embryonal development, the neural plate and neural groove form from specialized portions of the ectoderm known as neuroectoderm. The mature cellular elements of the CNS (neurons, astrocytes, oligodendrocytes, etc.) arise from pluripotential primitive cells of the neuroectoderm. The neural crest separates from the neural groove and gives rise to the dorsal root ganglia, sympathetic chain, adrenal medulla, the dura, and melanocytes.

Historically, neuroectodermal tumors have been classified according to their resemblance to the various immature and mature cellular elements of the nervous system. Thus, the tumor called "medulloepithelioma" exhibits morphologic features similar to the early neural tube epithelium, the primitive neuroectodermal tumors (PNETs) resemble the neuroectodermal precursor cell populations of fetal germinal matrix, astrocytomas show features of mature astrocytes, etc. Because the precursor populations in the developing nervous system are highly mitotically active, the tumors named for their resemblance to them tend to share this feature and are therefore all aggressive, malignant tumors (PNETs, for example, are all malignant), whereas tumors named for mature cell types often exhibit a broad spectrum of biologic behaviors ranging from indolent to highly malignant, thus necessitating the establishment of grading criteria in addition to simple classification. For example, the diffuse astrocytomas all share similarities to mature astrocytes, hence their classification as astrocytomas, but astrocytomas exhibit a wide range in clinical behavior from comparatively slow growing (low-grade astrocytoma, WHO grade II) to highly malignant (glioblastoma, WHO grade IV) and thus must be graded for prognosis and treatment purposes.

Note that, in contrast to most tumors of the systemic organs, such as lung, breast, and colon carcinomas, brain tumors are not staged and the TNM (Tumor size, lymph Node involvement, Metastases) staging system is not applicable.

> **Key Concept:** Tumors are named according to the phenotypic similarity of the tumor cells to normal cells and tissues of the adult and the developing nervous systems.

Primitive Neuroectodermal and Embryonal Tumors

This group of neuroectodermal tumors includes the classical PNETs, which are morphologically prototypical small blue cell neoplasms, and other malignant embryonal neoplasms that are viewed as equally primitive but are not small blue cell neoplasms, such as atypical teratoid/rhabdoid tumor.

Medulloblastoma

Medulloblastoma is the most common intracranial PNET and occurs in the cerebellum. The age distribution is bimodal, with the largest peak in childhood and a second peak in adults around 35–40 years of age. In children, medulloblastomas tend to be located in the midline vermis (Fig. 7-1), while in

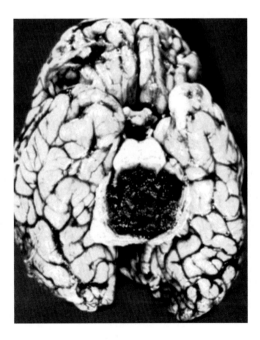

FIGURE 7-1. Medulloblastoma. Medulloblastoma that originated in the midline cerebellar vermis is seen filling the fourth ventricle.

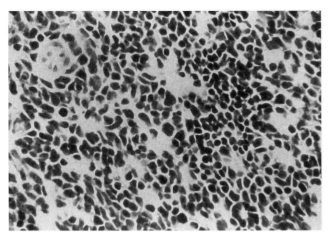

FIGURE 7-2. Medulloblastoma. Cerebellar medulloblastoma is the most common PNET and shows classical small blue cell tumor morphology. The clear areas are Homer Wright rosettes.

adults there is a predilection for lateral placement in the hemisphere and also for the desmoplastic variant. Medulloblastomas and pilocytic astrocytomas are the two most common brain tumors of childhood, each representing some 20–25% of all pediatric brain tumors with most series giving an edge to medulloblastoma. Treatment advances have been very successful with medulloblastoma, with a 50%, 10-year survival with multimodality therapy.

Histologically, medulloblastomas may show sheets of malignant small blue cells in the patternless variant or fields of Homer Wright rosettes may be present (Fig. 7-2). Mitotic figures are numerous and foci of tumor necrosis are present.

There are two major variants of medulloblastoma:

1. Desmoplastic medulloblastoma: Histologically, this variant superficially resembles a lymph node, with pale reticulin-free islands mimicking germinal centers. Desmoplastic medulloblastomas usually arise more laterally in the cerebellar hemisphere and in the adult cohort.
2. Medullomyoblastoma: This is a very rare variant of childhood; in addition to the medulloblastoma component, muscle differentiation is seen in the form of cross-striated strap cells and/or immunopositivity for muscle markers such as desmin.

Pineoblastoma

This is a PNET of the pineal gland and is discussed further under Pineal Tumors.

Ependymoblastoma

Ependymoblastoma is a PNET that displays diffuse ependymal differentiation in the form of large numbers of ubiquitously present, true ependymal rosettes.

Medulloepithelioma

Medulloepithelioma, like ependymoblastoma, is very rare. This malignant tumor recapitulates the architecture of the primitive developing neural tube with long epithelial surfaces and tubules. In the CNS, medulloepithelioma occurs in infants and children in which it pursues a rapidly malignant course. Together with ependymoblastoma, medulloepithelioma can also arise as a malignant neuroectodermal component of immature teratomas of the ovary and other organs.

Neuroblastoma

Cerebral neuroblastoma is a PNET that displays neuronal differentiation in the form of immunopositivity for synaptophysin and other neuronal markers.

Peripheral neuroblastoma arises in the sympathetic chain and adrenal medulla in childhood. The abdomen is the commonest location. This tumor may metastasize to bone. Neuroblastoma is associated with a paraneoplastic syndrome—opsoclonus (myoclonic encephalopathy/neuroblastoma syndrome). Molecular biological studies demonstrate amplification of N-myc present in over one-third of these tumors and, when present, the degree of amplification correlates with advanced stage and poor prognosis. The N-myc amplification site is usually on chromosome 2. N-myc amplification is seen as a variety of tumors, so presence of N-myc amplification per se does not assist in the differential diagnosis. In addition to N-myc amplification, other unfavorable prognostic indicators include late age of onset, diploidy rather than aneuploidy on DNA analysis, and reduced catecholamine metabolite production.

Rhabdomyosarcoma

Primary rhabdomyosarcoma of the brain parenchyma is rare but does occur. The histology can be very similar to that of the PNETs, i.e., a malignant small blue round cell tumor with high mitotic activity and focal necrosis, but somewhat more pleomorphic with a less uniformly monotontous composition. Elongated tumor cells with the characteristic cross-striations of skeletal muscle differentiation can be present but are not always seen. A suspected diagnosis is confirmed by demonstrating strong diffuse tumor positivity for desmin. When arising in the cerebellum, pure primary rhabdomyosarcoma must be distinguished from medullomyoblastoma, in which rhabdomyosarcomatous differentiation (desmin positive cells with or without the presence of strap cells) is found focally in an otherwise typical medulloblastoma (Fig. 7-3).

Retinoblastoma

Retinoblastoma is a PNET of the retina. These tumors are sporadic (60%) or autosomal dominant (40%; inheritance with 90% penetrance). Emergence of this tumor requires inactivation of the tumor suppressor Rb gene. This antioncogene resides on the q14 region of both chromosomes 13 in the normal diploid state. In the familial form, one of the loci is inactivated in the germ cell line, hence only one other locus must be inactivated to produce the tumor. In the sporadic form of the retinoblastoma, both Rb genes in a somatic cell of the retina must be inactivated to give rise to the tumor. In the familial disorder, bilateral retinoblastomas occur frequently and there is an increased incidence of osteosarcomas and other soft tissue sarcomas. Be aware of a rarity: "Trilateral retinoblastoma"—the occurrence of bilateral retinoblastomas and a pineoblastoma in the same person. The retinoblastoma contains Flexner–Wintersteiner rosettes; these resemble Homer Wright rosettes but have an internal membrane around the lumen, in contrast to Homer Wright rosettes where neuritic processes fill the lumen (Homer Wright rosettes may be seen in any PNET, including retinoblastoma).

Primary Rhabdomyosarcoma of the CNS

- **Rare but well documented**

- **Diffuse strong immunopositivity for desmin**

- **In cerebellum focal desmin positivity may be seen in a rare variant of medulloblastoma (medullomyoblastoma)**

FIGURE 7-3. Features of primary CNS rhabdomyosarcoma. In addition to PNETs, other types of malignant small blue cell tumors, such as rhabdomyosarcoma, can occasionally arise as primary neoplasms of the CNS.

Esthesioneuroblastoma

Esthesioneuroblastoma (olfactory neuroblastoma) arises from olfactory neuroepithelium. Involvement of the paranasal sinuses is common as is invasion upwards through the cribriform plate of the ethmoid into the anterior cranial fossa around the olfactory bulbs, gyri recti and orbitofrontal cortex. The surgical pathologist will frequently receive the olfactory bulbs for intraoperative frozen section examination to rule out the presence of invading esthesioneuroblastoma. For the surgical pathologist in this situation, having prior knowledge of the normal morphology of the olfactory bulb significantly decreases anxiety and is an aid to correct diagnosis.

Atypical Teratoid/Rhabdoid Tumor

Atypical teratoid/rhabdoid (ATRT) is a recently characterized malignant embryonal neoplasm (Fig. 7-4). These tumors may have fields of small blue cells with classical medulloblastoma features, but they also frequently have rhabdoid cells (cells with eccentric nuclei displaced by globular pink cytoplasm) and other neoplastic cells that are larger and more pleomorphic than typical PNET cells (Fig. 7-5). Most ATRTs occur in the posterior fossa but a significant number are supratentorial. This tumor has a grim prognosis and does not respond well to conventional PNET therapy. Most have LOH or partial deletion of chromosome 22, leading to loss of a tumor suppressor gene, hSNF5/INI1, which is a transcriptional activator. This genetic alteration is not seen in medulloblastomas.

Astrocytic Tumors: Diffuse and Circumscribed

Tumors with astrocytic differentiation can be separated into two categories: diffuse and circumscribed (Table 7-1). The diffuse astrocytomas, as the name states, diffusely infiltrate brain parenchyma and this is the primary obstacle to

TABLE 7-1. CLASSIFICATION OF ASTROCYTOMAS

Diffuse astrocytomas
   Low-grade astrocytoma
   Anaplastic astrocytoma
   Glioblastoma
Circumscribed astrocytomas
   Pilocytic astrocytoma
   Pleomorphic xanthoastrocytoma
   Subependymal giant cell astrocytoma
   Desmoplastic cerebral astrocytoma of infancy

Atypical Teratoid/Rhabdoid Tumor

- **Primarily in infants and young children**

- **75% in cerebellum; 25% in cerebrum**

- **Always positive for vimentin; most positive for epithelial membrane antigen and smooth muscle actin**

- **Variably positive for other antigens including epithelial markers (cytokeratins) and neuroectodermal markers (GFAP, neurofilament proteins)**

- **Cells are larger and more pleomorphic than those of a typical PNET such as medulloblastoma and more epithelioid than a typical malignant astrocytoma; the overall morphologic "gestalt" is that of a clearly malignant neoplasm that doesn't quite fit with either medulloblastoma or glioblastoma; ATRTs in the cerebellum are often misdiagnosed as medulloblastoma**

- **Recent genetic studies point to a mutation/deletion of the putative rhabdoid tumor suppressor gene INI1 (hSNF5) on chromosome 22q**

- **Malignant behavior with frequent dissemination and very poor prognosis**

FIGURE 7-4. Features of atypical teratoid/rhabdoid tumor.

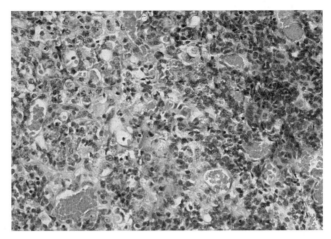

FIGURE 7-5. Atypical teratoid/rhabdoid tumor. In contrast to PNETs, ATRTs have a more pleomorphic cell population, with rhabdoid cells and other larger tumor cells intermixed with the small blue cell component.

Diffuse astrocytomas

- **Low-grade astrocytoma**
  - **Pleomorphism**
  - **No mitotic figures**

- **Anaplastic astrocytoma**
  - **Pleomorphism**
  - **Mitotic figures**
  - **Microvascular proliferation**

- **Glioblastoma multiforme**
  - **Above plus necrosis**
  - **Morphologic variants: small cell, giant cell, epithelioid**

- **Gliosarcoma**
  - **Glioblastoma plus sarcoma**
  - **Sarcoma component is negative for GFAP, positive for reticulin**
  - **Prognosis same as for glioblastoma**

FIGURE 7-6. Modified Ringertz classification of diffuse astrocytomas.

---

their successful treatment. They also tend to undergo anaplastic progression over time. Circumscribed astrocytomas, in contrast, can often be totally resected.

Diffuse Astrocytomas

Many grading systems have been proposed for the diffuse astrocytomas. Historically important systems included those of Kernohan and Ringertz. Currently, three systems are in use by pathologists throughout the world (Table 7-2; Figs 7-6, 7-7, and 7-8). Following is a summary of the main features of the five principal former and current grading systems:

A. Kernohan
 1. Four grades but only two prognostically significant groups (grades 1 + 2 and grades 3 + 4)
 2. Grades 1 and 2 are both low-grade (no mitotic figures permitted in grade 2)
 3. Grades 3 and 4 are both glioblastoma (necrosis present)
 4. This classification system has been abandoned

TABLE 7-2. GRADING SYSTEMS FOR THE DIFFUSE ASTROCYTOMAS

Kernohan (1949)	Ringertz (1950)	Modified Ringertz	St. Anne/Mayo (1988)	WHO (1993)
Astrocytoma grade I			Astrocytoma grade 1	
Astrocytoma grade 2	Astrocytoma	Low grade astrocytoma	Astrocytoma grade 2	Astrocytoma (grade II)
	Intermediate type	Anaplastic astrocytoma	Astrocytoma grade 3	Anaplastic astrocytoma (grade III)
Astrocytoma grade 3 Astrocytoma grade 4	Glioblastoma multiforme	Glioblastoma multiforme	Astrocytoma grade 4	Glioblastoma multiforme (grade IV)

St. Anne/Mayo ("Dumas-Duport")

- Objective criteria, based on simple presence or absence of 4 histologic features:
  - Pleomorphism
  - Mitotic figures
  - Microvascular proliferation (MVP)
  - Necrosis
- 0 features present = astrocytoma, grade 1
- 1 feature present (usually pleomorphism) = astrocytoma, grade 2
- 2 features present (usually pleomorphism + mitoses) = astrocytoma, grade 3
- 3 or 4 features present = astrocytoma, grade 4
  - Both grade 1 and grade 2 tumors are low-grade astrocytomas
  - Grade 1 tumors are very uncommon
  - Necrosis is not required for grade 4 astrocytoma (pleomorphism + mitoses + MVP)

FIGURE 7-7. The St. Anne–Mayo classification of diffuse astrocytomas.

B. Ringhertz
  1. Three-tiered system
  2. Necrosis permitted in intermediate grade tumors
C. Modified Ringertz (Nelson, Burger, Rubinstein)
  1. Three-tiered: low-grade astro, anaplastic astro (AA), glioblastoma
  2. The major "modification" of the original Ringertz system is the exclusion of necrosis from the intermediate group (AAs); i.e., an AA with necrosis is a GM according to modified Ringhertz criteria
  3. Necrosis is required for a diagnosis of glioblastoma
D. St. Anne–Mayo
  1. Objective criteria, based on simple presence or absence of four histologic features:
     a. Pleomorphism
     b. Mitotic figures
     c. Microvascular proliferation (MVP)
     d. Necrosis
  2. Zero features present = astrocytoma, grade 1
  3. One feature present (usually pleomorphism) = astrocytoma, grade 2
  4. Two features present (usually pleomorph + mitoses) = astrocytoma, grade 3
  5. Three or 4 features present = astrocytoma, grade 4
  6. Comments on the St. Anne–Mayo system:
     a. Grade 1 and grade 2 tumors are both low-grade astrocytoma
     b. Grade 1 tumors are very rare
     c. Necrosis is not required for grade 4 astrocytoma (pleomorph + mitoses + MVP is sufficient)
E. WHO
  1. Grade I astrocytic tumors = pilocytic astrocytoma and subependymal giant cell astrocytoma
  2. Grade II astrocytoma = low-grade astrocytoma (no mitoses present)
  3. Grade III astrocytoma = anaplastic astrocytoma
  4. Grade IV astrocytoma = glioblastoma
  5. Note that necrosis is *not* required for a diagnosis of glioblastoma by WHO criteria; vascular proliferation is sufficient (similar to St. Anne–Mayo criteria)

WHO

- Grade I astrocytic tumors = pilocytic astrocytomas and subependymal giant cell astrocytomas only
- Grade II astrocytoma = low-grade astrocytoma (no mitoses)
- Grade III astrocytoma = anaplastic astrocytoma
- Grade IV astrocytoma = glioblastoma

(Note: necrosis is not required for glioblastoma by WHO criteria; vascular proliferation is sufficient, similar to the St. Anne-Mayo criteria.)

FIGURE 7-8. The World Health Organization (WHO) classification of astrocytomas.

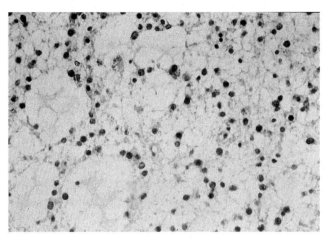

FIGURE 7-9. Low-grade astrocytoma. Note the diffuse infiltration of brain parenchyma; this innate property of diffuse astrocytomas presents a major problem to successful treatment.

Low-Grade Astrocytoma

Low-grade astrocytoma is characterized by increased cellularity compared to normal white matter (Fig. 7-9). Vascular proliferation and necrosis are not present, and mitotic figures are absent or very rare. There are three subtypes: fibrillary (most common variant), protoplasmic (originate in gray matter and have cytologic features resembling protoplasmic astrocytes), and gemistocytic (literally "stuffed cells"; gemistocytic astrocytomas are composed of neoplastic astrocytes with very large globular cytoplasm secondary to GFAP-positive glial intermediate filaments). The mean survival for low-grade diffuse astrocytoma is 36–48 months.

> **Caveat:**   Gemistocytic astrocytoma is classified by the WHO as a subtype of low-grade diffuse astrocytoma (WHO grade II). However, gemistocytic astrocytomas have tendency to rapidly progress to a higher grade (anaplastic astrocytoma or glioblastoma). In recognition of this behavior, many neuropathologists prefer to classify gemistocytic astrocytomas as anaplastic (WHO grade III).

Anaplastic Astrocytoma

Anaplastic astrocytoma (WHO grade III), is characterized by hypercellularity, pleomorphism, and mitotic figures. These tumors comprise 20–40% of all gliomas and have a median survival of 18 months, although similar to the glioblastoma, there is a strong age dependency of survival.

Glioblastoma

Glioblastomas represent 40–50% of all glial tumors. They can arise anywhere in the nervous system and at any age although they are most common in older adults over 50. One of the classic radiologic presentations is the "butterfly" pattern in which infiltrating tumor cells use the corpus callosum as a conduit to spread into the opposite hemisphere (Figs. 7-10 and 7-11). The "butterfly" pattern is a reflection of one of the most basic biologic properties of the diffuse astrocytomas: the ability to widely infiltrate the CNS. This is often reflected radiologically and on gross pathologic examination as diffuse enlargement of the infiltrated areas (Fig. 7-12). Histopathologically, microvascular proliferation and necrosis with tumor cell pseudopalisading characterize this

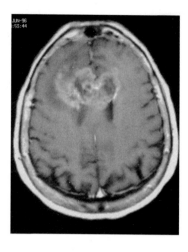

FIGURE 7-10. Axial MRI scan showing the classic contrast-enhancing "butterfly" pattern of glioblastoma involving the corpus callosum.

tumor (Fig. 7-13). The mean survival is approximately one year to 18 months, but is age dependent, with better survivals seen in patients under age 40 and less favorable survival in the elderly.

There are two major genetic subsets of glioblastoma: primary and secondary. Primary glioblastomas arise de novo and are characterized by epidermal growth factor receptor (EGFR) gene amplification and/or over-expression, *MDM2* gene over-expression, *p16* gene deletion, PTEN (MMAC1) mutation, and loss of chromosome 10. In contrast, secondary glioblastomas arise from anaplastic progression from lower grade astrocytoma and are characterized by *p53* gene mutation, 19q deletion, and 10q deletion. In addition to these major subsets, other pathways likely exist, including those for gliosarcoma and the giant cell variant of glioblastoma. This constitutes an area of active investigation and rapid advance—watch the literature!

There are several glioblastoma variants that warrant brief mention:

1. Gliosarcoma: This tumor has neoplastic glial and mesenchymal elements admixed. The diagnosis is currently made based on lack of immunopositivity of the suspected sarcomatous element for GFAP. Molecular genetic studies will very likely provide clarification in the near future.

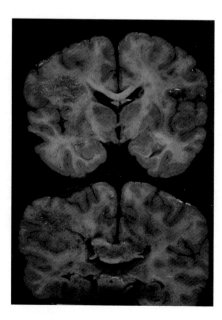

FIGURE 7-11. Classic "butterfly" glioblastoma of the splenium of the corpus callosum (seen in the lower panel of these two coronal sections). The "butterfly" pattern of tumor infiltration across the corpus callosum is characteristic but is not specific for glioblastoma; it can also be one of the radiologic presentations of primary CNS lymphoma!

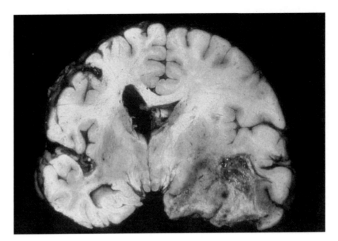

FIGURE 7-12. Glioblastoma. Diffuse enlargement of the temporal lobe is seen in this high-grade astrocytoma.

2. Giant cell glioblastoma: This tumor contains grotesque large neoplastic astrocytes. There is potential for diagnostic confusion with the more indolent but morphologically similar pleomorphic xanthoastrocytoma; however, giant cell glioblastomas will show the characteristic features of elevated mitotic rate, necrosis, and microvascular proliferation.

3. Epithelioid glioblastoma: This variant is often deceptively well circumscribed in young patients and has plump cells with distinct cytoplasmic borders mimicking epithelial tumors, particularly melanoma. They can cause considerable diagnostic confusion for those not familiar with their existence.

Circumscribed Astrocytomas

The circumscribed astrocytomas are a heterogeneous group of four different tumors (Fig. 7-14) that are united by the fact that they all show astrocytic differentiation (immuno-positive for GFAP) and, in contrast to the diffuse astrocytomas, do not widely infiltrate CNS parenchyma. The latter property often renders them surgically resectable. Because of the very significant differences in biology, prognosis, and therapy of the circumscribed astrocy-

---

Circumscribed Astrocytomas

- Pilocytic astrocytoma

- Pleomorphic xanthoastrocytoma

- Subependymal giant cell astrocytoma

- Desmoplastic cerebral astrocytoma of infancy

FIGURE 7-14. The four circumscribed astrocytomas. It is critical for the pathologist to be intimately familiar with the clinical, radiological, and histologic features of each of these tumors as their prognosis and treatment (surgical resection) are quite different from the diffuse astrocytomas.

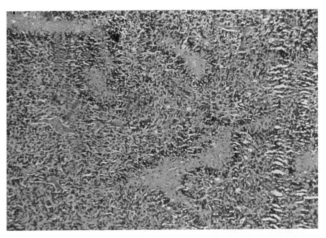

FIGURE 7-13. Glioblastoma. Necrosis with surrounding tumor cell pseudopalisading (right half of field) and florid microvascular proliferation (left half of field) are characteristic morphologic features of glioblastoma.

Circumscribed Astrocytomas

Shared features of the "circumscribed" astrocytomas:

- **Astrocytic differentiation (GFAP positive). Relatively circumscribed growth, with very limited infiltration of adjacent neural parenchyma compared to the diffuse astrocytomas**
- **Commonly invade overlying leptomeninges and subarachnoid space (JA, PXA, GG); this is not a negative prognostic factor!**
- **Histologic features mimic high-grade astrocytoma and can result in overgrading that results in inappropriate therapy (XRT, chemotherapy).**
- **Good prognosis compared to diffuse astrocytomas**
- **Treatment of choice is gross total resection with no radiotherapy or adjuvant chemotherapy**
- **In a small but definite percentage of cases, progression to high-grade astrocytoma occurs.**

FIGURE 7-15. Shared features of the circumscribed astrocytomas.

tomas compared to the diffuse astrocytomas (Fig. 7-15), it is critical that the correct diagnosis of these tumors be made.

Pilocytic Astrocytoma

Pilocytic astrocytomas constitute one of the two most common brain tumors of childhood (the other being medulloblastoma) and constitute approximately 20% of all brain tumors in children (Fig. 7-16). Cases in adults, even in the elderly, also occur. The most common sites of origin are the cerebellum, hypothalamic/third ventricular region, optic nerves, brainstem and spinal cord. The radiographic appearance is often the classic pattern of a cyst with an enhancing mural nodule, although solid tumors and tumors with multiple small intra-tumoral cysts are also seen. Histologically, pilocytic astrocytomas are characterized by highly spindled cells with elongated bipolar cytoplasmic cell processes (pilocytes), microcysts, eosinophilic granular bodies (EGBs), and Rosenthal fibers (Fig. 7-17).

Pilocytic Astrocytoma

- **20% of childhood brain tumors**
- **Cerebellum, hypothalamic/third ventricular region, optic nerves, cerebrum, brainstem, spinal cord**
- **MRI: in cerebellum, often cyst with contrast-enhancing mural nodule**
- **Biphasic architecture, pilocytic astrocytes, Rosenthal fibers, eosinophilic granular bodies**
- **Microvascular proliferation (contrast-enhancing)**
- **Nuclear atypia**
- **Commonly invade overlying leptomeninges**
- **Above three features can lead to overgrading as malignant astrocytoma**
- **Mitotic figures rare**

FIGURE 7-16. Major features of pilocytic astrocytoma.

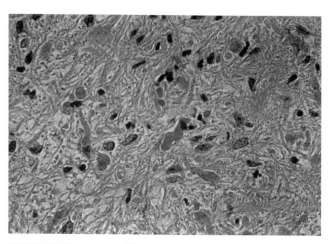

FIGURE 7-17. Rosenthal fibers in pilocytic astrocytoma. One of the morphologic hallmarks of pilocytic astrocytoma is the presence of Rosenthal fibers.

Subependymal Giant Cell Astrocytoma (SEGA)

- Intraventricular location (lateral ventricles)
- Resembles gemistocytic astrocytoma or ganglion cell tumor
- Spindle cell morphology also common
- Mitotic figures are rare.
- Although commonly associated with tuberous sclerosis, may be the presenting problem and in some cases no stigmata of TS are found; thus, a high index of suspicion is required as a history of TS is frequently lacking at presentation!
- Treatment is gross total resection.

FIGURE 7-18. Major features of subependymal giant cell astrocytoma.

TABLE 7-3. TUMORS WITH PROMINENT NUMBERS OF EOSINOPHILIC GRANULAR BODIES (EGBs)

Pilocytic astrocytoma (PA)
Pleomorphic xanthoastrocytoma (PXA)
Ganglioglioma (GG)

Pilocytic astrocytomas are indolent and potentially surgically curable if gross removal is possible (usually most successful in cerebellum, less so in optic nerve, and least successful in hypothalamic tumors).

Subependymal Giant Cell Astrocytoma

Subependymal giant cell astrocytoma (SEGA) is an intraventricular tumor associated with tuberous sclerosis complex that produces symptoms by obstructing CSF flow. Not infrequently, there is no history of tuberous sclerosis at the time of intraoperative frozen section diagnosis and the pathologist must be sufficiently familiar with the major clinicopathologic features of SEGA (Fig. 7-18) to have a high index of suspicion. Histologically, SEGAs resemble gemistocytic astrocytomas by virtue of their abundant eosinophilic cytoplasm. Some tumors show prominent large nucleoli and thereby mimic ganglion cell tumors. Often there are areas of highly spindled tumor cells interspersed with the epithelioid component. Despite all of the potential for misdiagnosis due to tumor mimicry, the diagnosis of SEGA will *never* be missed if the diagnostician is aware of the intraventricular location and the appropriate differential diagnosis for intraventricular tumors! The treatment for SEGA is surgical resection.

Pleomorphic Xanthoastrocytoma

Pleomorphic xanthoastrocytoma is a low-grade superficial cortical tumor of the young adults that histologically can be mistaken for glioblastoma due to its extreme pleomorphism. However, mitotic figures are rare compared to high-grade astrocytomas, necrosis is not a prominent feature, and EGBs are virtually always present and serve as a red flag to alert the pathologist to consider PXA high in the differential diagnosis (Table 7-3). Despite the frightening microscopic appearance, PXA has a comparatively good prognosis with surgical resection. One caveat is that approximately 15% of PXAs will ultimately progress to high-grade astrocytoma; thus, there is risk associated with residual tumor and patients in which gross total resection cannot be performed because of proximity to eloquent cortex or other reasons should be monitored closely clinically and radiologically for signs of recurrence or progression.

Desmoplastic Cerebral Astrocytoma of Infancy

Also called "superficial cerebral astrocytoma of infancy," desmoplastic cerebral astrocytoma of infancy (DCAI) is a circumscribed astrocytic neoplasm that arises very early in life and has a number of distinctive features (Fig. 7-19). The morphologic and clinical features overlap with those of desmoplastic infantile ganglioglioma (discussed under Mixed Glioneuronal Tumors). DCAIs are typically very large but the treatment is surgical resection, which can greatly extend survival. The DCAI is thus included with a number of other primary brain and spinal cord tumors for which the preferred treatment is gross total resection (Fig. 7-20).

Oligodendroglial Tumors

Oligodendroglioma is made up of uniform "fried egg" cells with cleared cytoplasm (perinuclear halos), distinct cell borders, and small bland hyperchromatic nuclei (Fig. 7-21). Delicately branching vessels ("chicken wire" pattern) are characteristic and micro-calcifications are also common. The "fried egg" appearance is a fortuitous fixation artifact that helps distinguish this glioma

Desmoplastic Cerebral Astrocytoma of Infancy (DCAI)

- Also called "superficial cerebral astrocytoma of infancy"

- Morphology and clinical features overlap with desmoplastic infantile ganglioglioma (the unifying term "desmoplastic neuroepithelial tumor of infancy" has been proposed but is not currently widely adopted).

- Presentation during infancy (first year of life)

- Very large tumors that in some cases occupy the majority of a hemisphere

- Invade overlying subarachnoid space (as also do JPA, PXA and GG)

- Remarkably good prognosis

- Treatment is gross total resection

FIGURE 7-19. Major features of desmoplastic cerebral astrocytoma of infancy.

from astrocytoma. Oligodendrogliomas frequently invade and diffusely infiltrate the cortex in which individual tumor cells tend to cluster around neuronal cell bodies (perineuronal satellitosis), blood vessels (perivascular satellitosis), and beneath the pia (subpial growth). These eye-catching architectural configurations, termed secondary structures of Scherer, serve as aids to diagnosis (Fig. 7-22).

The term anaplastic oligodendroglioma is applied to oligodendrogliomas with high mitotic activity and florid microvascular proliferation. Anaplastic oligodendrogliomas with foci of tumor necrosis with pseudopalisading were sometimes formerly classified as glioblastoma but in light of recent advances in our understanding of this tumor's molecular biology they are not reclassified today. Oligodendrogliomas frequently show LOH for chromosomes 1p

CNS Tumors Treated by Surgical Resection Alone

- Pilocytic astrocytoma
- Pleomorphic xanthoastrocytoma
- Subependymal giant cell astrocytoma
- Desmoplastic cerebral astrocytoma of infancy
- Dorsally exophytic brainstem glioma
- Myxopapillary ependymoma
- Subependymoma
- Dysplastic gangliocytoma of the cerebellum
- Central neurocytoma
- Paraganglioma of the filum
- Ganglioglioma
- Dysembryoplastic neuroepithelial tumor
- Hemangioblastoma

FIGURE 7-20. There are many brain and spinal cord tumors for which the preferred treatment at presentation is gross total resection when anatomically possible, without radiation therapy or chemotherapy. Because of the significant treatment and prognosis differences between this group of tumors and other, more aggressive, neoplasms, it is particularly important that the correct diagnosis be made. Thorough familiarity with the clinical, radiological, and histological features of each of these tumors greatly facilitates accurate diagnosis!

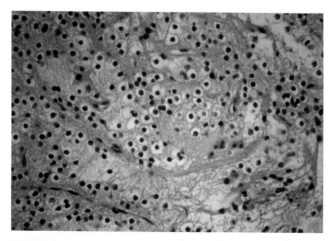

FIGURE 7-21. Oligodendroglioma. Note the prominent clearing of the cytoplasm around the nuclei (perinuclear halos, "fried egg" artifact).

Secondary Structures of Scherer

- "All those structures formed by the cells of a glioma which depend on the preexisting tissue elements"
- Gray matter:
  - Perineuronal satellitosis
  - Perivascular satellitosis
  - Subpial growth
  - Growth confined to the gray matter
- White matter:
  - Perifascicular growth
  - Intrafascicular growth
  - Interfibrillary growth
  - Growth confined to the white matter

FIGURE 7-22. Scherer described eight secondary structures. The most useful of these to the surgical pathologist during intraoperative frozen section diagnosis are perineuronal satellitosis, perivascular satellitosis, and subpial growth, which strongly suggest the presence of a diffusely infiltrating glioma.

Mixed Oligoastrocytoma

- "Compact" variant
  - Discrete, separate areas of astrocytoma and oligodendroglioma
- "Diffuse" variant
  - Intimately intermixed malignant astrocytes and oligodendrocytes
- "Tertium quid" (all malignant glial cells exhibit indeterminant morphologic features or features with characteristics intermediate between those of astros and those of oligos)

FIGURE 7-24. Three morphologic subtypes of mixed oligoastrocytoma.

Molecular Biology of Oligodendroglioma

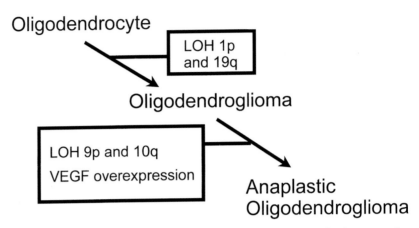

FIGURE 7-23. Molecular genetic alterations involved in the anaplastic progression of oligodendroglioma. LOH for 1p and 19q predict sensitivity to chemotherapy.

and 19q (Fig. 7-23). Tumors that exhibit these genetic features appear to respond to combination chemotherapy with such regimens as PCV (procarbazine, Cytoxan, vincristine).

Mixed oligoastrocytomas are composed of neoplastic oligodendroglial and astrocytic components in various combinations (Fig. 7-24). In the "compact" variant, there are discretely separate areas of astrocytoma and oligodendroglioma; in the "diffuse" variant, the oligo and astrocytic cells are intimately intermixed; and in a "tertium quid" variant, all of the cells exhibit mixed oligoastro features. The diagnosis of mixed oligoastrocytoma and anaplastic mixed oligoastrocytoma is quite subjective and is largely dependent on the relative weighting given various histologic features by the neuropathologist. This is an area in which help from molecular classification is greatly needed and should be shortly forthcoming.

Ependymal Tumors

There are a number of primary brain and spinal cord tumors that exhibit ependymal differentiation, ranging from benign incidental subependymomas to malignant ependymoblastomas (Fig. 7-25).

Classic Ependymoma

The histologic hallmark of ependymomas is the perivascular pseudorosette (gliovascular rosette; Fig. 7-26). True ependymal rosettes with central lumens and more elaborate canals and tubules can also be seen in some cases but are not as widespread as perivascular pseudorosettes (Fig. 7-27).

A large percentage of supratentorial ependymomas arise intraparenchymally without ventricular communication. In the posterior fossa, ependymomas are intraventricular and often fill the fourth ventricle (Fig. 7-28) and also spread to the subarachnoid space surrounding the brainstem via the lateral foramina of Luschka and median foramen on Magendie.

Anaplastic ependymomas are characterized by a high mitotic rate and florid microvascular proliferation. Areas of necrosis can be seen in both low- and high-grade ependymomas, and this feature does not have the same prognostic significance that it does in the diffuse astrocytomas.

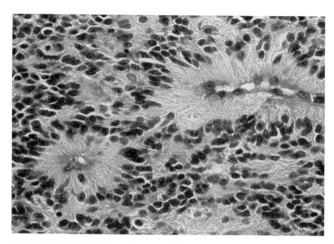

FIGURE 7-26. Perivascular pseudorosettes are the hallmark of ependymoma.

Ependymal Neoplasms

- **Classic ependymoma**
- **Papillary ependymoma**
- **Clear cell ependymoma**
- **Tanycytic ependymoma**
- **Myxopapillary ependymoma**
- **Subependymoma**
- **Ependymoblastoma**

FIGURE 7-25. The seven types of ependymal tumors.

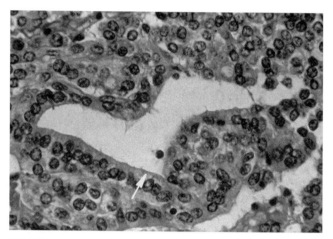

FIGURE 7-27. Epithelial surfaces (seen here), tubules, and true rosettes can also be seen in some ependymomas.

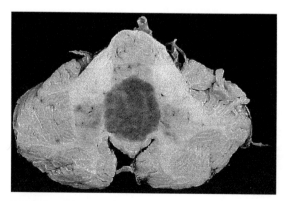

FIGURE 7-28. Ependymoma filling the fourth ventricle.

Myxopapillary Ependymoma of the Filum Terminale

- **Microcysts**
- **Mucin cuffs around blood vessels**
- **Often prominent highly spindled "pilocytic" glial background**

FIGURE 7-29. Major features of myxopapillary ependymoma.

Myxopapillary Ependymoma

This ependymoma variant arises in the filum terminale. Histologic hallmarks include mucin-containing microcysts, cuffs of mucin surrounding blood vessels, and an ependymal component that focally exhibits a highly spindled "pilocytic" morphology (Fig. 7-29). The principal entity in the radiologic differential diagnosis is paraganglioma of filum terminale (Fig. 7-30).

Papillary Ependymoma

Papillary ependymoma is often mentioned in the differential diagnosis of choroid plexus papilloma, but in reality it is relatively rare and virtually never closely mimics the distinctive papillary architecture of CP papillomas. The papillary cores of papillary ependymoma are composed of glial processes (GFAP-positive) as opposed to those of CP papillomas, which are composed of fibrovascular tissue.

Subependymoma

Subependymomas are benign gliomas of the lateral ventricle, fourth ventricle, and spinal cord. Lateral and fourth ventricular examples are often asymptomatic and only incidentally discovered on neuroradiological studies performed for other lesions or at autopsy (Fig. 7-31). However, some reach sufficient size to obstruct the foramen of Monro or the outlet foramina of the fourth ventricle and thus come to clinical attention by producing obstructive hydrocephalus. Spinal cord subependymomas usually become symptomatic. The treatment for symptomatic subependymomas is resection. Histologically, a characteristic lobulated pattern is seen with clusters of benign glial nuclei separated by a finely fibrillar matrix.

Tanycytic Ependymoma

This rare ependymoma variant is sometimes mistaken for schwannoma due to the sweeping fascicles of elongated bipolar cytoplasmic processes. Moreover, classic perivascular pseudorosettes are often not conspicuous. Ultrastructural examination is often required to confirm the diagnosis by demonstrating the presence of characteristic lumina filled with microvilli and occasional cilia, and surrounding prominent intercellular junctional complexes that seal the lumina.

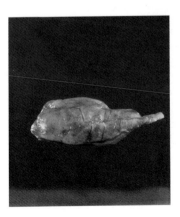

FIGURE 7-30. Fusiform "sausage-shaped" mass of the filum terminale. This gross appearance (also seen on MRI scans) is characteristic of two tumors of the filum: myxopapillary ependymoma and paraganglioma.

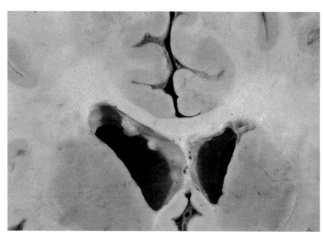

FIGURE 7-31. Subependymomas of the lateral ventricle. Subependymomas grow as exophytic excrescences into the ventricle. Small examples like these are asymptomatic; larger tumors can cause obstructive hydrocephalus.

Ependymoblastoma

Ependymoblastoma is a very rare PNET characterized histologically by profuse numbers of true ependymal rosettes. Ependymoblastoma is not infrequently identified as a component of immature teratomas arising in the ovary and other sites.

Clear Cell Ependymoma

This variant mimics oligodendroglioma and central neurocytoma, but the pathognomonic ependymal ultrastructural features (intercellular lumens filled with microvilli and occasional cilia, complex intercellular junctional complexes) are diagnostic.

Brainstem Gliomas

Just like astrocytomas of the cerebral hemispheres, those arising in the brainstem can be classified into two major types: diffuse and circumscribed (Fig. 7-32). The diffuse brainstem gliomas are typified by the classic pontine glioma, which infiltrates and expands the pons, in some cases with ventral exophytic growth engulfing the basilar artery (Fig. 7-33). Progression to high-grade astrocytoma (anaplastic astrocytoma or glioblastoma) is common, and the prognosis is poor. In contrast, the second type of brainstem glioma comprises the focal and dorsally exophytic gliomas. The most common histologic morphology in this group is that of pilocytic astrocytoma. Despite the oftentimes very large size and brainstem location, the treatment of choice is surgical resection and life can be greatly extended by this procedure in the hands of a skilled surgeon.

Other Gliomas

Gliomatosis Cerebri

In gliomatosis cerebri, malignant glial cells diffusely infiltrate extensive portions of the brain without forming an identifiable central mass or epicenter (Fig. 7-34). Usually the greater part of an entire hemisphere is involved and

---

Brain Stem Gliomas

- Classic pontine gliomas (malignant; diffusely infiltrating fibrillary astrocytomas; diffusely expand pons and engulf the basilar artery)
- Dorsally exophytic brain stem gliomas (low-grade; many are JPAs; comparatively circumscribed margins; gross total resection is preferred treatment; prognosis good, especially compared to classic pontine glioma)

FIGURE 7-32. Just as with supratentorial astrocytomas, there are two major classes of brainstem gliomas: diffuse (typified by the classic pontine glioma) and circumscribed (typified by the dorsally exophytic brainstem glioma).

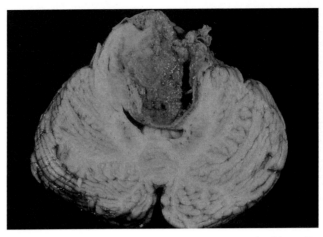

FIGURE 7-33. Pontine glioma. Pontine gliomas are highly malignant diffuse astrocytomas that infiltrate and expand the pons. Histologically, most are high-grade astrocytomas. In contrast to the focal and dorsally exophytic brainstem gliomas, which are treated with surgical resection, radiation therapy is usually used for pontine gliomas.

not infrequently there is also involvement of the contralateral hemisphere and brainstem. Further investigation of this neoplasm is needed.

Chordoid Glioma of the Third Ventricle

This recently described glioma (Fig. 7-35) arises in the region of the lamina terminalis, which forms the rostral wall of the third ventricle. Radiologically, the tumor forms a well-circumscribed ovoid mass. Histologically, the architecture resembles that of chordoma (hence the name) but the tumor cells are strongly positive for GFAP. Chordoid gliomas are histologically benign and

Gliomatosis Cerebri

- Diffuse glioma involving multiple lobes, usually the majority of an entire hemisphere; invades without forming mass or destroying architecture
- Contralateral hemisphere and brain stem involvement also seen
- Morphology of tumor usually astrocytic or undifferentiated glial, very rarely oligodendroglioma
- Two theories of origin:
  - Glioma with exceptional invasive properties
  - Simultaneous "field transformation" of glia throughout brain
- Historically, diagnosis made by whole brain neuropathological examination at autopsy
- Diagnosis today based on MR appearance plus biopsy confirmation of the presence of an infiltrating glioma
- In longer-surviving patients progression to glioblastoma (multiple foci of tumor necrosis) can be seen

FIGURE 7-34. Major features of gliomatosis cerebri.

Chordoid Glioma of the Third Ventricle

- Recently described (Brat et al, J Neuropath Exp Neurol 57:283,1998)
- Included in latest WHO classification of tumors of the nervous system
- Characteristic neuroanatomic location in the rostral 3rd ventricle
- Characteristic morphology consisting of cords of cells surrounded by mucinous matrix (hence, "chordoid")
- Strong positivity for GFAP; also focally positive for epithelial membrane antigen (EMA)
- Well-circumscribed, but usually attached to the hypothalamus (bad location)
- Low grade, but will recur following subtotal resection and location near hypothalamus can lead to significant morbidity

FIGURE 7-35. Major features of chordoid glioma.

the treatment is surgical resection; however, the anatomic area of origin makes gross total resection without adverse sequelae difficult.

Astroblastoma

The astroblastoma is a tumor with a very controversial history but the entity is formally recognized by the WHO as a brain tumor of uncertain histogenesis. The diagnosis is based primarily on a morphologic pattern consisting of tumor cells that form perivascular pseudorosettes with broad cytoplasmic processes extending from cell body to vessel wall. Behavior varies from indolent to highly malignant. Further investigation, particularly with respect to molecular characterization, is needed.

Choroid Plexus Tumors

The choroid plexus gives rise to several different types of tumors (Fig. 7-36). Choroid plexus papilloma recapitulates the papillary architecture of the choroid plexus but exhibits more exuberant growth and piling up of cells on the surface of the fronds (Fig. 7-37). These tumors produce ventricular obstruction or rarely CSF overproduction. Choroid plexus carcinoma, in contrast to papillomas, is characterized by high mitotic activity, nuclear and cellular pleomorphism, and at least focal loss of papillary architecture with areas of solid tumor. Carcinomas are rare and, in adults, metastatic carcinoma is far more common and must be excluded before rendering a diagnosis of choroid plexus carcinoma. In children the diagnosis is made with more confidence because the sources of metastatic carcinoma that are common in adults (lung, breast, kidney) are rare in children and thus do not complicate the differential diagnosis.

In the differential diagnosis of choroid plexus mass lesions, two additional entities must be included: choroid plexus meningioma and xanthogranuloma.

Neuronal Tumors

The normally post-mitotic mature neuron is incapable of division, but tumors with cellular constituents demonstrating neuronal differentiation can be seen

Choroid Plexus Neoplasms

- CP papilloma
  - Immunopositive for transthyretin (prealbumin)
- CP carcinoma
  - Loss of papillary architecture
  - Unfortunately, usually <u>negative</u> for transthyretin
  - Most confidently diagnosed in children; in adults most cases initially thought to be CP carcinoma turn out to be metastatic carcinoma!
- CP meningioma ("intraventricular" meningioma)
  - Arise from rests of arachnoid (meningothelial) cells normally present in the fibrovascular arachnoid stroma

FIGURE 7-36. The three major types of choroid plexus tumors.

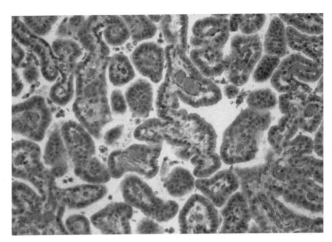

FIGURE 7-37. Choroid plexus papilloma.

Neuronal Tumors

- Of the 6 tumor types that exhibit purely neuronal differentiation, 4 are well-differentiated, benign lesions and only 2 are high-grade
- Well-differentiated
  - Gangliocytoma
  - Dysplastic gangliocytoma (Lhermitte-Duclos)
  - Central neurocytoma
  - Paraganglioma of the filum terminale
- High-grade
  - Ganglioneuroblastoma
  - Cerebral neuroblastoma

FIGURE 7-38. Six types of neuronal tumors.

Dysplastic Gangliocytoma of the Cerebellum (Lhermitte-Duclos)

- Mature ganglion cells of granular cell neuron origin (old misnomer: "Purkinjeoma")
- Borderline lesion between malformation and low-grade neoplasm; gross total resection is curative.
- 50% of patients have Cowden (multiple hamartoma) syndrome.

FIGURE 7-39. Major features of dysplastic gangliocytoma (Lhermitte-Duclos disease).

(Fig. 7-38). These may represent neoplastic stem cell differentiation along neuronal lines. Morphologic evidence of neuronal differentiation includes prominent rough endoplasmic reticulum (Nissl substance), neurotubule bundles and neurosecretory granules. The degree of phenotypic expression of differentiation hallmarks may be so subtle as to require electron microscopic or immunohistochemical study, or so conspicuous that tumor cells may be confused with mature resident neurons.

Of the six major types of tumors that show exclusively neuronal differentiation, the majority are low-grade (gangliocytoma, dysplastic gangliocytoma, central neurocytoma, and paraganglioma) and only two are high-grade (cerebral neuroblastoma and ganglioneuroblastoma).

Gangliocytoma

This quasi-hamartomatous lesion is composed of mature-appearing neurons (ganglion cells) only. Surgical resection is curative.

Dysplastic Gangliocytoma of the Cerebellum (Lhermitte–Duclos Disease)

The modifier "dysplastic" does not denote anaplasia but rather dysplasia in the sense of malformation. Dysplastic gangliocytomas (also known as Lhermitte-Duclos disease) arise in the cerebellum and typically present with motor or coordination problems. Magnetic resonance imaging (MRI) scans show enlarged folia. Histologically, the lesion is composed of large mature ganglion cells derived from granular cell precursors (an earlier erroneous assumption of a relationship to the Purkinje cells based on size of the ganglion cells led to the now abandoned misnomer "purkinjeoma"). An additional characteristic histologic feature is the abnormal presence of a layer of myelinated axons in the outermost molecular layer beneath the pia. There is an association with Cowden (multiple hamartoma) syndrome in approximately half of cases (Fig. 7-39). Surgical resection is curative.

Central Neurocytoma

Central neurocytomas (CNs) are low-grade neuronal tumors that were only first recognized in the early 1980s. Prior to that they were routinely misdiagnosed on light microscopic grounds as intraventricular oligodendrogliomas or clear cell ependymomas of the foramen of Monro. CNs grow exophytically

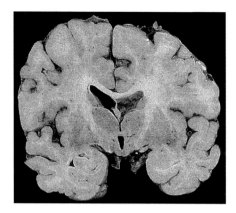

FIGURE 7-40. Central neurocytoma filling the lateral ventricle.

into the lateral ventricle (Fig. 7-40). Spread into the third ventricle is common and some cases even reach the fourth ventricle. A few cases appear to arise in the third ventricle but primaries of the fourth ventricle have not been reported. Histologically, the tumor is composed of uniform cells with regular round nuclei and often perinuclear halos ("fried egg artifact") that bear a striking resemblance to oligodendroglioma. Ultrastructurally and immunohistochemically the cells show unequivocal neuronal differentiation. The diagnosis is confirmed by demonstrating immunopositivity for synaptophysin. Surgical resection is the treatment (Fig. 7-41).

Paraganglioma of the Filum Terminale

This is one of two tumors unique to the filum terminale: paraganglioma and myxopapillary ependymoma. Paragangliomas are positive for synaptophysin and other neuronal and neuroendocrine markers, and about 10% of cases are positive for cytokeratin. Some examples show perivascular pseudorosettes very similar to ependymoma and that is the most common misdiagnosis made by those unfamiliar with this tumor. The diagnosis is confirmed by demonstrating immunopositivity for synaptophysin and the treatment is resection (Fig. 7-42).

Cerebral Neuroblastoma and Ganglioneuroblastoma

Cerebral neuroblastoma is a PNET with neuronal differentiation as assessed by strong diffuse tumor cell positivity for synaptophysin. Ganglioneuroblastomas, which are much more common outside of the CNS, also arise in the CNS and consist of a mixture of neuroblastoma and mature ganglion cells.

Mixed Glioneuronal Tumors

Desmoplastic Infantile Astrocytoma/Ganglioglioma

These tumors present in infancy as very large lesions of the cerebral hemisphere. Some are purely astrocytic in nature and show immunopositivity only for GFAP; other cases in which a neuronal component is recognized are classified as desmoplastic infantile gangliogliomas. The clinical behavior and treatment are identical and the two tumors likely represent a spectrum of the same entity. These tumors have a prominent spindled component with abundant interspersed collagen (desmoplasia) and they typically invade the overlying subarachnoid space. Despite the massive size and leptomeningeal invasion, the prognosis is comparatively good and the treatment is surgical resection.

Central Neurocytoma

- **Morphology closely mimics oligodendroglioma**
- **Uniform, rounded nuclei with perinuclear halos, delicate branching vascular pattern, microcalcifications**
- **Synaptophysin positive, GFAP negative**
- **Intraventricular location**
- **Good prognosis, but residual tumor will recur and intraoperative hemorrhage can be a problem**
- **Treatment is gross total resection**

FIGURE 7-41. Major features of central neurocytoma.

Paraganglioma of the Filum Terminale

- **Unique tumor arising from the filum, conus, or rarely a nerve root of the cauda equina**
- **Gross morphology (ovoid "sausage") and location (filum/conus) identical to myxopapillary ependymoma**
- **Mimics ependymoma with perivascular pseudorosettes**
- **Positive for the neuroendocrine differentiation markers synaptophysin and chromogranin**
- **Treatment is gross total resection**

FIGURE 7-42. Major features of paraganglioma of the filum terminale.

Ganglioglioma (GG)

- MRI: often classic cyst with enhancing mural nodule
- The "glioma" component is almost always astrocytoma; very rarely oligodendroglioma
- The glioma component frequently has a highly spindled, "pilocytic" morphology
- Eosinophilic granular bodies are prominent.
- Ganglion cells may be very sparse
- Often invade overlying subarachnoid space
- Treatment is gross total resection when possible
- Diagnostic pitfall: don't mistake entrapped normal neurons in cortex infiltrated by diffuse astrocytoma for neoplastic ganglion cells

FIGURE 7-43. Major features of ganglioglioma.

Dysembryoplastic Neuroepithelial Tumor (DNET)

- Clinical presentation in children with a history of seizures
- Low-grade, intracortical location, multinodular
- Prominent oligodendroglia-like cells (OLCs) mimic oligodendroglioma
- Prominent mucinous change in intracortical nodules results in "floating neurons"
- May be associated with dysplastic changes in surrounding cortex
- Gross total resection (and often even partial resection) is curative

FIGURE 7-44. Major features of DNET.

Ganglioglioma

Gangliogliomas are composed of a mixture of mature neuronal tumor cells (ganglion cells) and neoplastic astrocytes that often have a highly spindled "pilocytic" morphology (Fig. 7-43). EGBs, like those seen in other low-grade brain tumors, such as pilocytic astrocytoma and pleomorphic xanthoastrocytoma, are usually conspicuous. The clustered neuronal component may be scarce in some tumors. Temporal lobe is a very common location and often the MRI will show a cyst with enhancing nodule. The treatment is gross total resection when feasible. Similar to pleomorphic xanthoastrocytoma, there is a risk of progression to anaplastic astrocytoma or glioblastoma in residual tumor.

Dysembryoplastic Neuroepithelial Tumor

Dysembryoplastic neuroepithelial tumors (DNETs) are benign quasi-hamartomatous lesions of the superficial cerebral cortex that usually present in children with a history of seizures. Histologic examination shows multiple intracortical nodules composed of oligodendroglia-like cells and entrapped neurons "floating" in a mucinous-appearing background matrix. Adjacent cortex may show microdysgenesis. Surgical resection is curative (Fig. 7-44).

Primary Central Nervous System Lymphoma

Lymphoma can involve the CNS as either primary (Fig. 7-45) or metastatic disease. The vast majority of primary CNS lymphomas (PCNSLs) are diffuse large B-cell lymphomas, although occasional T-cell lymphomas do occur as well. The most common patient populations are the iatrogenically immunocompromised, AIDS patients (PCNSL is an indicator disease of AIDS), and the elderly. An initial dramatic response to corticosteroid administration may occur with pronounced radiologic shrinkage or even disappearance of the lesion in only a few days ("ghost tumor"), but recurrence is the rule. PCNSLs can present as solitary or multifocal lesions and can be in the superficial cortex or in a deep periventricular location (Fig. 7-46). Radiologic presentation

Primary CNS Lymphoma (PCNSL)

- Perivascular cuffing by malignant lymphocytes with expansion of the vascular wall (best appreciated with a reticulin stain; old name: reticulum cell sarcoma)
- Diffuse infiltration of brain parenchyma (like gliomas!)
- Majority are B-cell lymphomas
    - Immunopositive for leukocyte common antigen (LCA; CD45)
    - Immunopositive for the B-cell marker CD20 (L26)
    - Immunonegative for the T-cell markers CD3 (Leu-4) and UCHL-1
- Steroids: most PCNSLs show a dramatic initial response to steroid therapy, leading to the term "ghost tumor": shrinkage of the tumor on MRI scans; unfortunately, this response is only temporary, with recurrence as the rule
- A very small percentage are T-cell lymphomas

FIGURE 7-45. Major features of PCNSL.

as a classic "butterfly" lesion of the corpus callosum, virtually identical to that seen with some glioblastomas, also occurs. The contrast enhancement with lymphomas tends to be more solid and diffuse even compared to that of glioblastomas, but this is a relatively soft criterion.

Histologically, the hallmark of PCNSL is perivascular cuffing. Vascular mural infiltration and expansion is seen with reticulin staining (old name for PCNSL: reticulum cell sarcoma). PCNSLs diffusely infiltrate brain parenchyma just like gliomas. The diagnosis is confirmed by demonstrating immunopositivity for B-cell markers such as CD20 (Fig. 7-47). Reactivity for leukocyte common antigen (LCA, CD45) can be very weak in some cases so if PCNSL is suspected, the full panel of LCA, B-cell (CD20), and T-cell (CD3) markers should be performed either separately or in a combined screening cocktail.

Hemangioblastoma

Hemangioblastomas can arise sporadically or in association with von Hippel–Lindau disease (Fig. 7-48). The most common sites are the cerebellum

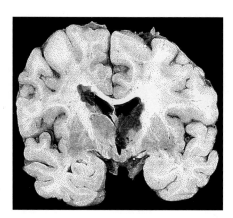

FIGURE 7-46. PCNSL: periventricular location is very common; PCNSL can present as solitary or multiple lesions, deep or superficial.

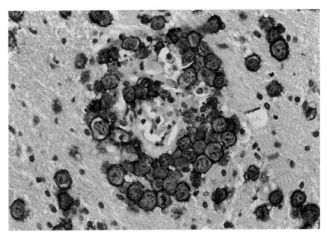

FIGURE 7-47. PCNSL: perivascular cuffing by lymphoma cells with diffuse invasion of the neuropil (CD20 immunostain).

Hemangioblastoma

- Cerebellum, spinal cord most common sites (supratentorial very rare and usually associated with von Hippel-Lindau)

- MRI: cyst with enhancing mural nodule

FIGURE 7-48. Features of hemangioblastoma.

MRI: Cyst with Enhancing Mural Nodule

- Pilocytic astrocytoma

- Pleomorphic xanthoastrocytoma

- Ganglioglioma

- Hemangioblastoma

FIGURE 7-50. Differential diagnosis of cyst with contrast-enhancing mural nodule.

---

and spinal cord. Cerebral hemangioblastomas are rare and usually associated with von Hippel–Lindau (see Appendix for summary of von Hippel–Lindau and other inherited cancer syndromes). MRI scans commonly show the classic pattern of a large cyst with a contrast-enhancing mural nodule (Fig. 7-49).

Differential Diagnosis

The radiologic pattern of a solitary large cyst with a focal contrast-enhancing mural nodule can be seen with a number of different tumors but is particularly characteristic of four tumors that should always be included in the differential diagnosis for this imaging pattern: hemangioblastoma, pilocytic astrocytoma, pleomorphic xanthoastrocytoma, and ganglioglioma (Fig. 7-50).

Histologically, hemangioblastomas are hypercellular, highly vascular tumors with clusters of foamy interstitial cells (the neoplastic element) separated by vascular channels (Fig. 7-51). Patients with von Hippel–Lindau must be followed closely as they may develop multiple CNS tumors and renal cell carcinoma. Metastatic renal cell carcinoma to the cerebellum is common and can closely resemble hemangioblastoma. In contrast to renal cell, however, hemangioblastoma is negative for epithelial membrane antigen (EMA).

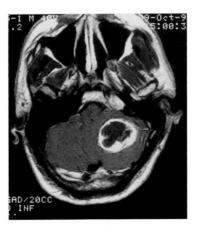

FIGURE 7-49. Hemangioblastoma: Axial MRI showing cyst with contrast-enhancing tumor.

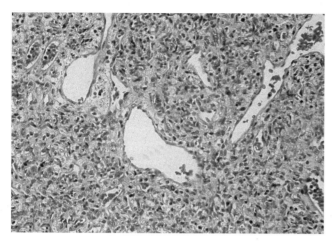

FIGURE 7-51. Hemangioblastoma: histology shows a highly vascular tumor.

Pineal Tumors

The pineal gland resides dorsal to the midbrain and is involved in the regulation of sexual maturation. If presentation occurs at the time of adolescence, tumors of this gland can result in loss of the normal pineal function in the control of maturation, resulting in sexual precocity. In patients of any age, the mass effect of an enlarged pineal can compress the midbrain, which produces disturbances of ocular movement and pupillary control (Parinaud's syndrome), and compress the aqueduct of Sylvius, which leads to obstructive hydrocephalus.

A number of different tumors can arise in the pineal (Figs. 7-52 and 7-53). The three major categories are (1) germ cell tumors, with germinoma being most common, (2) pineal parenchymal tumors (PPTs), and (3) astrocy-

Pineal Tumors

- Tumors of the pineal: germinoma, pineal parenchymal tumors (PPTs), astrocytoma, other germ cell tumors including mixed forms, rare meningiomas from surounding arachnoid cell nests

- GERMINOMA is the most common tumor of the pineal!
    - Biphasic cell population: small infiltrating lymphocytes and large neoplastic germinoma cells
    - Immunopositive for PLAP (placental alkaline phosphatase)

- Other germ cell tumors (immature and mature teratoma, choriocarcinoma, yolk sac tumor, embryonal carcinoma, mixed germ cell tumor) also occur in the pineal but are much rarer than germinoma

- The term "pinealoma" should be avoided; it was used in the past before a distinction was recognized between the pineal parenchymal tumors and germinoma (for example, hypothalamic germinomas were called "ectopic pinealomas")

FIGURE 7-52. Major features of pineal tumors.

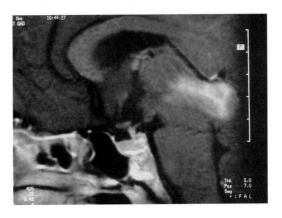

FIGURE 7-53. Pineal region mass. The differential diagnosis includes germinoma (and other germ cell tumors), pineal parenchymal tumor, astrocytoma, and metastasis.

tomas (from the indigenous pineal astrocytic population). In addition, metastasis to the pineal is not uncommon and should always be included in the differential diagnosis, and meningiomas can arise in the pineal region from the arachnoid nests in the leptomeninges that intimately surround the pineal (the velum interpositum).

Pineocytoma

Pineocytoma is the benign, low-grade variant of PPT. Pineocytomas are recognized by their large "pineocytomatous" rosettes, which resemble enlarged Homer Wright rosettes. Mitotic activity is very low, and surgical resection is the treatment of choice.

Pineoblastoma

Pineoblastomas are malignant primitive neuroectodermal tumors with high potential for dissemination through the neuraxis via the CSF. Aggressive treatment is warranted. Pineoblastomas are strongly positive for neuronal markers such as synaptophysin.

Mixed Pineocytoma/Pineoblastoma and PPT of Intermediate Differentiation

Mixed pineocytoma-pineoblastoma and intermediate differentiation PPTs also exist; these tumors have the potential for CSF dissemination similar to pineoblastoma and must be treated similarly.

Note that the terms "pinealoma" and "pinealocytoma" were historically used in the literature before a distinction between germinoma and the PPTs was made. For example, hypothalamic germinomas were called "ectopic pinealomas"! These two terms are therefore imprecise and ambiguous; don't use them!

Germinoma and Other Germ Cell Tumors

The most common pineal tumor is germinoma. Other germ cell tumors, including embryonal carcinoma, choriocarcinoma, mixed germ cell tumors, and mature and immature teratoma also arise in the pineal gland. The histology of germinoma is very distinctive. Two cell populations are typically seen: small dark reactive lymphocytes and very large atypical germinoma cells (Fig. 7-54).

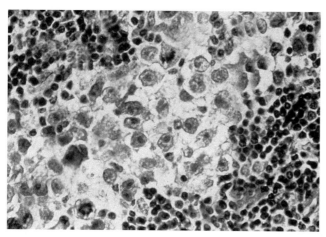

FIGURE 7-54. Germinoma. Histology shows characteristic bimodal cell population: small reactive lymphocytes and large neoplastic germinoma cells that have prominent nucleoli.

The germinoma cells are immunopositive for placental alkaline phosphatase (PLAP), which is sometimes performed to aid diagnosis. Additionally, in most cases of suspected germ cell tumor, immunostaining for beta-human chorionic gonadotropin (hCG; expressed in choriocarcinoma) and alpha-fetoprotein (AFP; expressed in yolk sac tumor) is performed to increase sensitivity of detection (Table 7-4). In positive cases, serum measurement of these markers is used to monitor for tumor recurrence.

Intraventricular Fetus-in-Fetu

Fetus-in-fetu entails the rare situation when one of what would have been two identical twins is completely encompassed by the second very early in development. In most cases of fetus-in-fetu, the included twin is located in the retroperitoneum of the thriving twin. Intracranial cases are exceptionally rare and only about a dozen or so bona fide examples have been reported in the world literature. Is the average (or even above average) clinician likely to encounter this entity? Unlikely. But exposure to the full spectrum of CNS diseases is not a bad thing.

Pituitary Tumors

Pituitary tumors may produce endocrine disturbances, neurological symptoms, or a combination of the two (Fig. 7-55). Since the pituitary gland regulates many other endocrine glands, the endocrine effects of pituitary disease can be far-reaching and complex. Because the pituitary resides at the base of the brain adjacent to the optic chiasm, cavernous sinuses and hypothalamus, the neurological manifestations secondary to tumor expansion and compression usually involve disturbances of vision, cranial nerves 3–6, and vegetative functions.

Pituitary Adenoma

Tumors produce endocrine symptoms and present as small lesions (microadenomas; less than 10 mm in diameter) early in the course of the disease if they hypersecrete; tumors that do not secrete hormones tend to present as large masses (macroadenomas) late in the disease course with compressive symp-

TABLE 7-4. MARKERS FOR GERM CELL TUMORS

Tumor	Marker
Germinoma	Placental alk phos (PLAP)
Yolk sac	Alpha fetoprotein (AFP)
Choriocarcinoma	Human chorionic gonadotropin (hCG)

Pituitary Adenoma Manifestations

- **Endocrinopathy - microadenoma**
- **Neurological - macroadenoma**
- **Both - macroadenoma**
- **Neither - incidentaloma**

FIGURE 7-55. Clinical abnormalities produced by pituitary adenomas.

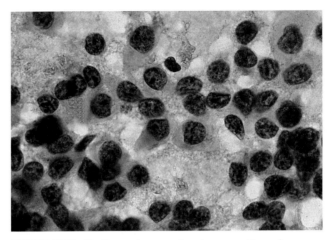

FIGURE 7-57. Pituitary adenoma: touch preparations show profuse shedding and are diagnostic.

Pituitary Adenomas

- Old tinctorial classification system (acidophiles, basophiles, chromophobes) has been supplanted by immunohistochemistry for pituitary hormones
- Common properties of all adenomas:
  - Shed cells profusely on "touch" preparation, which should be performed on all surgical specimens; especially critical for microadenomas!
  - Loss of normal lobular architecture best appreciated with a reticulin stain

FIGURE 7-56. Features of all pituitary adenomas.

toms. Pituitary adenomas may undergo hemorrhagic infarction, termed pituitary apoplexy, which is a surgical emergency requiring decompression.

Pituitary tumors are now classified by their hormonal products as assessed by clinical evaluation of serum levels and immunohistochemistry performed on resected adenoma tissue (Fig. 7-56). The older and now obsolete classification system was based on tinctorial properties, was imprecise, and is reproduced here for historical interest only:

1. Acidophil—GH ± prolactin; rare FSH or LH; acromegalic
2. Basophil—ACTH ≫ TSH; hyperadrenalism, Cushing's disease
3. Mixed acidophil-basophil—Several different hormonal possibilities
4. Chromophobe—Prolactin, null cell, rarely FSH/LH; amenorrhea-galactorrhea; impotence in men

Intraoperative diagnosis is greatly facilitated by performing a touch preparation (imprint) in which the tissue specimen is simply gently touched to a glass slide. Pituitary adenomas will shed cells copiously onto the glass slide (Fig. 7-57), in contrast to normal pituitary. The basis for this diagnostic property is the loss of normal acinar packaging of the adenohypophyseal cells. The acinar pattern of normal posterior pituitary is strikingly visualized with a reticulin stain (Fig. 7-58). In pituitary adenoma, growth of the tumor destroys the

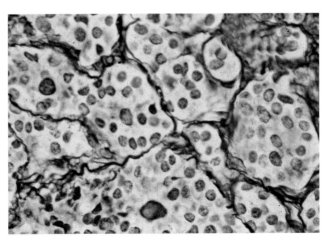

FIGURE 7-58. Normal pituitary: reticulin stain shows acinar pattern.

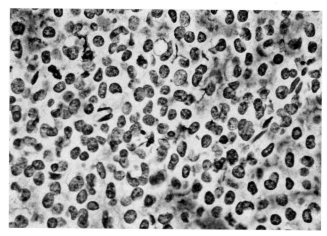

FIGURE 7-59. Pituitary adenoma: reticulin stain shows loss of acinar pattern.

fibrovascular septa that comprise the acinar walls; this effacement of the normal architecture is seen as loss of reticulin staining (Fig. 7-59). Without the encompassing acini, the loosely cohesive adenoma cells shed readily onto the glass slide.

Hyperprolactinemia is the most common hormonal abnormality associated with pituitary adenomas and may be due to primary hypersecretion or "stalk effect" in which the flow of dopamine (prolactin inhibitory factor) is impeded. The age of onset, tumor size, and type of clinical presentation of prolactinomas is different in men compared to women (Fig. 7-60). Treatment of a prolactinoma with bromocriptine may induce fibrosis in the tumor, rendering surgical resection and intraoperative surgical pathology interpretation difficult.

Pituitary adenomas are not infrequently detected in the absence of clinical manifestations on MRI scans performed for other reasons or at autopsy (Fig. 7-61). Such pituitary "incidentalomas" are usually very small microadenomas (less than 5 mm in diameter).

Pituitary Carcinoma

Carcinoma is diagnosed only if there is metastatic dissemination of the primary tumor; local invasiveness is common in adenomas and does not warrant

---

Pituitary Incidentaloma

- Usually detected by MRI performed for reasons unrelated to the sellar region
- Autopsy series: 5% - 27% incidental pituitary adenomas
- Subclinical adenomas usually less than 5 mm
- Size > 5 mm required to deviate stalk or cause unilateral gland enlargement

FIGURE 7-61. Major features of incidentally discovered pituitary adenomas (pituitary "incidentalomas").

Prolactin-Cell Adenoma

Women

- 25 years of age
- 70% microadenomas
- Endocrine presentation
  - Galactorrhea
  - Amenorrhea

Men

- 45 years of age
- 90% macroadenomas
- Neurological presentation
- Endocrine presentation
  - Loss of libido
  - Impotence

FIGURE 7-60. Major features of prolactinomas in women and men.

Molecular Biology of Pituitary Tumors

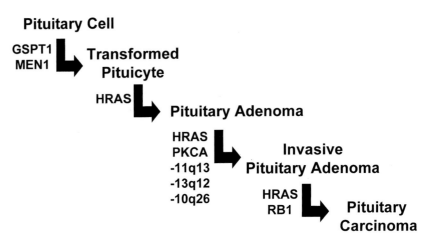

FIGURE 7-62. Some molecular alterations associated with pituitary adenoma and progression.

an increase in grade. If frankly malignant carcinoma is found in the pituitary, metastatic carcinoma from a systemic organ must be excluded. Breast carcinoma, in particular, shows a marked proclivity to metastasize to the pituitary. Progress is being made in the elucidation of the molecular pathogenesis of pituitary adenoma and carcinoma (Fig. 7-62). In particular, the Gsp gene may play an important role in some 40% of growth hormone-producing adenomas and the Ras oncogene may play a role in anaplastic progression. The MEN-1 gene, which has been cloned, is associated with familial adenomas.

In addition to pituitary carcinoma, there are a few other special features of pituitary adenomas that warrant brief mention (Fig. 7-63):

Pituitary adenomas sometimes present as acute hemorrhagic infarction (pituitary apoplexy), which requires surgical decompression.

Occasional prolactinomas form prominent amyloid bodies.

ACTH-producing adenomas often elicit a feedback regression of non-neoplastic ACTH cells resulting in the prominent cytoplasmic accumulation of keratin filaments; these cells have bright eosinophilic cytoplasm on H&E stains and are termed Crooke's cells (Crooke's hyaline change).

Lymphocytic Hypophysitis

Although lymphocytic hypophysitis is not a neoplasm, it does present as an intrasellar mass lesion that requires surgical decompression. Presentation is usually in women during pregnancy or shortly after delivery. The primary symptoms are secondary to pituitary insufficiency. MRI scans show an enlarged enhancing pituitary. Histologically, profuse numbers of lymphocytes are seen infiltrating the pituitary. The etiology is likely autoimmune.

Malformative Tumors and Cysts

Key Concept: Many of the tumors and cysts in this category arise from embryonal cell rests within the nervous system.

Unique Features of Some Pituitary Adenomas

- Occasional prolactinomas exhibit pathognomonic concentrically laminated amyloid bodies that are birefringent under polarized light
- Crooke's hyaline change may be seen in non-neoplastic corticotroph cells in patients that have an ACTH-producing adenoma (dense bundles of keratin filaments by electron microscopy)
- Pituitary apoplexy: hemorrhagic infarction of a pituitary macroadenoma
- Pituitary carcinoma: discontiguous dissemination within or outside of the CNS

FIGURE 7-63. Unique features of some adenoma subtypes.

Craniopharyngioma

Craniopharyngiomas occur in the suprasellar region and/or third ventricle. There are two subtypes: adamantinomatous and papillary (Fig. 7-64). The adamantinomatous variant occurs in children and adults, and exhibits a variety of distinctive histologic features, including peripheral columnar palisading of the epithelial cells, nodules of plump pale keratinocytes ("wet" keratin), calcification of the keratin nodules, loosely adhesive areas of epithelium ("stellate reticulum"), and viscous dark brown "machinery oil" fluid filling the cystic spaces. The papillary variant, in contrast occurs only in adults and is composed of only simple squamous epithelium, without any unique features of the adamantinomatous variant. The papillary variant may be somewhat less inclined to surround vessels, nerves, and other vital structures of the suprasellar region and therefore may be easier to resect. Any residual tumor will recur and ultimately lead to significant morbidity and eventual death.

Lipoma

Lipomas, which are composed of mature adipose tissue, can occur anywhere in the nervous system but show a predilection for midline sites, particularly the corpus callosum (Fig. 7-65). Other favored locations are the hypothalamus, cauda equina, and cerebellopontine angle (CPA).

Hypothalamic Neuronal Hamartoma

Hypothalamic hamartomas consist of disorganized hypothalamic gray matter in the region of the tuber cinereum. Some examples show extensive calcification. The tuber cinereum is also a common site for small lipomas.

Nasal Glial Heterotopia ("Nasal Glioma")

Despite the older designation "nasal glioma," this lesion is not a neoplasm but rather a heterotopic mass of disorganized glial tissue located in the nasopharyngeal region. It is exceptionally rare that they may give rise to a secondary neoplasm such as oligodendroglioma.

Rathke's Cleft Cyst

Rathke's cysts constitute one of the four main types of fluid-filled CNS cysts (Fig. 7-66). They presumably arise from remnants of the pharyngeal epithelial pouch (Rathke's pouch) that forms the adenohypophyseal pars intermedia. The cyst lining is ciliated pseudostratified columnar epithelium with goblet cells. They are common incidental findings on MRI scans and at autopsy but can also occasionally grow large enough to compress the pituitary and become symptomatic, necessitating surgical decompression. Rathke cyst should be included in the differential diagnosis of sellar region mass lesions (Fig. 7-67).

Epidermoid Cyst

Epidermoid cysts together with dermoid cysts comprise the epithelial inclusion cysts (Fig. 7-68). The lining of epidermoids is keratin-producing squamous epithelium (Fig. 7-69). The cyst contains white grumous flaky keratin, which is seen as anucleate flat squames by microscopy. Leakage of the cyst contents into the CSF produces severe chemical meningitis (a similar problem can arise with dermoid cysts).

Craniopharyngioma

* **Adamantinomatous (resembles ameloblastoma)**
  - **Palisading, "wet" keratin, calcification, "machinery oil" fluid**
  - **Children and adults**
* **Papillary**
  - **Well differentiated squamous epithelium with no keratin, palisading, or calcification**
  - **Adults**
  - **Better prognosis (less infiltrative and therefore more amenable to gross total resection)**

FIGURE 7-64. The two subtypes of craniopharyngioma.

Gross Differential Diagnosis Corpus Callosum Lesions

* **Agenesis**
* **Marchiafava-Bignami disease**
* **"Butterfly" glioblastoma**
* **Lymphoma**
* **Lipoma**

FIGURE 7-65. Differential diagnosis of corpus callosum lesions.

Common Sellar Region Masses

- Pituitary adenoma
- Craniopharyngioma
- Optic/hypothalamic glioma
- Meningioma
- Metastasis
- Rathke's cyst
- Hypophysitis
- Aneurysm
- Empty sella syndrome

FIGURE 7-67. Differential diagnosis of sellar region masses.

Epithelial Inclusion Cysts

- Epidermoid cyst
    - "Pearly tumor" (glistening white, lobulated)
    - Wall consists of keratinizing squamous epithelium
    - No adnexal structures (glands, hair follicles) in cyst wall
    - Cyst contents consists exclusively of sheets of anucleate squames
- Dermoid cyst
    - Similar to epidermoid, except cyst wall shows skin adnexae (sweat glands, hair follicles) and contents include hair
    - Rarely may contain teeth

FIGURE 7-68. The two types of CNS epithelial inclusion cysts.

TABLE 7-5. CYSTS WITH A CILIATED PSEUDOSTRATIFIED COLUMNAR EPITHELIUM WITH GOBLET CELLS

Colloid cyst
Rathke cyst
Neurenteric cyst

Cysts

- Arachnoid cyst
    - Sylvian fissure most common site
    - May occur at any site in the CNS where arachnoid is found
- Neurenteric cyst of spinal subarachnoid space
    - Variant: respiratory epithelial cyst
- Rathke cyst of sella turcica
- Colloid cyst of the 3rd ventricle
    - Cyst contents may include characteristic filamentous aggregates of degenerated protein and lipid that resemble actinomyces colonies
    - Patients frequently present with headaches
    - Some cases associated with "sudden death" (? acute hydrocephalus from "ball-valve" obstruction of intraventricular foramen?)

FIGURE 7-66. Four types of fluid-filled CNS cysts.

Dermoid Cyst

Same as an epidermoid cyst, but the lining has dermal skin appendages: hair follicles and sweat glands (Fig. 7-70). Hence the contents include hair as well as flaky keratin (and, rarely, teeth!).

Neurenteric (Enterogenous, Respiratory Epithelial) Cyst

Neurenteric cysts are thought to be derived from embryonic diverticular rests from the respiratory-gastrointestinal tract. The most common location is in the spinal canal anterior to the cord. The cyst wall consists of ciliated pseudostratified columnar epithelium with mucin-producing goblet cells (Figs. 7-71 and 7-72), very similar to the lining of Rathke cleft cysts of the pituitary and colloid cysts of the third ventricle (Table 7-5).

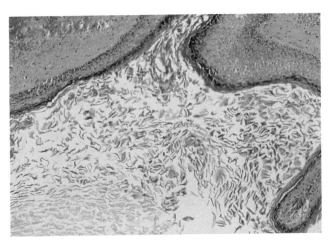

FIGURE 7-69. Epidermoid cyst.

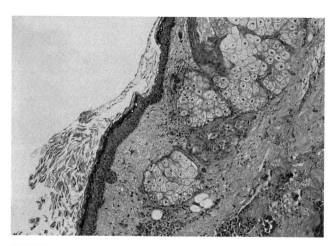

FIGURE 7-70. Dermoid cyst. Note sebaceous glands.

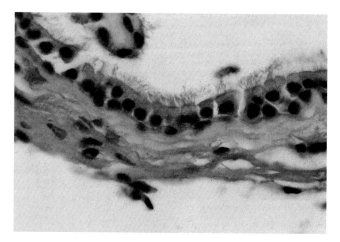

FIGURE 7-71. Neurenteric (respiratory epithelial) cyst. The lining is ciliated pseudostratified columnar epithelium with mucin-producing goblet cells. A similar lining is seen in Rathke cysts of the pituitary and colloid cysts of the third ventricle.

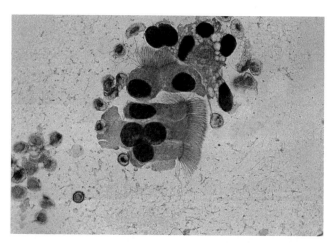

FIGURE 7-72. Neurenteric (respiratory epithelial) cyst. Ciliated epithelial cells from the cyst lining are seen on this touch (imprint) preparation.

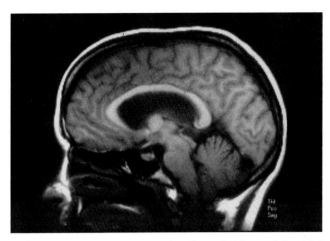

FIGURE 7-73. Mid-sagittal MRI showing colloid cyst of the third ventricle.

Colloid Cyst of the Third Ventricle

Colloid cysts arise in the rostral roof of the third ventricle close to the interventricular foramen of Monro (Figs. 7-73 and 7-74). The cyst lining is ciliated pseudostratified columnar epithelium with mucin-producing goblet cells (Fig. 7-75). Colloid cysts may produce positional hydrocephalus due to a "ball-valve" effect at the foramen of Monro, and some cases have been associated with sudden death, possibly due to acute obstruction.

Tumors of the Meninges

Meningioma

This tumor arises from arachnoid cells of the arachnoid (Fig. 7-76) and occurs primarily in older adults, although it may also occur in children. There is a female predominance, especially in the spinal canal. The most common sites are over the convexities and in relationship to the falx (Fig. 7-77; Table 7-6), but skull base meningiomas in aggregate account for roughly half of intracranial meningiomas. Rare intraventricular meningiomas arise from the normal arachnoid cell nests of the choroid plexus and must be included in the differential diagnosis of intraventricular tumors (Fig. 7-78). Menin-

TABLE 7-6. RADIOLOGIC (MRI) DIFFERENTIAL DIAGNOSIS OF A DURAL-BASED MASS LESION (MENINGIOMA AND ITS MIMICS)

Meningioma
Hemangiopericytoma
Solitary fibrous tumor
Rosai–Dorfmann disease
Granulocytic sarcoma ("chloroma")
Solitary dural metastasis

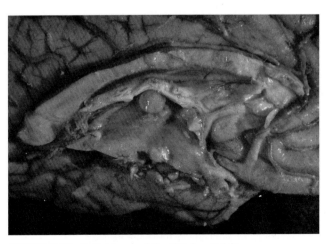

FIGURE 7-74. Colloid cyst of the third ventricle.

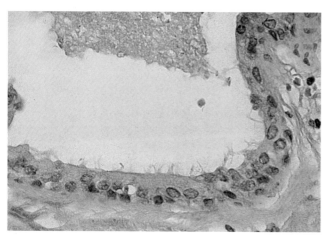

FIGURE 7-75. Colloid cyst lining: ciliated pseudostratified columnar epithelium with mucin-producing goblet cells. A similar lining is seen in Rathke cysts of the pituitary and neurenteric cysts of the spinal canal.

giomas can also arise from the arachnoid of the lumbar cistern and must be included in the differential diagnosis of solitary mass lesions at that site (Table 7-7). In short, meningiomas can arise in any location in which arachnoid cells are present, including ectopic rests that occasionally frequent the calvarium (intraosseous meningioma) and the soft tissues of the head and neck (ectopic meningioma).

Meningioma Histopathological Classification

There are thirteen morphological variants of meningioma that are recognizable based on their distinctive architectural features as seen on routine Hematoxylin-eosin stained sections (Table 7-8). Nine of these variants are benign low-grade (WHO grade I) tumors and simply must be recognized by the pathologist as being meningiomas to avoid confusion with other neoplasms. The remaining four variants exhibit more aggressive clinical behavior and are classified as either WHO grade II or III. In addition, any of the benign variants may warrant upgrading to atypical or anaplastic (malignant) if certain features are present as described below.

Meningioma

- **Originate from arachnoid (meningothelial) cells**
- **Common locations**
  - **parasagittal**
  - **convexity**
  - **sphenoid wing**
  - **spinal canal**
- **Other locations**
  - **optic nerve sheath**
  - **choroid plexus ("intraventricular")**

FIGURE 7-76. Origin and anatomic locations of meningioma.

Intraventricular Tumors

- **Choroid plexus papilloma/carcinoma**
- **Ependymoma**
- **Subependymoma**
- **Subependymal giant cell astrocytoma**
- **Central neurocytoma**
- **Intraventricular meningioma**

FIGURE 7-78. Differential diagnosis of intraventricular tumor.

TABLE 7-7. DIFFERENTIAL DIAGNOSIS OF A SOLITARY MASS IN THE LUMBAR CISTERN

Schwannoma
Meningioma
Myxopapillary ependymoma
Paraganglioma of the filum

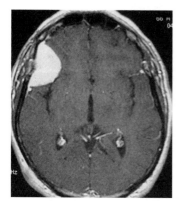

FIGURE 7-77. Meningioma. Note the extra-axial location and compression of underlying brain.

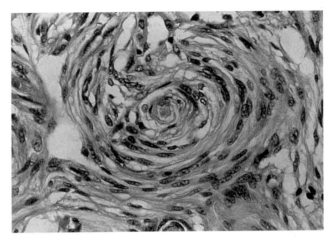

FIGURE 7-79. Meningioma, transitional subtype: characteristic meningothelial whorl.

TABLE 7-8. THIRTEEN HISTOLOGIC VARIANTS OF MENINGIOMA

Nine benign variants (WHO grade I)
  Meningothelial
  Fibrous
  Transitional
  Psammomatous
  Angiomatous
  Microcystic
  Secretory
  Lymphoplasmacyte-rich
  Metaplastic
Four variants with aggressive behavior (WHO grade II or III)
  Chordoid (WHO grade II)
  Clear cell (WHO grade II)
  Papillary (WHO grade III)
  Rhabdoid (WHO grade III)

The nine benign variants are:

A. Classical
   1. Meningothelial (syncytial): sheets of nuclei with indistinct cell boundaries
   2. Fibrous (fibroblastic): highly spindled and fascicular
   3. Transitional: classical meningothelial whorls (Fig. 7-79)
B. Psammomatous: profuse psammoma bodies (Fig. 7-80)
C. Angiomatous: highly vascular
D. Microcystic: prominent microcysts
E. Secretory: "pseudopsammoma bodies" are spherical, intracytoplasmic, eosinophilic inclusion bodies that are positive for carcinoembryonic antigen (CEA) and PAS; the meningioma cells that produce the pseudopsammoma bodies are strongly positive for keratin
F. Lymphoplasmacyte-rich: prominent chronic inflammatory cell infiltrate of lymphocytes and plasma cells

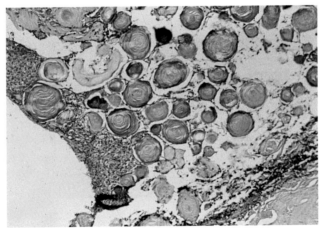

FIGURE 7-80. Psammomatous meningioma.

G. Metaplastic: focal formation of bone, cartilage, or fat

The four aggressive variants are:

A. Chordoid (WHO grade II): cords of cells in mucinous matrix mimic chordoma
B. Clear cell (WHO grade II): round nuclei with prominent cytoplasmic clearing mimic oligodendroglioma or ependymoma
C. Papillary (WHO grade III): aggressive variant; pseudopapillae with cytoplasmic processes extending to blood vessels mimic the perivascular pseudorosettes of ependymoma; more common in young patients
D. Rhabdoid (WHO grade III): aggressive meningioma with rhabdoid morphology

Atypical Meningioma

In addition to the four aggressive morphological variants listed above, a meningioma of any morphologic subtype warrants upgrading to Atypical Meningioma (WHO Grade II) if the following features are present:

Brain invasion, or
Maximal mitotic rate of 4/10 HPF or greater, or three of the following five features:
 Sheeting (patternless) architecture
 Hypercellularity (>53 nuclei per HPF diameter)
 Macronucleoli
 Small cell formation
 Micronecrosis with pseudopalisading

Anaplastic ("Malignant") Meningioma

Traditionally, brain-invasive meningiomas have been termed "malignant." Recent studies, however, indicate that brain-invasive meningiomas are equivalent to "atypical" meningiomas in terms of propensity for recurrence and aggressive growth, but may not be significantly worse; it is therefore recommended that brain-invasive meningiomas be classified as "atypical" rather than anaplastic.

A meningioma of any morphological subtype should be upgraded to Anaplastic Meningioma if either of the following two features are present:

Maximal mitotic rate of 20/10 HPF or greater
Highly anaplastic features resembling sarcoma, carcinoma, or melanoma

Note that, in contrast to invasion of the underlying brain parenchyma, which warrants a diagnosis of atypical meningioma, invasion of the overlying cranial bone is frequently encountered with benign meningiomas and is *not* a negative prognostic factor per se.

Caveat concerning the term "benign meningioma": Even though ordinary low-grade meningiomas show "benign" histological features and are slow growing, they may cause significant morbidity and eventually death when arising or recurring in areas not amenable to gross total resection, as is the case for many skull base meningiomas.

Hemangiopericytoma

Hemangiopericytomas are dural-based tumors that were formerly considered variants of meningioma but for the reasons listed in the accompanying figures should be diagnosed as hemangiopericytomas (Fig. 7-81 and 7-82). Histolog-

Hemangiopericytoma

- The term "angioblastic meningioma" should be avoided; it is an archaic term that includes highly vascular ("angiomatous") meningiomas, hemangiopericytomas, and dura-based hemangioblastomas.
- Hemangiopericytomas are not variants of meningioma!
- It is important to correctly diagnose hemangiopericytoma because the recurrence rates and metastasis rates are higher for hemangiopericytomas compared to meningiomas
- Morphologic features of hemangiopericytoma:
- Rich reticulin pattern surrounding individual cells
- Typical branching vascular pattern ("staghorn" pattern)
- Negative for EMA (in contrast to meningiomas)
- By ultrastructural examination, large numbers of desmosomes linking cell processes are not seen in hemangiopericytomas (as compared to their abundance in meningiomas)

FIGURE 7-81. Major features of hemangiopericytoma.

ically, these tumors are highly vascular, with the characteristic branching "staghorn" vessel pattern.

Meningioangiomatosis

Meningioangiomatosis is a relatively rare cause of seizures in children (Fig. 7-83) and consists of a proliferation of meningothelial cells and fibroblasts in the

---

Meningioangiomatosis

- Presents primarily during childhood
- Hamartomatous lesion of the cerebral meninges and vasculature of the superficial cortex
- Associated with NF type 2
- Sporadic
- Clinical history of seizures
- Proliferation of spindled cells in subarachnoid space that form cuffs around penetrating blood vessels of the cortex
- Cells exhibit features of either meningothelial cells or fibroblasts

FIGURE 7-83. Major features of meningioangiomatosis.

Hemangiopericytomas Are Not Meningiomas

- Hemangiopericytomas have different light microscopic, ultrastructural, and immunohistochemical features compared to meningiomas
- The features of meningeal hemangiopericytomas are identical to those of hemangiopericytomas arising elsewhere in the body
- The clinical behavior of hemangiopericytomas is unequivocally more aggressive than that of benign meningiomas
- There is no female predilection for hemangiopericytomas like that seen for meningiomas
- There is no association with prior radiation therapy like that seen with meningiomas
- The cytogenetic and molecular biologic evidence linking a large percentage of meningiomas with a tumor suppressor gene on chr. 22 is not found with hemangiopericytomas

FIGURE 7-82. Hemangiopericytomas are not meningiomas!

subarachnoid space with spread into the underlying cortex along the perivascular Virchow–Robin spaces. Surgical resection is curative.

Tumors of Nerve Sheath Cells

Schwannoma (Neurilemoma, Neurinoma, Acoustic Neuroma)

Schwannomas most commonly arise on CN VIII, but may be seen on other cranial nerves and spinal roots or rarely within brain parenchyma or other tissues of the body where the tumor presumably arises from Schwann cells or Schwann cell progenitors in nerves surrounding blood vessels or in the nerves providing primary innervation of the tissue. Histopathological examination demonstrates dense (Antoni A) and loose (Antoni B) tissue architecture. Organized linear palisades of nuclei in Antoni A tissue are called "Verocay bodies" (Fig. 7-84). Schwannomas arise eccentrically within the nerve, displacing the axons and thereby rendering nerve-sparing surgical resection possible in some cases. Malignant progression of schwannomas is *exceptionally rare,* and the term "malignant schwannoma" should not be used as a generic substitute for malignant peripheral nerve sheath tumor (MPNST)!

Neurofibroma

Neurofibromas have axons diffusely incorporated within the tumor parenchyma that consists of a mixture of Schwann cells, fibroblasts, perineurial cells, and mast cells (Fig. 7-85). These tumors usually arise on peripheral nerves and roots where they may lead to gross enlargement of individual nerve twigs. Neurofibromas may be sporadic or associated with neurofibromatosis. They may undergo malignant progression, giving rise to MPNST (also called "neurofibrosarcoma" or "neurogenic sarcoma"), especially in the large plexiform neurofibromas of NF1 (Fig. 7-86). Central neurofibromatosis (NF2) features bilateral eighth nerve schwannomas; the gene resides on chromosome 22q12. Chromosome 22 thus provides a genetic link between many cases of meningioma, schwannoma, and neurofibroma (Fig. 7-87). Peripheral neurofibromatosis (NF1) features PNS neurofibromas; the gene resides on chromosome 17q12. See the Appendix for further information on these diseases and other inherited cancer syndromes.

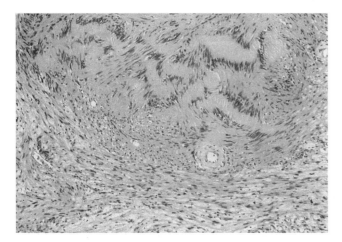

FIGURE 7-84. Schwannoma: Antoni A tissue with Verocay bodies (nuclear palisades).

Molecular Biology of Meningioma, Schwannoma, and Neurofibroma

- Loss of all or part of chromosome 22 in most meningiomas

- Mutation on chromosome 22 in neurofibromatosis, type 2, associated schwannomas and neurofibromas

- The common gene codes for "merlin" a cytoskeletal to membrane linking protein

FIGURE 7-87. Molecular biologic link between meningioma and the nerve sheath tumors.

Triton Tumors

- Tumor with both muscle and neural differentiation

- Strict sense: MPNST with rhabdomyosarcomatous differentiation

- Broad sense: any tumor with muscle and neural differentiation, including neuromuscular hamartoma ("benign Triton tumor"), medulloblastoma with rhabdomyosarcoma (medullomyoblastoma), and rhabdomyosarcoma with focal neural differentiation

FIGURE 7-88. Definition and spectrum of Triton tumors.

Peripheral Primitive Neuroectodermal Tumor (pPNET) / Ewings Sarcoma

pPNETs comprise a spectrum of small blue cell tumors ranging from neoplasms originating in peripheral nerves that show neuronal differentiation to skeletal and extraskeletal Ewings sarcoma (Ewing's sarcoma can be considered as an undifferentiated form of pPNET)

FIGURE 7-89. pPNET/Ewings sarcoma.

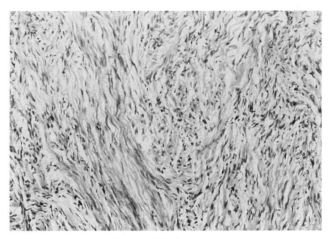

FIGURE 7-85. Neurofibroma histology.

Triton Tumors

Triton tumors (named for experiments performed by Piera Locatelli in the 1920s with the Triton salamander in which re-implanting the proximal end of a sectioned sciatic nerve into the dorsal surface induced supranumery limb formation) show both muscle and neural differentiation (Fig. 7-88). In the strict sense they are a combination of MPNST with a rhabdomyosarcoma component. In a broader sense, the term has been used for any tumor with muscle and neural differentiation, including neuromuscular hamartoma ("benign Triton tumor"), medulloblastoma with rhabdomyosarcoma (medullomyoblastoma), and rhabdomyosarcoma with focal neural differentiation.

Peripheral Primitive Neuroectodermal Tumors

Peripheral PNETs (pPNETs) constitute part of a spectrum of malignant small blue cell tumors that includes skeletal and extraskeletal Ewing's sarcoma (Fig. 7-89). pPNETs are genetically distinct from CNS PNETs (cPNETs) (Fig. 7-90). pPNETs are immuno-positive for antibodies (such as HBA-71) that recognize epitopes on the cell surface glycoprotein p30/32. p30/32 is a product of the *MIC2* gene. Although most pPNETs arise extracranially within peripheral nerves or in body soft tissues, they can also present as primary CNS malignancies in the cranial or spinal leptomeninges, particularly the cauda equina and lumbar cistern.

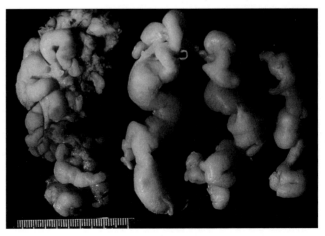

FIGURE 7-86. Plexiform neurofibroma.

Central PNETs (cPNETs) and Peripheral PNETs (pPNETs) Are Completely Different, Unrelated Entities!!

- Immunohistochemically, pPNETs are positive with HBA-71 (and antibodies directed against CD99) that recognizes an epitope of the cell surface glycoprotein p30/32, which is a product of the MIC2 gene. A t(11;22)(q24;q12) translocation is present in over 80% of pPNETs.

- These molecular and immunohistochemical features are characteristic of pPNETs only, NOT cPNETs!

- pPNETs may rarely arise as primary intraspinal neoplasms of the cauda equina/lumbar cistern region or even more rarely of the intracranial subarachnoid space; the molecular alterations are identical to those of other pPNETs (and are not those of cPNETs); pPNETs arising within the lumbar cistern must be distinguished from "drop" metastases from an intracranial cPNET such as medulloblastoma.

FIGURE 7-90. cPNET versus pPNET.

Extra-CNS Regional Tumors

A number of tumors arise in the bone and soft tissues that surround the nervous system and can secondarily involve the nervous system by compression and/or invasion, of which the most important are:

Chordoma: The sacrum and clivus are the most common anatomic sites of origin; physaliphorous ("bubble-bearing") cells constitute the hallmark histologic feature; chordomas arise from notochord remnants that normally exist as small nests in the sacrum and clivus and as the nucleus pulposus of intervertebral disks; chordomas are relentlessly locally invasive.

Glomus jugulare tumor = chemodectoma = paraganglioma

Chondroma (enchondroma, enchondrosis): benign; most common origin is anterior to the pons.

Chondrosarcoma and Osteosarcoma: malignant bone and cartilaginous tumors can arise from either cranium or vertebrae.

METASTATIC DISEASE

Extracranial Dissemination of Brain Tumors

Extracranial spread of primary brain tumors is uncommon but may be seen with any anaplastic glial tumor or PNET, and is also seen with meningiomas. Spread is most commonly associated with prior surgery. Spread via intracranial shunts is another route for dissemination.

Metastasis to the Central Nervous System

Metastatic disease is a major clinical problem in contemporary neuro-oncology. The salient points concerning metastases to the CNS are succinctly summarized in the accompanying figures (Fig. 7-91 through 7-98).

Metastatic Tumors

- Most frequent site: gray-white junction of cerebral hemispheres in distribution territory of middle cerebral artery
- Most common metastases in older adults:
  - Lung
  - Breast
  - Melanoma
  - Renal
  - Gastrointestinal tract

FIGURE 7-91. The most common metastatic tumors.

CNS Clear Cell Tumors

- Oligodendroglioma
- Central neurocytoma
- Clear cell ependymoma
- Clear cell meningioma
- Metastatic renal cell

FIGURE 7-92. Differential diagnosis of clear cell tumors.

Common Tumors That Rarely Metastasize to Brain Parenchyma

- Prostate
- Cervical
- Sarcomas in general
- Squamous cell carcinoma of skin

FIGURE 7-93. Tumors that rarely metastasize to CNS parenchyma.

Hemorrhagic Metastases

- Renal
- Melanoma
- Choriocarcinoma

FIGURE 7-96. The metastatic tumors that are most likely to bleed.

Lobar Hemorrhage

- Amyloid angiopathy
- AVM
- Hypertension
- Trauma
- Oligodendroglioma/GBM
- Metastases (renal, melanoma, choriocarcinoma)

FIGURE 7-97. The differential diagnosis of cerebral hemisphere lobar hemorrhage should include hemorrhagic metastasis.

Multiple Tumors

- Metastases
- Multifocal
  - Glioblastoma multiforme
  - Primary CNS lymphoma
- Genetic predisposition
  - Neurofibromatosis: neurofibroma, schwannoma, meningioma
  - Tuberous sclerosis: subependymal giant cell astrocytoma
  - Von Hippel-Lindau: hemangioblastoma, renal cell carcinoma
- Multiple masses are not always neoplastic!

FIGURE 7-98. Multiple mass lesions in the brain are very often metastases, but other possibilities must be included in the differential diagnosis.

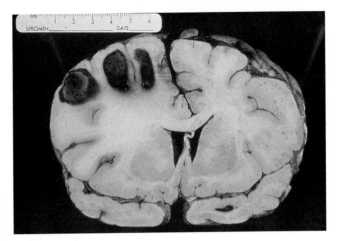

FIGURE 7-94. Metastases, illustrated here with metastatic melanoma, are frequently multiple and located at the gray-white junction.

Treatment Effects

Each of the three major therapeutic modalities used to treat brain tumors—surgery, radiation therapy, and chemotherapy—has side effects that both the primary clinician and pathologist must be familiar with. The most important are:

Radiation therapy: delayed radiation necrosis (Fig. 7-99).

Radiation therapy: secondary tumors (Fig. 7-100). The most common radiation-induced tumors of the brain and spinal cord are meningiomas, sarcomas, and high-grade gliomas.

Chemotherapy: chemonecrosis. Chemonecrosis is most commonly seen with methotrexate administered intrathecally, particularly when used in combination with radiation therapy.

Surgery: textilomas (gossypibomas). Mass lesions that arise secondary to foreign body reaction to hemostatic agents, including gelatin foam (Gelfoam),

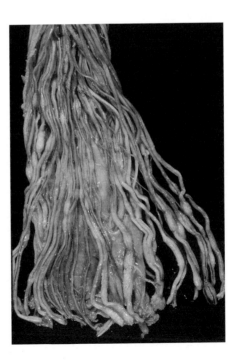

FIGURE 7-95. "Drop" metastases from a supratentorial brain tumor appear grossly as lumpy nerve roots of the cauda equina.

oxidized cellulose (Surgicel, Oxycel), and microfibrillar collagen (Avitine), can simulate recurrent tumor clinically (mass effect secondary to inflammation and edema) and on neuroimaging studies (contrast enhancement).

Preoperative embolization: embolization-induced atypia in meningiomas. Highly vascular tumors such as renal cell carcinomas, hemangioblastomas, hemangiopericytomas, and angiomatous meningiomas are often embolized to decrease bleeding at surgery. In some meningiomas, embolization is associated with a reactive atypia that could be mistaken for anaplastic progression by those not familiar with this phenomenon.

BIBLIOGRAPHY

Kleihues P, Cavenee WK, eds. *Pathology and genetics of tumours of the nervous system,* 2nd ed. New York: Oxford University Press, 2000.

APPENDIX

Throughout this chapter, many different tumors have been described that can arise either sporadically or in association with a specific heritable genetic defect. The following figures provide a summary of the major genetic associations of nervous system tumors and the clinicopathologic features of the inherited cancer syndromes (Figures 7-101 through 7-113).

Chromosomal Alterations

• Oligodendroglioma	• LOH 1p, 19q
• Ependymoma	• LOH 22
• Medulloblastoma	• LOH 17p, DM's NMYC
• Meningioma	• LOH 22
• Schwannoma	• LOH 22
• Astrocytoma	• LOH 17 p53 LOH 22
• Anaplastic Astrocytoma	• LOH 13 Rb, 16p, 9q, 19q
• Glioblastoma	• LOH 10 + EGF amp
• ATRT	• LOH 22

FIGURE 7-101. Major chromosomal alterations of brain tumors.

Delayed Radiation Necrosis

- Primarily affects white matter with relative sparing of cortex and other gray matter structures
- Optic nerves/chiasm and spinal cord particularly vulnerable
- Fibrinoid necrosis of blood vessel walls
- Associated "geographic zones" of bland parenchymal necrosis with secondary mineralization
- Telangiectasias
- Thick-walled hyalinized vessels

FIGURE 7-99. Major features of delayed radiation necrosis.

Secondary (Radiation-Induced) Tumors

- Average latency of approximately 10 years (related to dose)
- Therefore most commonly seen in patients with longer survivals, such as patients radiated for benign diseases (e.g., tinea capitis) or low-grade tumors (e.g., pituitary adenoma, PXA)
- Meningiomas
- Sarcomas
- Malignant astrocytomas

FIGURE 7-100. Major features and types of secondary (radiation-induced) tumors.

Inherited Cancer Syndromes

- NF1
- NF2
- Von Hippel-Lindau
- Tuberous sclerosis
- Sturge-Weber
- Li-Fraumeni syndrome
- Cowden syndrome
- Gorlin syndrome
- Turcot syndrome

FIGURE 7-102. Inherited cancer syndromes.

NF1: At Least Two of the Following Must Be Present:

- 6 or more cafe-au-lait spots with a diameter greater than 5 mm in prepubescent patients or 15 mm in postpubescent patients
- 1 plexiform neurofibroma or 2 neurofibromas
- Axillary or inguinal freckling
- An NF1-associated bone lesion (e.g., sphenoid dysplasia)
- Optic glioma
- 2 or more Lisch nodules
- A first degree relative (parent, sibling or child) with NF1

FIGURE 7-104. Diagnostic criteria for NF1.

NF1 (Classic Von Recklinghausen's Disease, "Peripheral NF")

- 90% of NF cases are NF1
- Common disorder; prevalance 1/3,000
- AD, chr 17q (encodes protein neurofibromin)
- Neurofibromin is a *ras* GTPase activator protein
- Cafe-au-lait spots
- Plexiform neurofibromas; multiple neurofibromas
- Axillary / inguinal freckling
- Iris hamartomas (Lisch nodules)
- Osseous dysplasias
- Optic gliomas (JPA of optic nerves)
- JPAs of 3rd vent and cerebellum
- High-grade astrocytomas of brain and spinal cord
- Focal signal hyperintensities in basal ganglia and other sites
- MPNSTs develop from neurofibromas in about 5% of patients

FIGURE 7-103. Major features of NF1.

NF2 (Bilateral Acoustic NF, "Central NF")

- Uncommon disorder; prevalance 1/40,000
- AD, chr. 22q (codes for protein merlin/schwannomin)
- Classic tumor suppressor gene; schwannomin is a member of the protein 4.1 family of cytoskeleton-associated proteins.
- NF2 tumors derived from the Nerves, Coverings and Lining of the CNS (schwannomas, meningiomas, ependymomas of spinal cord)
- Bilateral vestibular schwannomas
- Schwannomas of other cranial and spinal nerves
- Schwannosis of spinal nerve roots and cord
- Multiple meningiomas
- Meningioangiomatosis
- Ependymomas of spinal cord
- Astrocytomas and JPA also occur in NF2 but are rare.
- Neurofibromas (?); many reported neurofibromas upon review are actually schwannomas
- Plexiform neurofibromas do not occur in NF2
- Calcifications of cerebral and cerebellar cortices
- Cataracts (juvenile posterior subcapsular lenticular opacities)
- Note: NF2 patients also have cafe-au-lait spots but not as many and not as large as in NF1 patients

FIGURE 7-105. Major features of NF2.

A Dx of NF2 Can Be Made in Any One of Four Ways:

- Bilateral vestibular schwannomas
- A unilateral vestibular schwannoma and a first degree relative with NF2
- A first degree relative with NF2 and any two of the following:
  - Neurofibroma
  - Meningioma
  - Glioma
  - Schwannoma
  - Posterior subcapsular lens opacity (juvenile cataract)
  - Cerebral calcification
- Two of the following:
  - Unilateral vestibular schwannoma
  - Multiple meningiomas
  - One of the following: neurofibroma, schwannoma, glioma, posterior subcapsular lens opacity, cerebral calcification

FIGURE 7-106. Diagnostic criteria for NF2.

Tuberous Sclerosis

- AD, TSC1 (9q34); TSC2 (chr 16p); 60% sporadic as new mutations
- "Adenoma sebaceum" (angiofibromas) of face
- Pulmonary lymphangiomatosis
- Subungual fibromas
- Cardiac rhabdomyoma
- Renal angiomyolipoma
- Cortical glioneuronal hamartomas (tubers), ependymal hamartomas ("candle gutterings")
- Subependymal giant cell astrocytoma

FIGURE 7-107. Major features of tuberous sclerosis.

Von Hippel-Lindau Disease

- AD, chr 3p25
- Retinal angioma (von Hippel lesion)
- Cerebellar (Lindau tumor) and spinal cord hemangioblastomas
- Cerebral hemangioblastomas do occur but are much rarer than cerebellum and spinal cord tumors
- Renal angiomatosis
- Renal cell carcinoma
- Pheochromocytoma
- Cysts of kidneys, pancreas
- Cystadenoma of the epididymis

FIGURE 7-108. Major features of von Hippel–Lindau disease.

Sturge-Weber (Encephalofacial Angiomatosis)

- Vast majority of cases sporadic; etiology unknown
- Hemiparesis, epilepsy, mental retardation within first year of life or early childhood
- Pathologic findings are almost always unilateral:
  - Nevus flammeus or port wine stain of face, esp. in distribution of ophthalmic branch of trigeminal nerve
  - Ipsilateral leptomeningeal venous angiomas
  - Calcification of superficial cortex underlying angioma (distinctive gyriform pattern of calcification seen on neuroimaging studies referred to as "tram tracks" or "railroad tracks")
  - Secondary ischemic cortical atrophy

FIGURE 7-109. Major features of Sturge–Weber disease.

Li-Fraumeni Syndrome

- *TP53* germline mutation
- AD, multiple neoplasms in children and young adults
- Sarcomas, breast cancer
- CNS: diffuse astrocytomas most common (low-grade, AA, GBM); medulloblastoma and supratentorial PNETs less common

FIGURE 7-110. Major features of Li–Fraumeni syndrome.

Cowden Syndrome

- "Multiple hamartoma syndrome", AD

- Oral mucosa fibromas, multiple trichilemmomas, hamartomatous colon polyps, thyroid neoplasms, breast cancer

- CNS: dysplastic gangliocytoma of the cerebellum (Lhermitte-Duclos disease)

- Approximately 50% of patients with dysplastic gangliocytoma have stigmata of Cowden syndrome

FIGURE 7-111. Major features of Cowden syndrome.

Gorlin (Nevoid Basal Cell Carcinoma Syndrome)

- AD, nevoid basal cell carcinomas, jaw keratocysts, palmar and plantar pits, ovarian fibromas

- CNS: approximately 5% develop cerebellar medulloblastoma (especially desmoplastic medulloblastoma)

FIGURE 7-112. Major features of Gorlin syndrome.

Turcot

- At least 3 different genetic diseases that share the combination of coexisting multiple colorectal tumors (polyps or carcinomas) and a malignant brain tumor:

- FAP-associated Turcot
  - Familial adenomatous polyposis (FAP) (germline mutation of the *APC* gene) with medulloblastoma

- HNPCC-associated Turcot
  - Hereditary non-polyposis colorectal carcinoma (HNPCC) syndrome with glioblastoma (germline mutation of one of two DNA mismatch repair genes, *hMLH1* or *hPMS2*)
  - Approximately 50% of patients in this Turcot subgroup have cafe-au-lait spots

- Non-FAP, non-HNPCC Turcot
  - Some patients with coexisting colon and brain tumors do not have a demonstrable mutation of the *APC, hMLH1,* or *hPMS2* genes; the genetic defect in this group remains to be determined

FIGURE 7-113. Major features of Turcot syndrome.

8

DEMYELINATING DISEASES

PERSPECTIVE

1. Intact myelin is required for saltatory action potential conduction; loss of myelin renders an axon electrically nonfunctional even though it is physically intact. If conduction is possible at all, the conduction velocity is dramatically slowed. Conduction velocity can be measured both in the central and peripheral nervous system to assess the degree and location of demyelination.
2. Demyelinating disorders can affect central myelin alone, peripheral myelin alone, or both central and peripheral myelin simultaneously.

OBJECTIVES

1. Understand the function of myelin, and the electrophysiological consequence of myelin loss. Know the difference between central and peripheral myelin.
2. Learn that diseases may afflict central myelin, peripheral myelin, or both central and peripheral myelin.
3. Know the gross and microscopic features of multiple sclerosis (MS) and how these correlate with the clinical course of the disease.
4. Understand the molecular basis of metachromatic leukodystrophy, Krabbe's leukodystrophy, and adrenoleukodystrophy. Describe the clinical and pathological features of these disorders.
5. Learn that Guillain–Barré syndrome is a common disease of peripheral myelin characterized by ascending and potentially life-threatening paralysis.

Myelin sheaths are multilaminar sheets of complex proteolipids wrapped spirally around axons in the central and peripheral nervous system (Fig. 8-1). In the peripheral nervous system, the Schwann cells form myelin, and in the CNS, myelin is formed by the oligodendrocytes. A Schwann cell generally myelinates only one axon, whereas the oligodendrocyte may myelinate up to 50 axons. There are differences in the chemical composition of central versus peripheral myelin, and there is even some regional variation in myelin composition in the CNS. Central myelin contains five major proteins—proteolipid, myelin basic protein (MBP), 2'–3' cyclic nucleotide phosphohydrolase, and myelin-associated and myelin-oligodendrocyte glyco-protein. Myelin makes saltatory conduction possible. Axonal depolarization occurs at the nodes of Ranvier (gaps between successive myelin sheaths) permitting rapid signal conduction. Additionally, ion channels are concentrated at the nodes of Ranvier; therefore, the neuron need not concern itself with manu-

(Fig. 8-2)

Central Versus Peripheral Myelin

- **Central myelin**
  - **Oligodendroglia**
  - **Multiple axons invested**

- **Peripheral myelin**
  - **Schwann cell**
  - **Single axon invested**

FIGURE 8-1. Central versus peripheral myelin.

Neuropathology of White Matter Disorders

- **Idiopathic demyelinating diseases**
- **Post-infectious demyelination**
- **Dysmyelinating diseases**
- **Acquired metabolic demyelination**
- **Infectious demyelination**
- **Toxic demyelination**

FIGURE 8-2. Central demyelination can result from a variety of causes.

facturing channels for the entire axonal membrane surface. If an axon loses its myelin, its conduction velocity drops dramatically; indeed, conduction through the demyelinated area may cease altogether even though the axon remains intact.

Disorders that damage the oligodendroglia or Schwann cells with their myelin sheaths directly are said to result in primary demyelination (Fig. 8-2). The axons are relatively preserved, and if remyelination occurs (as it does in the peripheral nervous system, and to a lesser degree in the CNS), then normal function can be restored.

The maintenance of the myelin sheath depends in part on the integrity of the axon; disorders that damage the axon may lead to loss of the myelin sheath. This is secondary demyelination. The best example of this process is Wallerian degeneration (axonal and myelin degeneration distal to an axonal transection site). These conditions are not really disorders of myelin and will not be discussed further here. A variety of inheritable metabolic disorders result in impaired myelin metabolism and are referred to as "dysmyelinating disorders" or "leukodystrophies."

Myelin stains are used to evaluate these disorders morphologically. The stains include Luxol Fast Blue (LFB), and the eponymic stains of Weil, Weigert, and Woelke. Normal myelin will be blue or black when exposed to these stains, and areas of myelin loss will be pale. Myelin stains have two major uses: (1) detection of primary demyelinating disorders and (2) disclosure of tract degeneration evinced by secondary demyelination. In addition, Sudan Black and Oil Red O stains are used to demonstrate myelin breakdown products as these dyes are soluble in neutral lipid. Detailed analysis of myelin breakdown is possible using selected histochemical techniques, and classical descriptions of myelin disorders derive, in large measure, from these methods. Myelin is degraded initially into phospholipids that are Luxol-chloroform positive, glycolipids that are PAS positive, and cholesterol that is Feigin stain positive, with spontaneous formation of lipid complexes having the appearance of Maltese crosses. Phospholipids and glycolipids are stripped of their fatty acid constituents, which then react with glycerol from phospholipids and cholesterol to form triglycerides and cholesterol esters, respectively. Triglycerides and cholesterol esters are both neutral lipids that stain with Sudan black and are therefore called "sudanophilic." Acquired or hereditary disorders of myelin where complete myelin degradation occurs normally will lead to accumulation of sudanophilic myelin breakdown products, while leukodystrophies with defective myelin catabolism lead to accumulation of more complex lipids, including phospholipids, glycolipids and cholesterol. When stained with toluidine blue or cresyl violet, these complex lipid products assume a reddish hue; this spectral shift from the anticipated blue color of these dyes (orthochromasia) is called "metachromasia." Metachromasia can be seen early in massive normal myelin catabolism induced by myelin destruction or may be observed in hereditary myelin dyscatabolism such as metachromatic leukodystrophy resulting from arylsulfatase deficiency.

PROTOTYPICAL DISORDERS OF CENTRAL MYELIN

Inflammatory: MS, disseminated leukoencephalomyelitis

Infectious: Progressive multifocal leukoencephalopathy (PML)

Leukodystrophies: Alexander's disease, Canavan's disease, Krabbe's disease, adrenoleukodystrophy, Pelizaeus–Merzbacher disease (peripheral myelin also often involved in the leukodystrophies)

Disorders of Central Myelin

Multiple sclerosis (MS) is a depressingly common disease afflicting predominantly persons between age 20 and 40 years, with a slight female predominance. Foci of demyelination occur throughout the neuraxis, and episodes of demyelination are separated by periods of remission that may last weeks, months, or years. This dissemination in time (attack–remission–relapse–remission) and space (multiple sites in the CNS) is essential for the confident diagnosis of the disease, although there is great variability in the severity of attacks and duration of remissions. The long myelinated pathways (motor and sensory tracts, cerebellar tracts, optic nerves-tracts-radiations, and the medial longitudinal fasciculus) are interrupted to variable degrees by areas of demyelination leading to weakness, sensory alterations (including numbness and paresthesias), incoordination, visual disturbances (including central scotomata), and diplopia due to oculomotor incoordination. Remissions are rarely complete, and patients accumulate deficits as new areas are demyelinated. Depending on the tempo of the disease progression, the patient may become completely disabled with blindness, ataxia, and weakness, and as the white matter bundles connecting cortical regions become involved, intellectual impairment may ensue. Other patients will have mild, infrequent attacks with excellent remissions; these patients can lead relatively normal, productive lives but must live with the possibility that an attack of major severity may occur at any time.

Examination of the brain and spinal cord reveals irregular light pink to gray areas of demyelination called "plaques," which range in size from several centimeters to areas scarcely visible to the unaided eye (Fig. 8-3). Plaques grossly have a predilection for the white matter surrounding the ventricles (especially the angles of the lateral ventricles), but they may occur anywhere in the CNS. Areas with incomplete loss of myelin or with partial replacement of myelin by remyelination are called "shadow plaques."

Microscopically, myelin loss occurs around small veins and venules accompanied by lymphocytes and monocytes; these microscopic foci of demyelination may coalesce, forming macroscopic plaques with the inflammatory cells being seen at the interface of the plaque with normal surrounding tissue (Fig. 8-4 and 8-5). Within the plaque, the oligodendrocytes are destroyed, reactive astrogliosis and macrophage infiltration ensue, and the axons passing through the plaque are spared to some degree, but axonal loss is increasingly being recognized in the pathogenesis of MS. New, active plaques tend to be pink with faint borders grossly, and microscopically exhibit an intense inflammatory response. Old, inactive plaques are gray and firm, are sharply demarcated, and have a gliotic background traversed by axons but are devoid of oligodendrocytes. Sometimes, the border between plaque and surrounding normal tissue is indistinct, shading gradually from abnormal to normal; such border areas are known as shadow plaques and are areas of partial demyelination (and possibly remyelination). Relapses of MS coincide with reduction in circulating suppresser lymphocytes (T5/8); and within active plaques, helper T4 lymphocytes are seen at the expanding border of the lesion, whereas T5/8's are seen in the central portion. Important MS variants include Devic's disease (neuromyelitis optica/optic system and spinal cord demyelination) and Balo's disease (concentric sclerosis) (Fig. 8-6 through 8-11).

The cause of MS is unknown, but any hypothesis regarding the disease must account for the epidemiological observations that MS occurs at a higher rate at higher latitudes and that an individual's latitude-related risk becomes fixed by adolescence. These observations suggest an early exposure to the etiologic agent. Family clustering suggests a common exposure and/or familial

---

Idiopathic Central Demyelinating Disease

Multiple sclerosis
- **Gross neuropathology**
  - **Plaques may occur anywhere there is myelin**
    - **Periventricular, subpial, junctional**
  - **Well defined, clearly demarcated, gelatinous**
  - **Grey due to loss of lipid in myelin**
  - **May be symmetrical**
  - **Acute plaque may be pink**

FIGURE 8-3. The most common CNS disorder is multiple sclerosis.

Idiopathic Demyelinating Disease

Multiple sclerosis
- **Microscopic neuropathology**
  - **Perivascular lymphocytic infiltrate**
  - **Loss of oligodendroglia**
  - **Myelin sheath stripping**
  - **Macrophage infiltration**
  - **Astrogliosis**
  - **Relative sparing of axons**

FIGURE 8-4. Multiple sclerosis is the most common idiopathic central demyelinating disease.

Multiple Sclerosis Pathology

- **Demyelination**
- **Infiltration by polyclonal mature lymphocytes**
- **Angiocentric infiltration**
- **Macrophage infiltration to carry off debris**
- **Gliosis**
- **Creutzfeldt astrocyte very suggestive**

FIGURE 8-5. Microscopic histopathology of multiple sclerosis.

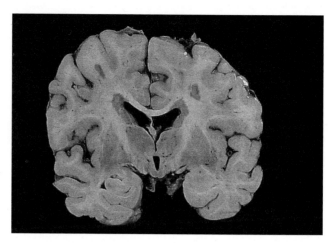

FIGURE 8-6. Multiple sclerosis with periventricular plaques appearing grey due to loss of myelin.

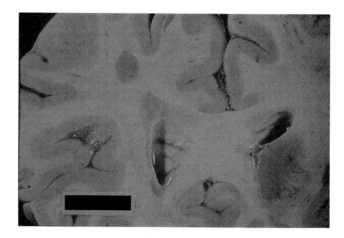

FIGURE 8-7. Multiple sclerosis with periventricular plaques appearing grey due to loss of myelin coupled with a plaque in the centrum semiovale.

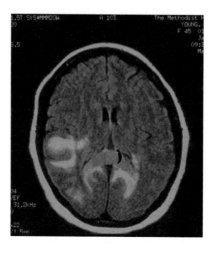

FIGURE 8-8. MRI showing multiple irregular white matter signal abnormalities compatible with either multiple sclerosis or post-infectious leukoencephalitis.

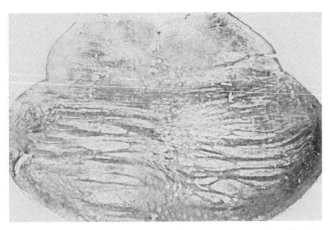

FIGURE 8-9. Normal appearance of the pons when viewed without myelin stains.

predisposition. Infectious agents have been carefully sought, and to date, no definite agent has been identified. MS is best regarded as an autoimmune disease in which the oligodendroglia are the target. HLA A3, B7, and DW2 are over-represented in MS populations.

The diagnosis of the disease rests on clinical evidence of neurological symptoms disseminated in time and space. There are no definitive laboratory studies, although reduced central conduction velocities as measured by evoked responses (indicating demyelination) and cerebrospinal fluid (CSF) findings, including elevated lymphocytes, increased protein, the presence of oligoclonal bands (oligoclonal IgG in the CSF), and the presence of MBP from the breakdown of myelin, all support the diagnosis. None of these laboratory abnormalities is diagnostic of MS as they may occur in other conditions. Magnetic resonance imaging (MRI) is extremely valuable for detecting lesions proving multisite involvement and has proven extremely valuable in showing the nearly continuous ebb and flow of plaque development and involution (often asymptomatic) in patients with MS.

Acute disseminated encephalomyelitis is a set of disorders differing only in severity characterized by an immune-mediated, monophasic, attack on central

---

Multiple Sclerosis Variants

- **Classic MS (Charcot)**
- **Acute MS (Marburg)**
- **Neuromyelitis optica (Devic's disease)**
- **Concentric sclerosis (Balo's)**

FIGURE 8-11. There are several variants of multiple sclerosis that are regarded by some as separate unique diseases.

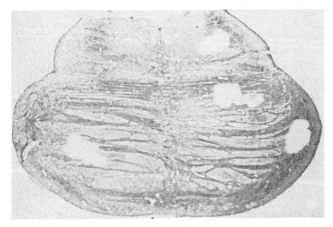

FIGURE 8-10. Several demyelinating plaques can now be seen in the pons when a myelin stain is used. Note that the plaques do not follow a vascular or functional territory.

Post-Infectious Demyelination

- Acute disseminated encephalomyelitis
  - Monophasic T-cell mediated hypersensitivity
  - Perivenular lymphocytes
  - Marked swelling
  - Scattered small foci of hemorrhage
- Acute hemorrhagic leukoencephalopathy
  - Hyperacute ADE
  - Swelling with multiple hemorrhages

FIGURE 8-12. Post-infectious demyelinating diseases.

Infectious Demyelination

Progressive multifocal leukoencephalopathy (PML)

- Glial infection by JC virus (DNA virus)
- Oligodendroglia
  - Large intranuclear viral inclusions (ground glass nuclei)
  - Oligodendroglial cytolysis and myelin destruction
- Astroglia
  - Large bizarre nuclei
  - Pleomorphic cytoplasm

FIGURE 8-13. If the oligodendrocyte is infected by the JC virus, progressive multifocal leukoencephalopathy ensues.

myelin (Fig. 8-12). The disease follows exposure to antigen either as a viral infection or by vaccination; symptoms usually develop within days of the exposure with headache, neck stiffness, lethargy, coma, and death in a substantial number of patients. Survivors may be severely impaired. It is believed that the inciting antigen and myelin share common antigenic sites, so, as the foreign antigen comes under attack, so also does the myelin. Examination of the brain shows multiple foci of perivenular demyelination with lymphocytic cuffing and axonal preservation. The terms "acute disseminated encephalomyelitis" or "postinfectious/postvaccinal encephalomyelitis" are used to describe this milder form of the disease; if focal hemorrhage and necrosis is seen, then the term "acute necrotizing hemorrhagic leukoencephalitis" is used.

Progressive multifocal leukoencephalopathy (PML) is a papovavirus (JC virus) induced demyelinating disease predominantly in immunocompromised hosts (indicator disease for AIDS) (Fig. 8-13). Intranuclear inclusions with virions are present in oligodendroglia, and in areas of demyelination, reactive astrocytes have large bizarre nuclei and cytoplasm. The JC virus is a DNA virus that is symbiotic with immunocompetent individuals residing in the bone marrow and secreted in the urine. Up to 40% of the general population is seropositive for this virus, which produces disease only in the immunocompromised person in whom spread to the CNS occurs. There is presently no effective therapy for this infection, but immunological reconstitution may permit host control of the disease. The virus is oncogenic in rodents, producing astrocytomas; the bizarre morphology of astrocytes in human infections suggests anomalous growth control and rare instances of coexisting PML and astrocytoma have been reported. (These reports are too few to really substantiate the hypothesis that JC virus is oncogenic in humans.) Please note that the letters JC are the initials of the first patient with PML and have nothing to do with Jakob–Creutzfeldt disease, as is erroneously stated in several textbooks!

In addition to demyelination from autoimmune, osmotic, and infectious causes, demyelination can result from exposure to a variety of toxins (Fig. 8-14 and 8-15).

DISORDERS OF PERIPHERAL MYELIN

Prototypical Disorders of Peripheral Myelin

Inflammatory: Guillain–Barré syndrome
Infectious: Rabies, diphtheria
Hereditary demyelinating neuropathies: Charcot–Marie–Tooth

Acute idiopathic polyneuritis (Guillain–Barré syndrome) is similar to perivenous encephalomyelitis in that it tends to follow viral infections or vaccinations, but the immune-mediated demyelination is confined to the peripheral nervous system. Antecedent antigen exposure can be documented in only about 50% of cases. Patients develop weakness with minimal or no sensory symptoms; the weakness is mild initially and may be so subtle that the patient's complaints are attributed to malingering, but progression to profound weakness with involvement of the respiratory muscles may occur within hours to days. Patients have died at home and on hospital wards from respiratory insufficiency in cases where the diagnosis was not suspected or the tempo of progression underestimated. Patients suspected of having early Guillain–Barré should be hospitalized, preferably in the intensive care unit or respiratory care unit. Use of plasmapheresis early in the course may reduce the severity and duration of symptoms. Early symptoms include mild weakness and loss of distal deep tendon reflexes. The weakness may commence in the lower extremities and then spread to involve the trunk and arms, hence the term "ascending paralysis" often applied to this condition. Nerve conduction velocities are reduced, and CSF examination discloses marked protein elevation with relatively few cells (both of these studies may be normal early in the disease) (Fig. 8-16). Patients tend to recover almost completely in the weeks to months following the illness. Pathologically, the condition is characterized by focal accumulations of lymphocytes and macrophages throughout the peripheral nerves. The myelin lamellae are split and digested by the macrophages, leaving the Schwann cells and axons intact; remyelination and functional recovery then ensue. Uncommonly, the disease may assume a recurring or progressive form. With repeated bouts of demyelination and remyelination of peripheral nerves, concentric arrays of Schwann cells and collagen surround individual axons; this ineffectual thickening of the myelin sheath is referred to as "onion-bulbing." This may be seen in recurrent acquired demyelinating disorders as well as the hereditary hypertrophic neuropathies (Dejerine-Sottas sensory neuropathy and the hypertrophic form of Charcot-Marie-Tooth neuropathy) and Refsum's disease. A less common axonal form of fulminant Guillain–Barré occurs in association with *Campylobacter jejuni* infection.

Paralytic rabies accounts for 10–20% of cases of rabies and may initially mimic Guillain–Barré by presenting with ascending, demyelinative neuropathy; the situation may become clear as encephalitis ensues.

Diphtheria pharyngitis results from *Corynebacterium diphtheriae* infection. The organism may elaborate an exotoxin that impairs protein synthesis in Schwann cells leading to a predominantly cranial demyelinating neuropathy in the weeks following the primary infection.

The hereditary demyelinating neuropathies are characterized by continuous demyelination with remyelination. The Schwann cells in a futile attempt at construction of compact myelin, encircle the axon but are separated by extracellular matrix, resulting in grossly apparent thickening of the peripheral nerves. The concentrically arrayed Schwann cells can be viewed by electron microscopy or high magnification light microscopy in plastic embedded sections, and in a vegetable analogy used so frequently in pathology, are said to exhibit "onion-bulbing" (Figs. 8-17 and 8-18).

Acquired Metabolic Demyelination

- Central pontine myelinolysis (CPM)
  - rapid correction of hyponatremia (8 mEq/L/day x 5 d)
  - 40% may not have hx of hyponatremia
- Multifocal necrotizing leukoencephalopathy (MNL)
- Marchiafava-Bignami disease

Osmotic demyelination syndromes or osmotic myelinolysis

FIGURE 8-14. Central demyelination can result from systemic metabolic derangements such as hyponatremia.

Toxic Demyelination

- Irradiation damage: white matter necrosis
- Triethyltin
- Hexachlorophene
- Cyclosporin
- Amphotericin

FIGURE 8-15. Central demyelination can also be the consequence of irradiation or toxic effects of compounds.

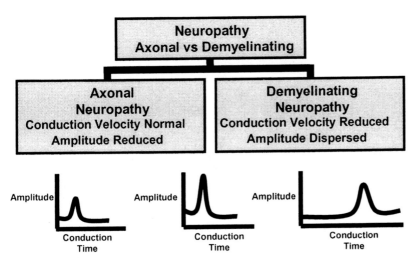

FIGURE 8-16. Peripheral demyelination results in a neuropathy with dramatically reduced nerve conduction velocities in contrast to axonal neuropathies where conduction velocity is preserved but amplitude is diminished.

Onion Bulb Formation in Demyelinating Neuropathy
Repeated Demyelination & Remyelination

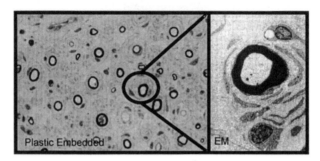

Image Courtesy of Dr. Hannes Vogel, BCM Neuropathology

FIGURE 8-17. Hereditary dysmyelination of the peripheral nerve in Charcot-Marie-Tooth disease leading to "onion-bulbing" from repeated bouts of demyelination and remyelination. In the electron micrograph on the right, the Schwann cells surround the axon in concentric layers. Onion bulbing can be seen in any condition with demyelination and remyelination such as chronic relapsing inflammatory polyneuropathy.

INBORN ERRORS OF MYELIN AFFECT BOTH CENTRAL AND PERIPHERAL MYELIN

Leukodystrophies

Leukodystrophies are hereditary disorders of myelin metabolism that tend to present in childhood, although adult forms are being increasingly recognized (Fig. 8-19 through 8-21). These diseases always involve central myelin and in several diseases, peripheral myelin is involved as well. These are also known as the dysmyelinating disorders. Biopsy is rarely indicated, and is usually done when these disorders are mistaken for neoplastic diseases. The leukodystrophies are not inflammatory disorders, but are included here to complete the discussion of diseases of myelin. There is an inflammatory component to some of these disorders, including Krabbe's disease, in which multinucleate giant

---

Leukodystrophies

- Metachromatic leukodystrophy
- Krabbe's globoid cell leukodystrophy
- Adrenoleukodystrophy
- Alexander's disease
- Canavan's disease

FIGURE 8-19. The major leukodystrophies.

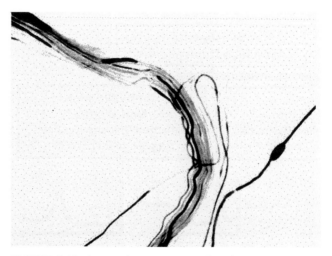

FIGURE 8-18. A teased nerve preparation showing a tomaculum—a sausage-like swelling—of the myelin around an axon. Tomaculous neuropathy predisposes to pressure palsies and results from triplication of the Charcot-Marie-Tooth gene.

cells are present, and adrenoleukodystrophy, where considerable white matter inflammation can be seen leading to contrast enhancement and the potential for this disorder being mistaken for a tumor.

Metachromatic leukodystrophy is an autosomal recessive deficiency of aryl-sulfatase A (cerebroside sulfatase) leading to the accumulation of galactosyl-3-sulfidate. The term "metachromatic" derives from the observation that tissue stained with cresyl violet is brown rather than the normal violet tint. The material is seen in neurons, macrophages, Schwann cells, and the free tissue spaces as well as in extraneural tissues. The brain on coronal sections shows shrunken, yellow, white matter with sparing of the subcortical myelin. The disease usually has its onset clinically in the first 4 years of life with progressive motor impairment, mental deterioration, and peripheral neuropathy. The diagnosis is made by measuring urinary arylsulfatase A activity which is diminished or absent in the disease. Peripheral nerve biopsy may show myelin breakdown and sulfatide accumulation but is rarely indicated (Fig. 8-22).

Krabbe's disease is an autosomal recessive deficiency of galactocerebroside β-galactosidase leading to accumulation of galactocerebroside. The gross appearance is like metachromatic leukodystrophy (MLD), but microscopically, metachromasia is absent, and instead, large, multinucleate histiocytic cells (globoid cells) are seen in addition to demyelination (Fig. 8-23). The peripheral nervous system is less involved than in MLD. Symptoms begin in early infancy, and death occurs within a year.

Adrenoleukodystrophy/adrenomyeloneuropathy is an X-linked recessive disorder with central and peripheral demyelination and adrenal insufficiency. In younger patients the central involvement is more marked and the term "adrenoleukodystrophy" is applied to this relentless, lethal disorder. The parieto-occipital demyelination with contrast enhancement may lead to the clinical misdiagnosis of glioma. The adult form tends to involve the spinal cord and peripheral nerves, hence the term "adrenomyeloneuropathy." Transitional forms have been seen, and both disorders have been seen in the same unlucky families implicating a common biochemical basis. Female carriers (heterozygotes) are particularly likely to exhibit the adult form of the disorder. These patients have elevated plasma long chain fatty acid esters, and they are unable to β-oxidize long-chain fatty acids in peroxisomes. This is not due to deficiency of peroxisomal acyl coenzyme A synthetase, as was originally be-

Leukodystrophies According to Cellular Derangement

- **Lysosomal disorders**
  - Metachromatic leukodystrophy
  - Krabbe leukodystrophy
- **Peroxisomal disorder**
  - Adrenoleukodystrophy
- **Mitochondrial disorder**
  - Canavan's disease
- **Cytoskeletal disorder**
  - Alexander's disease

FIGURE 8-20. Leukodystrophies can be classified according to affected cellular organelle.

Morphology of Leukodystrophies

Disorder	Feature
Krabbe's disease	Globoid cells
Metachromatic leukodystrophy	Metachromasia
Canavan's disease	Spongiform white matter
Alexander's disease	Rosenthal fibers

FIGURE 8-21. Morphology of the leukodystrophies.

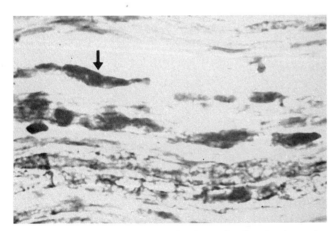

FIGURE 8-22. Metachromatic leukodystrophy showing irregular globular accumulations of abnormal myelin breakdown products that show a spectral shift (metachromasia) when stained with cresyl violet or toluidine blue.

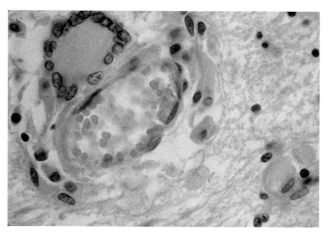

FIGURE 8-23. Krabbe's disease showing a multinucleated giant cell (globoid cell) most commonly seen in the perivascular regions of the white matter.

lieved, but results from a defect in a 70-Kd peroxisomal membrane protein (PMP), which imports acyl coenzyme A synthetase into the peroxisome.

Canavan's disease (spongiform leukodystrophy; spongy degeneration of the white matter; Canavan–Van Bogaert–Bertrand disease) is an autosomal recessive disorder with onset in infancy manifesting with megacephaly, hypotonia, developmental delay then regression. Spasticity may develop late in the illness. This disorder is associated with a point mutation of aspartylacylase leading to elevated urinary and CSF *N*-acetyl-aspartic acid (NAA). The CNS white matter bears the brunt of the disease with no peripheral nerve involvement (Fig. 8-24).

Alexander's disease is a leukodystrophy that is appropriately regarded as a disorder of astrocytes in view of prominent Rosenthal fibers around blood vessels in the white matter (Fig. 8-25). This disorder presents with megacephaly with developmental regression, seizures, and spasticity in the infantile form. Adult forms clinically resembling MS have been rarely seen. The infantile form of this disorder results from mutations of the glial fibrillary acidic protein (GFAP) gene on chromosome 17.

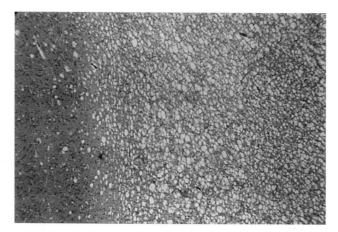

FIGURE 8-24. Canavan's disease showing bubbly spongiform change in the white matter. This appearance results in this condition sometimes being called "spongiform leukodystrophy."

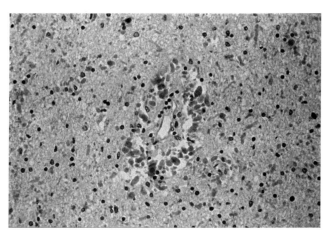

FIGURE 8-25. Alexander's disease is characterized by incredibly abundant perivascular and subpial Rosenthal fibers.

Pelizaeus–Merzbacher disease is a rare, X-linked, recessive disorder with onset in infancy with nystagmus, ataxia, and myoclonic seizures and death occurring within 3 years. "Tigroid" pattern of demyelination is seen. Point mutations of the proteolipid protein (PLP) gene have been described leading to defective myelin maturation and maintenance. This protein constitutes about 50% of central myelin proteins and less than 1% of peripheral myelin, hence the dominance of central symptoms.

BRAIN BIOPSY IN DEMYELINATING DISORDERS

Brain biopsy is not normally used in the diagnostic evaluation of patients with demyelinating disorders. Demyelinating lesions may, however, be biopsied due to imaging features or clinical manifestations mimicking neoplastic conditions (Figs. 8-26 through 8-28). The following demyelinating diseases are particularly likely to lead to biopsy:

Acute MS plaque with intense imaging enhancement, edema, rapid clinical progression, and no previous history of MS may be mistaken for tumor.

Adrenoleukodystrophy leads to strikingly asymmetrical enhancing demyelination in the parietal and occipital lobes with involvement of the corpus callosum. This may lead to the misimpression of glioblastoma multiforme (butterfly spread) of this region.

Large focal tumor-like areas of demyelination have been described in patients with MS or as the sole manifestation of acute disseminated encephalomyelitis. These lesions are extremely worrisome on imaging and mimic either intrinsic gliomas or metastases. They may be cystic and though they are usually solitary they may be multiple. They respond well to corticosteroids and are compatible with protracted survival. Some have unfortunately been mistaken for tumors and treated with irradiation therapy. These lesions often have a rim of enhancement that has a break or discontinuity leading to a C-shaped pattern of enhancement that can be extremely useful in distinguishing this lesion on neuroimaging from neoplasm or abscess, both of which tend to have continuous rims of enhancement.

The gliosis and lymphocyte infiltration seen in demyelination can even mimic tumor histologically, but the most significant indication that the process is nonneoplastic is the presence of abundant macrophages often containing lipid. Extreme caution is indicated in diagnosing neoplasm in the presence of macrophages.

Demyelinating Disorders Mimicking Tumor

- Active plaques can enhance and exert mass effect

- Parietal-occipital demyelination in ADL can enhance and be mistaken for posterior butterfly GBM

- Large focal tumor-like demyelinating plaques of Kepes

FIGURE 8-26. Demyelinating disease can be mistaken for tumor leading to therapeutic misadventures.

PCNSL Mimicking M!

- Steroid responsive
- Steroids may lyse tumor cells ing gliosis and reactive lymph cytes and macrophages
- Multifocality of PCNSL leads dissemination in space

FIGURE 8-27. Primary CNS lymphoma is notorious for mimicking multiple sclerosis.

Lesions That May Mimic Demyelinating Disease

- Infarct during subacute phase with macrophage infiltration and gliosis
- Acute encephalitis
- Primary CNS lymphoma

FIGURE 8-28. There are some conditions which may mimic multiple sclerosis.

Brain or nerve biopsy in the leukodystrophies have been replaced by molecular genetic and biochemical assays. This diagnostic category, however, must be borne in mind in patients with progressive cognitive and motor decline, and these diseases are occasionally encountered on biopsy.

BIBLIOGRAPHY

Kepes J. J. Large focal tumor-like demyelinating lesions of the brain: intermediate entity between multiple sclerosis and acute disseminated encephalomyelitis? A study of 31 patients. Ann. Neurol. 33:18–27 1993.

9

INFECTIOUS DISEASES

PERSPECTIVE

1. Many of the infections of the nervous system are devastating or lethal if untreated. The clinical course may be swift and ferocious, or indolent and progressive, and can mimic many other disorders. You must be vigilant and complete in your diagnostic evaluation, and emphatic in your therapeutic response.
2. The clinical context of infections of the nervous system is crucial. The patient's age, socioeconomic situation, sexual behavior, immune status, and travel history are very important in assessing CNS infections. AIDS, iatrogenic immunocompromise, economic stagnation, and trans-global travel and immigration have changed the face of infectious diseases in the past decade.

OBJECTIVES

1. Learn the clinical features of meningitis, which organisms produce meningitis at different ages, and the fact that the clinical features of meningitis change with age.
2. Understand the value of the cerebrospinal fluid (CSF) examination in infections.
3. Learn about granulomatous meningitis, the causative organisms, the clinical courses of these illnesses.
4. Describe the evolution and final gross and microscopic features of brain abscesses.
5. Learn about the major viral infections of the CNS, including herpes simplex, arbovirus, rabies, poliomyelitis, and HIV.
6. Name and discuss the nervous system manifestations of AIDS.
7. Understand *Toxoplasmosis gondii* infections of the brain, and know that these infections are usually opportunistic.
8. Understand the neurological diseases associated with prions and their modes of transmission. Know what precautions should be taken in handling prion-infected tissues.

Infections can affect different compartments of the nervous system leading to varied clinical and pathological manifestations. Furthermore, some organisms are predisposed to invade particular regions of the nervous system. The site and nature of the inflammatory reaction leads to several different names used to describe these infections. These are the basic definitions:

Meningitis: Purulent exudate in the subarachnoid space; parenchymal involvement may follow with cerebral edema, vasculitis with thrombosis or hemorrhage and infarction, and cerebritis. Long-term complications can include effusions and obstruction of CSF flow with hydrocephalus.

Empyema: Pocket of pus in epidural or subdural space usually related to trauma or spread from contiguous infection in sinuses or ear.

Cerebritis: Purulent parenchymal infection which is usually bacterial; the tissue is soft and soupy and the borders of the infection cannot be easily discerned.

Brain abscess is formed when cerebritis is walled off; many polymorphonuclear cells within necrotic core surrounded by a dense fibrovascular capsule and gliotic rind.

Encephalitis: Parenchymal infection, usually viral; with necrosis, perivascular lymphocytic cuffing, microglial nodules or stars; intranuclear or cytoplasmic inclusions may be seen, as may gliosis, demyelination, status spongiosus.

BACTERIAL INFECTIONS

Empyema is a localized collection of purulent material most commonly resulting from extension of a bacterial infection from the skull (osteomyelitis) or an infected sinus (sinusitis or mastoiditis) (Fig. 9-1). Such infections may complicate head injury with skull fractures as well as neurosurgical craniotomy sites.

The bacterial agents causing meningitis vary as a function of patient age. In the neonate (age of less than 2 months), the organisms of primary concern are Group B Streptococcus and *Escherichia coli*, but *Listeria monocytogenes* must be borne in mind. In infants and small children 3 months to 3 years of age, the organisms are *Haemophilus influenzae, Streptococcus pneumonia,* and *Neisseria meningitidis.* The introduction of the *H. influenzae* vaccine has resulted in a remarkable reduction in meningitis caused by this organism; therefore, the classical organisms in meningitis in childhood are not seen as frequently, and when a case of bacterial meningitis is encountered, one must consider other organisms. In patients 3 years of age or older, the common organisms are *Streptococcus pneumoniae* and *N. meningitidis.* In the elderly, *Streptococcus pneumoniae* and Gram-negative organisms are the major causes of bacterial meningitis. Polymorphonuclear cells predominate in the CSF, although early in the disease or in partially treated meningitis, lymphocytes may domi-

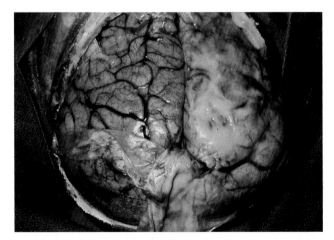

FIGURE 9-1. Empyema is a localized collection of purulent material on the surface of the brain.

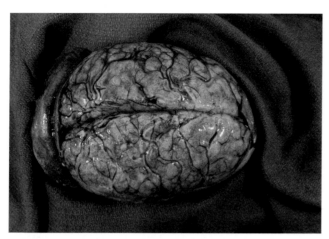

FIGURE 9-2. Gross appearance of bacterial meningitis with clouding of the leptomeninges over the cerebral convexities.

nate. Organisms can sometimes be seen on Gram stains of the CSF. Bacterial antigens can be rapidly detected, permitting very rapid diagnosis, and cultures are usually promptly positive unless the patient has been partially treated or the organism is unusual. There are no reliable specific gross or microscopic features other than identification of the organism in sections that permit differentiation of the bacterial meningitis on pathological grounds alone. Grossly, bacterial meningitis is characterized by purulent material in the subarachnoid space (Fig. 9-2 through 9-5).

A very fundamental question remains: Is it the presence of the organisms themselves that is so destructive, or is it the inflammatory reaction they incite? Evidence is compelling that the polymorphonuclear cells recruited to the infection induce damage to the surrounding parenchyma by the release of cytotoxic free radicals and recent microdialysis studies have shown that the excitatory amino acids are also released into the brains of animals with experimental bacterial meningitis. If free radicals are quenched with free radical scavenging drugs or excitotoxicity is blocked by the use of NMDS receptor blockers, the tissue injury in animals is reduced despite the fact that increased numbers of bacteria are present (since the polymorphonuclear cells are no longer effective in killing the organisms). While it is obviously essential to eliminate the or-

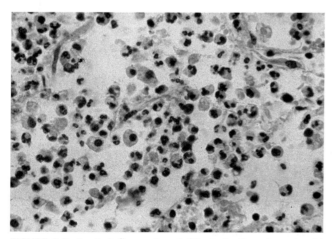

FIGURE 9-3. Acute inflammatory infiltrate in the subarachnoid space in bacterial meningitis.

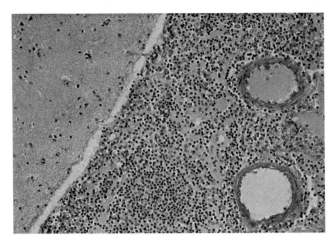

FIGURE 9-4. Vessels in the subarachnoid space in bacterial meningitis may become inflamed and thickened leading to infarcts in their territories.

Bacterial Meningitis

- Neonate   Group B Strep, E. coli, Listeria

- Childhood   Meningococcus, pneumococcus

- Adolescence Meningococcus

- Adult   Pneumococcus

- H. influenza has dramatically declined due to vaccine.

FIGURE 9-5. Organisms responsible for bacterial meningitis vary according to the patient's age.

ganisms using antimicrobials, we must remain mindful of the damage wrought by the host reaction to the bacteria.

Bacterial brain abscesses are multiple in 15% of cases, occur at the gray-white junction similar to metastases, and are produced by multiple microaerophilic organisms ("sterile" if cultures are not handled properly for anaerobic culture). Consider Staphylococcus if there are multiple hemorrhagic abscesses and the course is fulminant. Cerebritis precedes the walling off which forms an abscess; in cerebritis there is intense gliosis and a dense polymorphonuclear infiltrate. Fibroblasts and proliferating blood vessels form the wall of the abscess. In the parenchyma adjacent to the abscess wall there is marked reactive gliosis and edema. Extreme cellularity and vascularity of the abscess wall may look like tumor both radiographically and pathologically (Figs. 9-6 and 9-7). Fungal and toxoplasmosis abscesses are increasingly common and will be discussed below.

GRANULOMATOUS INFECTIONS AND INFLAMMATORY CONDITIONS

Granulomatous inflammatory conditions are characterized by multinucleate giant cells (epithelioid syncytial macrophages) often accompanied by lympho-

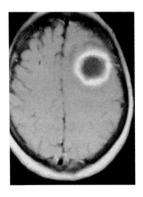

FIGURE 9-6. Magnetic resonance imaging of a bacterial abscess showing a smooth-walled ring enhancing lesion.

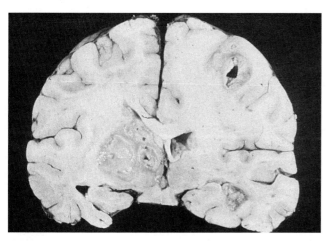

FIGURE 9-7. Bacterial brain abscesses are composed of a centrally necrotic core, a tough fibrovascular rind, and rim of gliosis. They may be multiple in up to 15% of cases.

cytes and plasma cells (Fig. 9-8). These conditions are more chronic in their clinical and pathologic courses than the more acute bacterial infections discussed above. Granulomatous infections are classically produced by mycobacteria, fungi and spirochetes, but granulomatous inflammation can also occur idiopathically in sarcoidosis involving the CNS or in response to foreign material. These infections produce inflammatory exudates at the base of the brain rather than over the convexities as is seen in bacterial meningitis. The basilar location of the inflammation leads to cranial neuropathies and obstruction of CSF flow from the fourth ventricle with resultant hydrocephalus. Parenchymal involvement takes the form of granulomata that can mimic multiple neoplasms on imaging.

Tuberculosis (Mycobacterium tuberculosis) produces caseating granulomata along vessels in the meninges, and in the brain parenchyma. Granulomata consist of caseating necrosis with multinucleate giant cells accompanied by lymphocytes and plasma cells. Tissue granulomata rupture into CSF to produce meningitis. Vessel wall thickening and arterial occlusion lead to cranial nerve palsies and stroke; subarachnoid basal fibrosis may also lead to cranial

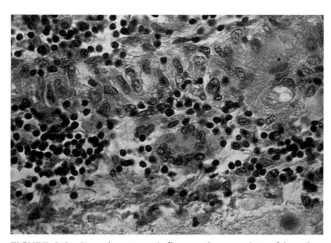

FIGURE 9-8. Granulomatous inflammation consists of lymphocytes, plasma cells and the multinucleated giant cell that gives this form of inflammation its name.

nerve palsies and communicating hydrocephalus. Tuberculoma is a very common CNS mass in areas where TB is common; in children, tuberculomas are more common in the posterior fossa where they mimic tumors. Pott's disease is TB of the vertebral body and may produce gibbus deformity of the spine. If one sees plasma cells in CSF, consider TB. Systemic *M. avium–intracellulare* is increasingly seen in AIDS and other immunocompromised patients, but MAI meningitis remains very rare, and in most instances *M. tuberculosis* is the causative organism of tuberculous meningitis. Mycobacterial infections can now be diagnosed using polymerase chain reaction (PCR) of CSF or tissue—a procedure that is clearly advantageous since cultures often take several weeks for positive growth.

Sarcoidosis produces noncaseating granulomata at the base of the brain producing cranial nerve palsies and hypothalamic dysfunction and may mimic TB; rarely but sometimes occurs in absence of systemic sarcoidosis.

Neurosyphilis produces meningovascular and parenchymatous involvement, which may coexist. Chronic leptomeningeal inflammation with lymphocytes and plasma cells with spinal arachnoiditis and meningeal thickening are common. The inflammation may involve blood vessels to produce endarteritis obliterans (Heubner's arteritis) leading to infarcts in the supplied territories. Many of the classical eponymic brainstem stroke syndromes resulted from neurosyphilis. The dorsal root entry zones (zones of Hitzig) of the spinal cord may undergo degeneration with ascending degeneration of the dorsal columns leading to tabes dorsalis. In the cerebral cortex, there is marked microglial proliferation ("rod cells") with iron deposition (Perl's stain for Fe). The inciting treponemes themselves may be seen with silver stains. Neurosyphilis pursues a more virulent course and may be less responsive to therapy in AIDS patients.

FUNGAL INFECTIONS

Fungi exist as yeast forms or hyphae or a combination (Fig. 9-9 through 9-11).

Yeast forms: Cryptococcosis, Coccidioidomycosis, Histoplasmosis, Blastomycosis
Hyphae: Mucormycosis, Aspergillosis
Hyphae and Yeast: Candida

Many of the mycotic infections of the CNS are opportunistic, reflecting the basically indolent saprophytic lifestyle of these organisms. A few fungi are sufficiently virulent, however, to produce disease in immunocompetent individuals. Fungi-invading tissue may assume either a round to oval, often budding, yeast form or a branching hyphal form, and in some infections both

Fungal Infections

- **Yeast**
  - **Cryptococcus**
  - **Coccidioidomycosis**
  - **Histoplasmosis**
  - **Blastomycosis**

- **Hyphae**
  - **Aspergillosis**
  - **Mucormycosis**

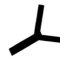

FIGURE 9-9. Fungi exist in two forms—yeast and hyphae. The fungi causing disease can sometimes be provisionally identified based on their microscopic appearance.

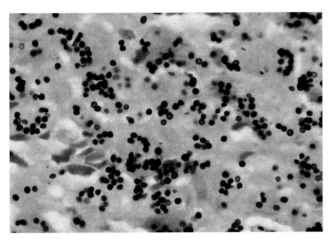

FIGURE 9-10. Yeast-form fungi appear as small, sometimes budding organisms. The Gomori methenamine silver stain highlights these organisms as black dots on a pale green background. In this example, the organism is Coccidioidomycosis.

yeast and hyphae are seen. This morphological dichotomy permits tentative identification of organisms in tissue sections although definitive identification requires antigenic, PCR, or culture confirmation (Figs. 9-12 and 9-13).

Yeast-form CNS fungal infections include the following.

Cryptococcosis is produced by budding yeast forms 4–10 μm in diameter endowed with thick carbohydrate capsules, which blunt host immune detection and response, so one may see a minimal inflammatory response in the CSF although hypoglycorrhachia and elevated protein are frequently present (Fig. 9-14). In addition to meningitis, numerous cortical and subcortical microabscesses may be present. The capsules of the organisms in aggregate impart a slimy (stewed okra) feel to the brain at gross examination. Sometimes, larger abscesses—cryptococcomas—may mimic tumors or abscesses caused by other organisms. These are common in the immunocompromised but may also occur in the immunocompetent. Cryptococcal antigen in CSF is a very

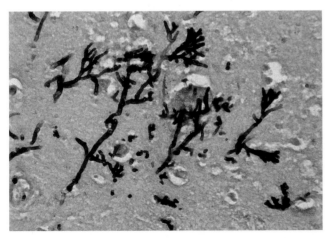

FIGURE 9-11. Hyphae are seen in fungal infections such as Aspergillosis and Phycomycosis (Mucormycosis). Pseudohyphae are also seen in Candida infections along with yeast forms of the organism.

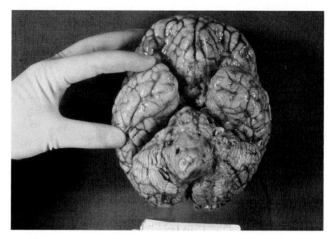

FIGURE 9-12. Granulomatous infections tend to produce an inflammatory exudate at the base of the brain. This leads to multiple cranial nerve dysfunction and obstruction of CSF egress from the fourth ventricle leading to hydrocephalus with headache.

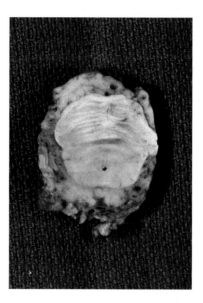

FIGURE 9-13. Granulomatous inflammation surrounding the pons in a case of fungal meningitis.

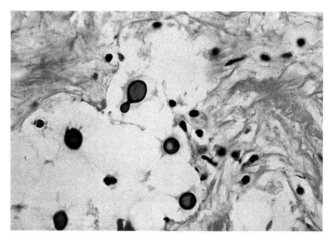

FIGURE 9-14. Cryptococcosis organisms are budding yeast forms of variable size, but are among the largest yeast forms seen. The organism has a coat which may be highlighted by the India ink preparation.

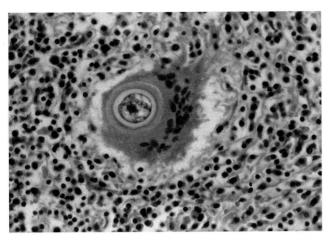

FIGURE 9-15. Coccidiomycosis produces small yeast forms as well as striking large spherules called "sporangia" or "endospores."

good diagnostic method; the India ink preparation is useful, but the novice may mistake lymphocytes for cryptococcal yeast forms.

Coccidioidomycosis is a yeast form occurring endemically in the arid regions of the Southwest and San Joaquin Valley in California (Fig. 9-15). Usually, an asymptomatic pulmonary infection occurs with uncommon dissemination. A combination of suppurative and granulomatous inflammation is seen sometimes in combination with arteritis, which may be complicated by infarction. The organism appears in tissue sections as small yeast forms accompanied by much larger spherical endospores (Fig. 9-15).

Histoplasmosis is endemic in the Mississippi basin and usually results in asymptomatic pulmonary infections, but rare CNS dissemination of this small yeast form residing in macrophages may occur. The infection may take the form of chronic meningitis or multiple granulomata. The organisms are very small (2–5 μm; smaller than an erythrocyte!) and, in contrast to other yeast forms, reside within the cytoplasm of macrophages, where they appear as multiple minute dots (Fig. 9-16). They can be seen best with periodic acid–Schiff–stained and Gomori methenamine silver–stained sections.

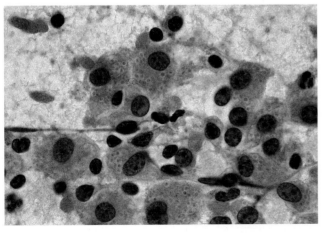

FIGURE 9-16. Histoplasmosis organisms are extremely tiny round to ovoid yeast residing within the cytoplasm of macrophages.

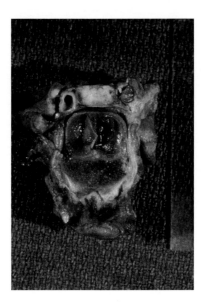

FIGURE 9-17. Mucormycosis involving the sphenoid sinus and carotid artery. The carotid artery on the right in the cavernous sinus is occluded.

Blastomycosis is an uncommon cause of mycotic meningitis. The organisms are solitary broad-based budding yeast forms that are encapsulated, resembling cryptococcus.

Hyphae are seen in the following CNS fungal infections.

Mucormycosis (Phycomycosis) is an angioinvasive, nonseptate, irregular, broad hyphal fungus commonly afflicting poorly controlled diabetics or immunocompromised patients (Figs. 9-17 through 9-20). The large vessels at the skull base, orbit, and neck are subject to invasion with distal infarction and hemorrhage. Black nasal mucosa indicating mucosal infarction is sometimes seen and can be used for diagnosis.

Aspergillosis is an angiocentric septate hyphal fungus seen predominantly in the immunocompromised host. The hyphae are narrow and more regular compared to Mucormycosis, and they branch at regular acute angles allowing provisional identification on microscopy. The angioinvasion by septate hyphae produces multiple gray necrotic abscesses within the parenchyma (Figs. 9-21 and 9-22). The lung is the primary site of infection, but the brain is the second most commonly involved organ.

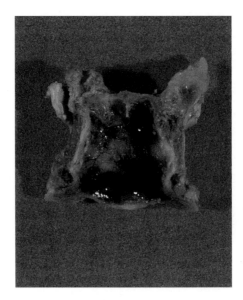

FIGURE 9-18. Respiratory mucosa in Mucormycosis showing the dark infarcted mucosa.

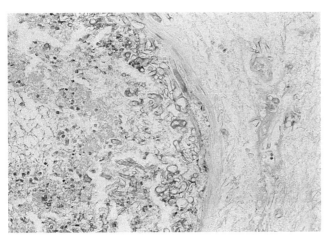

FIGURE 9-19. Mucormycosis in a blood vessel. Note the clublike hyphae branching irregularly.

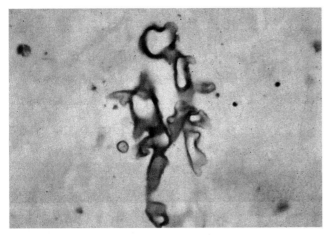

FIGURE 9-20. Mucormycosis. An irregular hyphal form.

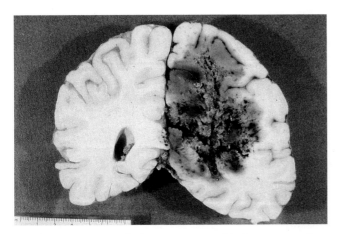

FIGURE 9-21. Aspergillosis. Gross image with shaggy necrosis.

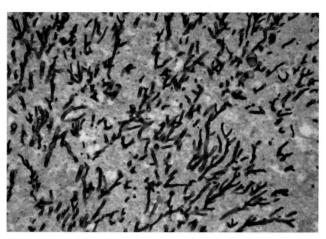

FIGURE 9-22. Aspergillosis with delicate acutely branching septate hyphae.

Candida is a ubiquitous opportunistic fungus producing both yeast and pseudohyphae; the simultaneous occurrence of these two forms is strongly suggestive of this diagnosis. The infection may be granulomatous but is more commonly acute with lymphocytes, plasma cells and polymorphonuclear cells. This infection is very common in immunocompromised patients, producing numerous microabscesses. Concurrent systemic involvement is common.

PROTOZOAN INFECTIONS

Toxoplasmosis is a ubiquitous protozoan to which most (50–100% depending on geographic location) of us have protective antibodies and cellular immunity. Immunocompromised patients lose the ability to contain the proliferation of these organisms. The major routes of exposure are fecal contamination from infected domestic cats and consumption of inadequately cooked meat contaminated by the organism. The infection can occur in the congenital form or in acquired forms in immunocompetent and immunocompromised individuals. If a nonimmune pregnant woman acquires the infection in the first or second trimester, her fetus has a significant probability of developing congenital toxoplasmosis characterized by chorioretinitis, microcephaly, and cerebral periventricular mineralization, with blindness and severe psychomotor retardation occurring as the clinical counterparts in the most severely affected. Acquisition of the infection by a mature immunocompetent individual is usually unaccompanied by symptoms but may occasionally be heralded by fever and lymphadenopathy. Reactivation of infection or new acquisition by an immunocompromised individual can, however, be devastating and in the nervous system is characterized by foci of necrotizing encephalitis with surrounding edema (Figs. 9-23 and 9-24). In tissue, small comma-like tachyzoites and large cysts (bradyzoites) are seen in association with chronic inflammation, tissue necrosis, and vasculitis. Toxoplasmosis is the single most frequent cause of multiple intracranial masses in AIDS patients and is an indicator disease of AIDS. The cysts are by far the most eye-catching microscopic feature of this infection which may also have geographic necrosis, acute and chronic inflammatory cell infiltrates, and fibrinoid necrosis of blood vessels (Fig. 9-25).

Naegleria produces primary amebic meningoencephalitis, a fulminant and rapidly fatal meningitis with diffuse brain swelling. Brain inoculation occurs via the nasal route by swimming in stagnant fresh water pools. The brain

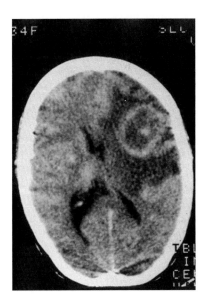

FIGURE 9-23. Magnetic resonance imaging of toxoplasmosis abscess.

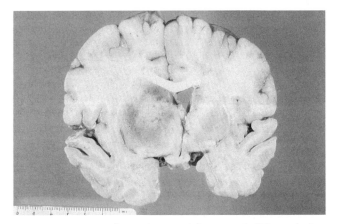

FIGURE 9-24. Toxoplasmosis necrotizing encephalitis producing a basal ganglion mass.

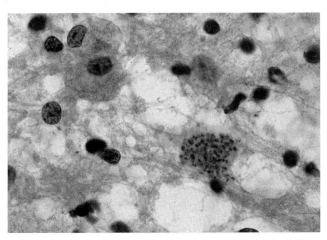

FIGURE 9-25. Toxoplasmosis with cyst form and background of inflammation.

is swollen and soft and frequently hemorrhagic, but despite the chaos wrought by the organism on the parenchyma, the leptomeninges are rarely very cloudy.

Acanthamoeba produces granulomatous amebic encephalitis, a subacute usually fatal illness characterized by multiple granulomatous abscesses usually seen in the immunocompromised host. In this setting, the primary differential diagnosis is between toxoplasmosis, bacterial abscess, primary CNS lymphoma and granulomatous amebic encephalitis.

Entamoeba histolytica leads to amebic brain abscess from spread from a gastrointestinal or hepatic locus. Amoebae in tissue sections can be difficult to distinguish from foamy macrophages.

Malaria is caused most commonly by *Plasmodium falciparum*. During attacks of cerebral malaria, CSF examination shows elevated protein and pressure, but pleocytosis is uncommon. In fatal cases, the brain is diffusely swollen and may be otherwise unremarkable, but one may see microinfarcts with gliosis (Durck's granulomata) in white matter or numerous small hemorrhages. Both the infarcts and microhemorrhages may be due to obstruction of blood flow in small vessels due to parasitemia. Severity of cerebral malaria is also related to tumor necrosis factor release from the host immune system.

VIRAL INFECTIONS

Viruses produce an astonishing range of neuropathological conditions, including banal aseptic meningitis, acute and chronic encephalitis, and demyelinating disease, and they are oncogenic in animals producing astrocytomas.

Viral CNS infections may present with *aseptic meningitis* characterized by fever, headache and lymphocytic CSF pleocytosis with mildly elevated protein and usually normal glucose. *Echovirus* and *Coxsackie* give rise to most late summer and fall aseptic meningitis. Mumps and LCM account for most aseptic meningitis in winter and early spring. Aseptic viral meningitis is usually self-limited and benign.

Parenchymal viral infection, however, is more sinister and is often manifested by headache, fever, altered mental status and seizures. Tissue destruction can occur and vigorous influx of lymphocytes and monocytes as well as activation of astrocytes are common. Foci of cellular death are often decorated by hordes of macrophages clearing out the debris; these collections are called "microglial nodules" or "microglial stars." Tissue destruction, lymphocyte infiltration, microglial and macrophage activation, and gliosis are all relatively nonspecific features of viral encephalitis (Figs. 9-26 through 9-28). They are reassuring to find on brain biopsy for this condition in that these abnormalities indicate that lesional tissue has been obtained. Some of the viral encephalitides, however, produce characteristic viral inclusions either in the nucleus or cytoplasm that allow the morphological differential diagnosis to be narrowed. The viral infections producing intranuclear neuronal viral inclusions (Cowdry A) include the herpes infections—herpes simplex, simiae and zoster, as well as other viruses producing subacute sclerosing panencephalitis (SSPE), and cytomegalovirus (Fig. 9-29). Intranuclear viral inclusions in oligodendroglia (ground glass inclusions) are seen in progressive multifocal leukoencephalopathy produced by a DNA virus (the JC virus). Finally, intracytoplasmic viral inclusions, called "Negri bodies," are seen in neurons infected with rabies.

Herpes simplex is the most common cause of sporadic, nonepidemic viral encephalitis and is characterized by destructive, hemorrhagic lesions with predilection for temporal and basal frontal lobes; Cowdry A inclusions may be

---

Viral Encephalitis Histopathology

- **Lymphocyte perivascular cuffing**
- **Microglial nodules**
- **Gliosis**
- **Necrosis**
- **Inclusions**
  - **Intranuclear**
    - **Cowdry A**
    - **Cowdry B**
    - **Ground glass**
  - **Cytoplasmic**
    - **Negri bodies**

FIGURE 9-26. Histopathology of viral encephalitis.

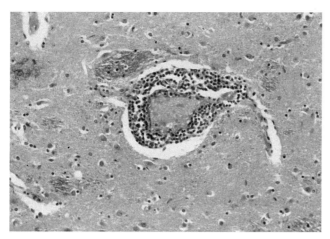

FIGURE 9-27. Lymphocytic cuffing in viral encephalitis.

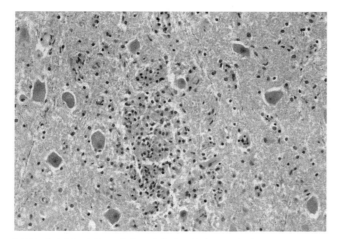

FIGURE 9-28. Microglial nodule in viral encephalitis.

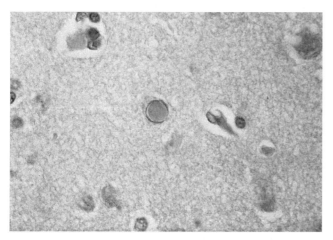

FIGURE 9-29. Cowdry A intranuclear inclusion in Herpes encephalitis.

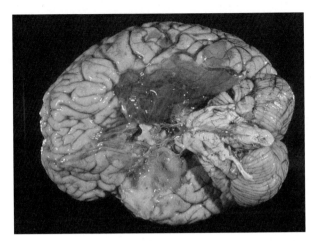

FIGURE 9-30. Asymmetrical temporal lobe damage in herpes encephalitis.

seen (Fig. 9-30). This virus is easily cultured from tissue. Therapy should not be withheld pending biopsy results in clinically suspected cases. In fact the role of brain biopsy is disputed with some arguing for empirical anti-viral therapy with the biopsy being reserved for atypical cases and to rule out other diagnostic possibilities. PCR detection of herpes genomic material in the CSF may obviate the need for biopsy. Herpes encephalitis in the newborn is a widely destructive process in contrast to its focal counterpart in the adult.

Epidemic viral encephalitis is principally caused by the *arboviruses (arthropod borne)* harbored by wild birds and transmitted by mosquitoes; eastern equine encephalitis is least common but most lethal; western equine encephalitis is next most common but rather benign; St. Louis encephalitis is most common and is particularly dangerous in elderly persons. These infections do not produce viral inclusions, and the tissue destruction is not focal, as in herpes encephalitis.

AIDS has a variety of neurological manifestations ranging from aseptic meningitis, encephalitis, opportunistic infections, immunocompromised related lymphoma, myelopathy, and myopathy (Fig. 9-31). AIDS encephalopathy (more properly known as AIDS encephalitis) is incompletely understood but common, and is characterized by gliosis, microglial nodules and foamy perivascular multinucleate macrophages; mild cortical atrophy with ventricular enlargement and myelin pallor are common gross findings (Fig. 9-32). HIV is present in the brain particularly in association with the macrophages. The neuropathological findings are subtle relative to the severity of clinical manifestations of this disorder. In children with AIDS, calcification of vessels and parenchyma of the basal ganglia is common in contrast to adults where these findings are rare. In the spinal cord one may see vacuolar myelopathy which looks similar to subacute combined degeneration. The middle and lower thoracic cord are usually most severely involved, and the white matter of the ascending posterior tracts tends to be most damaged although white matter anywhere in the spinal cord may be involved. The cause of the myelopathy is unclear, and HIV has not been consistently demonstrated in the involved regions. Opportunistic infections may coexist, especially cytomegalovirus, progressive multifocal leukoencephalopathy, and toxoplasmosis, complicating interpretation. A minority of AIDS patients develops peripheral neuropathy, but myopathy is common and may result from HIV myositis or AZT toxicity. AZT myopathy is characterized by mitochondrial abnormalities including bizarre shapes, enlargement, and paracrystalline inclusions.

CNS Indicator Diseases of AIDS

- **Toxoplasmosis**

- **Progressive multifocal leukoencephalopathy**

- **CNS Lymphoma**

FIGURE 9-31. Indicator diseases of AIDS.

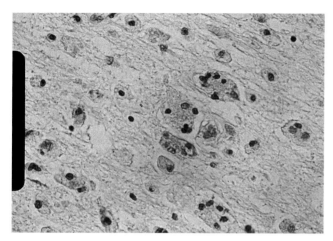

FIGURE 9-32. Multinucleated giant cells in AIDS encephalitis.

Rabies is a neuronotropic lethal infection with retrograde transport of virus to CNS from replication sites in skeletal muscle at the site of the infecting bite. The virus spreads trans-synaptically throughout the nervous system and is then transported diabolically down axons to the salivary glands in preparation for the next transmission. The transport is not, however, selective to the salivary glands but rather throughout the peripheral nervous system; therefore, viral particles can be detected in skin biopsies or corneal scrapes bearing sensory nerve terminals. In addition to nonspecific inflammatory changes, the pathognomic eosinophilic Negri bodies (intracytoplasmic intra-neuronal inclusions) are seen (Fig. 9-33). In many cases in the United States and other industrialized countries, the infecting animal bite is never identified, but skunks and bats are the largest endogenous reservoirs of this infection. The infection usually manifests as a rapidly progressive encephalitis; however, in about 15% of cases, the disease is called "dumb" rabies and is characterized by flaccid paralysis mimicking Guillain–Barré syndrome. Iatrogenic transmission has occurred with corneal transplantation. Such catastrophes (as well as the occasional iatrogenic transmission of prion diseases by the same route) have resulted in the laudable rule in transplantation medicine that patients dying of strange neurological diseases are not suitable donors.

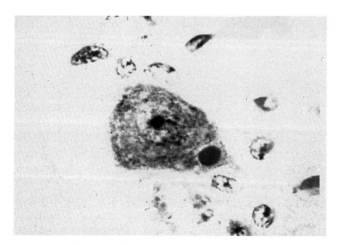

FIGURE 9-33. The Negri body of rabies is an intracytoplasmic in-traneuronal inclusion.

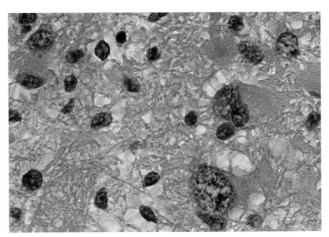

FIGURE 9-34. Histopathology of progressive multifocal leukoencephalopathy

Poliomyelitis is also neuronotropic and attacks anterior horn cells (often asymmetrically). Widespread CNS involvement is common but not invariable. Cowdry B inclusions are sometimes seen during the acute phase of the infection.

Subacute sclerosing panencephalitis (SSPE) is due to infection early in life by a replication-defective measles virus leading in a few years to a gradually progressive cognitive deterioration often accompanied by myoclonus and periodic discharges on EEG. This infection is disappearing with effective measles immunization. In the brain there is neuronal loss and marked gliosis with demyelination, Cowdry A inclusions bearing virions are seen in neurons and glia (especially oligodendroglia). CSF measles titers are high and oligoclonal bands are present.

Progressive multifocal leukoencephalopathy (PML) is a papovavirus (JC virus) induced demyelinating disease predominantly in immunocompromised hosts (indicator disease for AIDS). Intranuclear inclusions with virions are present in oligodendroglia and in areas of demyelination reactive astrocytes have large bizarre nuclei and cytoplasm (Fig. 9-34). Patchy areas of demyelination occur as the oligodendroglia fail to maintain myelin. The JC virus is oncogenic in rodents, producing astrocytomas; the bizarre morphology of astrocytes in human infections suggest anomalous growth control and rare instances of coexisting PML and astrocytoma have been reported (these reports are too few to really substantiate the hypothesis that JC virus is oncogenic in humans).

PRION DISEASES

Creutzfeldt–Jakob disease (corticostriatospinal degeneration, subacute spongiform encephalopathy; CJD) is the most common sporadic form of human prion disease. Kuru is rapidly disappearing with cultural changes among with Fore people who were once devastated by this disease transmitted by ritualistic cannibalism. Familial forms have been described and have provided unique insights into the molecular pathogenesis of this very important set of disorders. Like oncogenes, mutations of the normal cellular prion protein gene (function unknown), lead to disease. Abnormal prion protein differs from oncogene products in that the prion protein programs its own creation from normal cellular proteins.

The transmissible "agent" is a small protein designated "prion protein" (PrP^{sc}) for prion protein scrapie (scrapie being the first prion disease described—a neurodegenerative disease in sheep). There is a gene sequence on chromosome 20 for an analogue of prion protein present in normal cells designated PrPc for prion protein cellular. The function of this normal protein is not precisely known but evidence implicates a role in cellular copper homeostasis. Much like the oncogene story, it appears that mutations of the normal cellular PrPc lead to disease, and studies of familial spongiform disorders have disclosed point mutations in this gene. The sporadic forms are much more common, however, and similar point mutations have not been detected in these cases. The biologically remarkable aspect of these diseases is the fact that the abnormal protein appears to "instruct" normal protein to change so that it is functionally similar to the abnormal protein; that is, post-translational alteration of the cellular protein leads to production of more abnormal protein. The crucial molecular event appears to be the conversion of two alpha coils of the protein's secondary structure to beta-pleated sheets that facilitate polymerization of the protein. There are naturally occurring polymorphisms of the normal cellular PrPc, and some of these normal structural variants appear to be more susceptible to the "instructions" to form anomalous products than other variants. The distribution of cellular PrPc polymorphisms in a population may determine that population's risk for spongiform encephalopathies. It is possible that, like cancer, a mutation in a single cell could lead to catastrophic disease if that cell begins to produce mutant PrP which sets into motion a self-regenerating cascade of anomalous PrP production in its neighbors. Alternatively, inoculation with a minute amount of pathological PrP permits transmission from host to host. The elucidation of the molecular details of prion protein action has been one of the major scientific developments of the late 20th century (Figs. 9-35 through 9-39).

The microscopic alterations consist of spongy change in neuropil, neuronal loss, and gliosis (Figs. 9-40 and 9-41). The spongiform change is not pathognomic and similar spongy change may be seen following anoxia and in some cases of Alzheimer's disorders and diffuse Lewy body disease.

The Gerstmann–Straussler syndrome is a variant of subacute spongiform encephalopathy characterized by cerebellar ataxia, dementia, Kuru-like amyloid plaques, and spongy change. Brain biopsy is not essential in a typi-

Prion Biology

- **Normal cellular isoform PrP^c**
- **Coded on Chromosome 20**
- **Function unknown**
- **Expressed in high levels in neurons**
- **Cell surface molecule**
- **Transgenic knock-out mice normal until old age then become ataxic. These animals cannot be infected.**

FIGURE 9-35. Prion biology.

Molecular Pathology of Prions

The essential molecular event is conversion of alpha-helices of normal PrP to beta-sheets of abnormal PrP.

FIGURE 9-36. Molecular pathology of prions.

Pathologic PrP Isoforms: Prions

- **Abnormal PrP isoforms cause normal PrP secondary structure to change to abnormal isoform**
- **The abnormal isoform in turn provokes more transformation of PrP^c to PrP^{sc}**

FIGURE 9-38. Prion protein isoforms.

Pathologic PrP Isoforms: Prions

- **Hereditary spongiform encephalopathies result from mutations of PrP^c gene**
- **The resulting abnormal PrP isoforms form poorly soluble protein aggregates**
- **Fatal familial insomnia, familial CJD, and Gerstmann-Straussler-Scheinker disease arise from such mutations**

FIGURE 9-39. Pathological prion protein isoforms.

Prion Proteinopathies

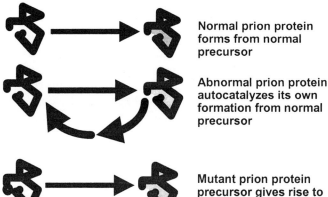

Normal prion protein forms from normal precursor

Abnormal prion protein autocatalyzes its own formation from normal precursor

Mutant prion protein precursor gives rise to abnormal prion protein

FIGURE 9-37. Molecular mechanism of prion action.

Histopathology of Prion Diseases

- Spongiform change
- Gliosis
- PrP immunoreactive plaques
- Absence of inflammation
- Changes are patchy and may be missed on biopsy

FIGURE 9-40. Histopathology of prion disorders.

Human Prion Diseases

- Kuru
- Creutzfeldt-Jakob disease
- New variant Creutzfeldt-Jakob disease
- Gerstmann-Straussler-Scheinker disease
- Fatal familial insomnia

FIGURE 9-42. The classical human prion diseases. New variant CJD has recently been added to the list of human prion diseases and represents dissemination of bovine spongiform encephalopathy to humans.

Prion Susceptibility Genetics

- There is genetic polymorphism of the normal cellular PrP gene
- PrP codon 129 may code for valine or methionine
- Homozygotes at codon 129 are more susceptible to prion diseases
- 49% of Caucasians are homozygotes

FIGURE 9-43. Prion susceptibility genetics.

Prion Disease Transmission

- Ritualistic cannibalism
- Iatrogenic
  - Dural grafts
  - Intracerebral electrodes
  - Cadaveric pituitary growth hormone
  - Corneal transplantation
- Unsuspected contact

FIGURE 9-44. Prion disease transmission.

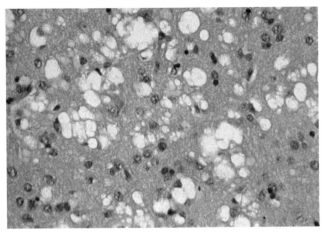

FIGURE 9-41. Spongiform change in Creutzfeldt–Jakob disease.

cal case of prion disease, and if such a procedure is contemplated, all members of the diagnostic team must be alerted to the biohazard potential. Detection of spongy change alone is not sufficient for a neuropathological diagnosis of prion disease, but must be corroborated with Western blot or immunohistochemical demonstration of abnormal prion protein. The required antibodies are not widely available, necessitating shipping of the biopsy material to one of the research facilities engaged in prion research and surveillance. If a familial prion proteinopathy is suspected, molecular genetic analysis of DNA from lymphocytes can be performed. CSF 14-3-3 protein analysis is also useful in the antemortem diagnosis of sporadic CJD. This protein is a neuronal structural protein that is elevated in a variety of CNS tissue destructive processes such as stroke or trauma, but in the appropriate clinical setting of rapidly progressive dementia, an elevated CSF 14-3-3 level has relatively high specificity and sensitivity (Figs. 9-42 through 9-44).

Iatrogenic transmission has occurred via corneal transplants, pituitary growth hormone extracts, dura implants, and depth electrode reuse (Fig. 9-45 and 9-46). The infectious protein is very robust, and is not inactivated by most conventional disinfectants. The agent is also durable; contaminated tissues retain infectivity for years. Instruments should be decontaminated with 2N sodium hydroxide, in contrast to the previous recommendation, that Clorox (sodium hypochlorite solution) be used (Figs. 9-47 and 9-48).

There is much concern about bovine spongiform encephalopathy (BSE; "mad cow disease") in Europe where the sheep prion disease scrapie apparently made a species jump following the feeding of sheep offal to cattle. Several cases of "new variant CJD" (nvCJD or vCJD) have been described in the United Kingdom and other European countries, and these cases appear to be BSE transmitted to humans. These patients were much younger than conventional CJD, had predominantly psychiatric initial symptoms, did not have periodic discharges on EEG, and had more protracted courses than usual. At autopsy, spongiform changes were mild, but "florid" PrP immunoreactive plaques were seen. Variant CJD appears to represent transmission of BSE to humans since the neuropathology of BSE in nonhuman primates is identical to that seen in these cases and molecular identity of the BSE prion and the prion in vCJD has been demonstrated (Fig. 9-49). CJD, vCJD, Gerstmann–Straussler disease, kuru, and fatal familial insomnia are the currently recognized human prion diseases.

METAZOANS

Cysticercosis (T. solium; pig tapeworm) may lead to multiple cysts up to 1 cm in the parenchyma, intraventricularly, or in the basal cisterns. Grossly and on imaging the scolex of the worm can be seen as a punctate structure asymmetrically situated in the cyst. Microscopically one may see the scolex, cuticle or internal organs of the organism. The dead organism incites a vigorous host immune response that may convert an asymptomatic infection to one characterized by headache and seizures. The structure of the deceased worm may be less easily discerned microscopically and may be calcified. Treatment with the currently available highly effective anti-cysticercosis drugs may result in a massive increase in dead worm burden leading to massive cerebral edema.

Echinococcosis (T. echinococcus or *Echinococcus granulosus*; dog tapeworm) produces cerebral cysts that are usually solitary and may be huge, in contrast to the smaller multiple cysts of cysticercosis. The brain lesion is frequently accompanied by hepatic cysts.

Trichinosis (Trichinella spiralis) usually infects skeletal and cardiac muscle producing an acute eosinophilic myositis during the invasive phase whereupon the larva may then die and calcify, producing fibrosis and low-grade inflammation. The infection may rarely encroach on the CNS, producing lymphocytic-eosinophilic aseptic meningitis.

BRAIN BIOPSY IN INFECTIOUS DISORDERS

Brain biopsy is the procedure of last resort in the diagnosis of CNS infections, but in those situations where other techniques fail to provide diagnostic information, direct acquisition of tissue may permit the kind of emphatic pathogen-directed therapy required in the management of infections. Biopsy is rarely needed in bacterial meningitis, but may be helpful in chronic fungal or mycobacterial meningitis if other diagnostic techniques fail. Parenchymal involvement by these types of organisms as well as viruses and metazoans may require biopsy if other techniques do not provide definitive information. Intraparenchymal infections leading to abscesses, cerebritis, or granulomata may mimic neoplasms and sometimes resolution of this dilemma can be obtained only with biopsy. Immunocompromised individuals fall prey to a variety of infections and neoplasms that may disguise themselves as one another, and so require direct scrutiny. Empirical treatment of brain masses in AIDS patients with anti-toxoplasmosis drugs may no longer be appropriate since more effective therapy for primary CNS lymphoma has emerged rendering such therapeutic nihilism suspect.

While the emergence of new infections and therapeutics have expanded the role of brain biopsy to some extent, the development of PCR directed molecular diagnostics of infections is curtailing some older indications and is enhancing the power of the procedure when it does become necessary (Fig. 9-50). Generally speaking, detection of infectious agent genomic material in the CSF by PCR is indicative of active CNS infection. Detection of herpes viral DNA in CSF by PCR has proven to be very sensitive and specific for this infection. This fact, as well as the safety of current anti-herpes therapy, has largely obviated the need for brain biopsy in the context of possible herpes encephalitis. Caution is warranted in interpreting viral PCR positivity in brain parenchyma as it is becoming very clear that viral latency is the norm rather than the exception for herpes and JC virus (the agent responsible for progressive multifocal leukoencephalopathy). The viral ecology of the CNS is an area of great interest and activity, and will require several years to sort out. The po-

---

Prion Disease Transmission

- **Familial**
  - Mutant PrP
- **Sporadic**
  - Unsuspected contact with abnormal PrP
  - Somatic cell mutation with propagation
- **Infectious**
  - Contact with abnormal PrP isoform

FIGURE 9-45. Prion disease transmission.

Diagnosis of Prion Diseases

- **Spongiosis and gliosis are suggestive but not specific**
- **Demonstration of abnormal PrP isoform by immunohistochemistry or Western blotting required for firm Dx**
- **Genotyping is possible on familial cases; no biopsy required**

FIGURE 9-46. Diagnosis of prion diseases.

Brain Biopsy Precautions

- **Prion precautions in all dementia cases, but especially if**
  - Rapid progression
  - Ataxia
  - Myoclonus
  - Oculomotor disturbances
- **Why are you doing the biopsy?**

FIGURE 9-47. Brain biopsy precautions.

Prion Decontamination: Surfaces and Instruments

- **Not destroyed by formalin, alcohol, halogens, UV irradiation, or gas sterilization**
- **2 N Sodium hydroxide for 1 hour**
- **Undiluted sodium hypochlorite (Clorox) for 1 hour (?)**
- **Autoclave 132 degrees Celcius at 20 PSI for at least 1 hour**

FIGURE 9-48. Prion decontamination.

Variant CJD: BSE in Humans

- Young age of onset
- Slower progression
- Initial psychiatric sx and peripheral pain then dementia
- Myoclonus and periodic EEG not seen
- "Florid" PrP plaques on histology
- Histology identical to primates inoculated with BSE

FIGURE 9-49. Variant Creutzfeldt–Jakob disease is bovine spongiform encephalopathy in humans.

PCR for Infectious Disorders

PCR + in CSF indicates active infection

PCR + in brain parenchyma may or may not indicate active infection

JC and herpes can be detected in brain of normals

FIGURE 9-50. Polymerase chain reaction can be used for diagnosis of infections of the nervous system.

Brain Biopsy: Indications

Almost always:

- Mass lesion

After exhaustive evaluation:

- Multifocal atypical process
- Diffuse process

FIGURE 9-51. Brain biopsy indications.

Stereotactic Brain Biopsy

Excellent for deep or small lesions

Tiny specimen obtained

Stereotactic approach with open biopsy good for subcortical discrete lesions

May be done under local anesthesia

FIGURE 9-52. Advantages of stereotactic brain biopsy.

tential role of viruses in neurodegenerative disorders is being revisited now that PCR techniques are available, but extreme care to use controls and avoidance of cross-contamination is absolutely essential. Nevertheless, articles are appearing implicating viruses in a variety of chronic neurological disorders (echovirus 7 in ALS, for example). Detection of fungal, mycobacterial, and protozoan genetic material in parenchyma by PCR can probably be safely viewed as indicative of infection, and detection in CSF is almost certainly indicative of active infection.

BRAIN BIOPSY IN GENERAL MEDICAL NEUROPATHOLOGY

When to Consider Brain Biopsy

Brain biopsy is an invasive and expensive diagnostic procedure associated with a small but definite risk of morbidity and mortality. This diagnostic procedure is rightfully regarded as the last resort in a diagnostic evaluation of a patient with serious neurological disease. Refinements of imaging techniques and developments in molecular diagnostics have dramatically reduced the indications for this procedure. These advances have simultaneously improved the ease, precision, and power of the brain biopsy when it does become necessary.

Patients who are candidates for brain biopsy are those with focal, multifocal, or diffuse brain disease which defies conventional complete evaluation (Fig. 9-51). Those with focal or multifocal disease often have processes in the differential diagnosis which include neoplasm, infection, vascular, or demyelinating disease. Major therapeutic decisions hinge on precise diagnosis, and sterotactic biopsy of one of the affected areas will often lead to unambiguous diagnostic information.

Patients with diffuse disease are more problematic as a discrete target for biopsy is not evident. Furthermore, these patients tend to be diagnostic dilemmas whose clinical, imaging, or laboratory data fail to fit well into a specific diagnostic category. Such patients usually present with progressive cognitive decline and/or multifocal symptoms. Imaging does not show discrete mass lesions but may be normal or demonstrate leptomeningeal thickening or enhancement, or may show parenchymal patchy signal abnormalities. The CSF examination may be abnormal, but sufficiently nonspecific that a precise diagnosis cannot be reached. Diagnostic considerations often include diffuse neoplasm or meningeal carcinomatosis, chronic infection, vasculitis, or neurodegenerative disease. The diagnostic yield is lower because the tissue acquired may not be affected with the disease, or the changes wrought may be nonspecific.

Technique

For focal disease the stereotactic biopsy is appropriate (Fig. 9-52). Under local or general anesthesia a frame is attached to the patient's head, and the geometric relationship of the frame to the lesion to be biopsied is ascertained by computed tomography (CT) or magnetic resonance imaging (MRI). Using computer-generated coordinates, the lesion is biopsied using a small cannula. Intraoperative neuropathological consultation is essential to be assured that lesional tissue has been acquired, and in some instances, a provisional diagnosis can be rendered on frozen section or cytological imprints. If an inflammatory/infections process is seen, appropriate microbiological processing can be initiated. Stereotactic biopsies are very small (usually 2 mm thick cores having a length of 8—10 mm) so that they may not be completely representative of the lesion being biopsied.

Open biopsy is more appropriate for diffuse processes because more tissue can be acquired. The procedure is usually done under general anesthesia. Dural and arachnoid biopsies can be obtained as the brain is approached, and the brain and its overlying structures can be examined for gross abnormalities. A properly done open brain biopsy yields a 10 mm long, 10 mm deep, 5 mm wide contiguous piece of cerebral cortex and underlying white matter. The right frontal lobe is usually chosen for biopsy in diffuse processes, but if there are clinical, electrophysiological, or imaging data suggestive of a focal area of more intense involvement, then this more involved area should be biopsied unless it is functionally eloquent. Intraoperative neuropathological consultation is essential for optimal handling of open brain biopsies.

A few pragmatic points should be borne in mind before performing a brain biopsy. The neurologist, neurosurgeon, neuroradiologist, and neuropathologist should discuss the case, differential diagnosis, and specimen handling prior to the biopsy. The neurosurgeon should be experienced in stereotactic brain biopsy if that technique is to be used, and the neuroradiological backup should be trustworthy. A neuropathologist should do the tissue handling and histopathological interpretation; general pathologists are rarely capable of comfortably dealing with these especially crucial specimens. The biopsy should be scheduled early in the day and preferably early in the week for optimal specimen handling. Histopathological, microbiological, and molecular diagnostic services depend on a cadre of experienced and dedicated laboratorians operating under very real fiscal and logistic restraints, and full diagnostic power of laboratory services can only be provided during normal operating hours in most institutions. Delays in processing due to late tissue acquisition may reduce diagnostic yield (Fig. 9-53 and 9-54).

RISKS

The risks associated with brain biopsy include the complications of general anesthesia, hemorrhage at the biopsy site, and development of seizures from the injury induced by the biopsy. Stereotactic biopsy under local anesthesia reduces the anesthetic risk. Patients with coagulation defects should have these abnormalities corrected prior to biopsy.

Stereotactic Brain Biopsy

Diagnosis obtained in 90% - 95%

Diagnosis in tumors approaches 100%

Diagnostic accuracy very dependent on proper sampling--go for the edge

Complications: 1% - 10%
  0.04% - 5% hemorrhage
  Death: 0.2%

FIGURE 9-53. Risks and benefits of stereotactic brain biopsy.

Stereotactic Brain Biopsy

Unexpected Diagnosis in 12%

  Multicentric glioma

  Inflammatory or demyelinating lesions

  Benign cysts

  Stroke

FIGURE 9-54. Unexpected findings on brain biopsy.

10

VASCULAR DISORDERS

PERSPECTIVE

1. In the final analysis, blood vessels have a limited repertoire of behaviors; they can either plug up, producing ischemia, or they can leak producing hemorrhage.
2. Atherosclerosis is the primary pathological substrate of cerebrovascular disease.
3. The distribution of ischemic injury in the brain may be determined by the large and variable arterial vascular territories, borderzone or watershed supply territories, small vessel disease, and neurochemical factors related to excitotoxicity and local metabolic demand.

OBJECTIVES

1. Learn about atherosclerosis as the primary cause of ischemic cerebrovascular disease.
2. Distinguish between focal and global ischemia, and learn the pathological evolution of cerebral infarcts.
3. Understand the contribution of excitotoxicity to ischemic injury.
4. Learn the significance of transient ischemic attacks as harbingers of stroke.
5. Learn the differences in etiology, clinical features, pathology, and prognosis of intraparenchymal versus subarachnoid hemorrhage.
6. Understand that chronic hypertension alters cerebral blood vessels so as to predispose to intraparenchymal hemorrhage in the basal ganglia, pons, and cerebellum.
7. Learn that intraparenchymal hemorrhages outside of the standard hypertensive hemorrhage locations may still be due to hypertension but may result from amyloid angiopathy, bleeding diathesis, or hemorrhagic tumor.
8. Learn that nontraumatic subarachnoid hemorrhage most commonly results from rupture of aneurysms on the proximal arterial tree of the brain. Subarachnoid hemorrhage often produces the worst headache the patient has ever experienced and is often fatal.
9. Understand that subarachnoid and intraparenchymal hemorrhage may arise from vascular malformations.

Vascular disorders of the nervous system lead to either (1) globally or focally inadequate blood flow (ischemia), which, if sufficiently protracted, leads to tissue necrosis (infarction), or (2) rupture of vascular structures, leading to hemorrhage.

Atherosclerosis is the primary pathological substrate of occlusive cerebrovascular disease. Atherosclerosis is a disease of large and medium sized muscular arteries in which the fundamental lesion is the atheroma or plaque (Fig. 10-1). "Atheroma" is derived from the Greek word for gruel, reflecting the friable grumous appearance of the plaque. These lesions are gray-white to yellow and protrude into the vascular lumen. They gradually enlarge, may calcify, and if they ulcerate, intraluminal thrombogenesis may be triggered leading to emboli or thrombosis of the vessel. The vessels involved in descending order of frequency are abdominal aorta, proximal coronary arteries, popliteal arteries, descending thoracic aorta, internal carotid arteries, and the vessels of the circle of Willis. Bifurcations and ostia are particularly prone to atherogenesis.

The typical uncomplicated plaque has a vascular luminal surface fibrous cap composed of smooth muscle cells, macrophages, and fibroblasts. Beneath the cap is a necrotic center filled with lipid debris, cholesterol crystals, calcium, and lipid-filled foam cells. The smooth muscle cells of the media may be encroached upon by the plaque, and the wall of the vessel weakened. Ulceration, thrombosis, or hemorrhage within a plaque warrant the designation "complicated" atheroma.

Theories about the pathogenesis of atherosclerosis currently focus on the vascular injury theory. Endothelial injury by any of a large variety of mechanisms (mechanical, toxic, viral infection, hemodynamic) leads to invasion of the intima by monocytes from the circulation and smooth muscle cells from the media. The smooth muscle cells, in particular, proliferate and may undergo transformation to fibroblasts and foam cells. This proliferative response is driven by growth factors released by damaged endothelial cells and macrophages. The macrophages may further damage the vessel by releasing cytokines and by oxidizing lipids, leading to a self-perpetuating injury site. Many details remain to be worked out, but it appears that there are multiple cellular and molecular targets for therapeutic intervention in this devastating disease. While atherosclerosis is the most common cause of carotid artery compromise, other processes such as arterial dissection can also lead to stroke (Fig. 10-2).

The distribution of ischemic injury in the brain may be determined by the large and variable arterial vascular territories, borderzone or watershed supply territories, small vessel disease, and neurochemical factors related to excitotoxicity and local metabolic demand. The brain accounts for about 20% of basal cardiac output and body oxygen consumption. Aerobic glycolysis is vir-

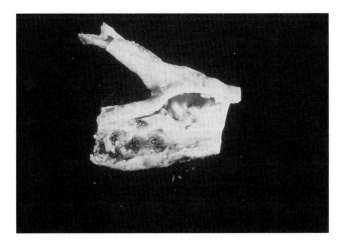

FIGURE 10-1. Carotid endarterectomy specimen showing the atherosclerotic plaque.

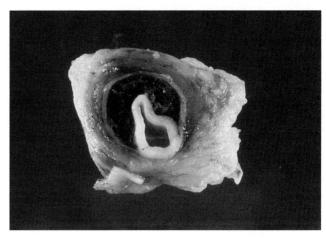

FIGURE 10-2. Common carotid dissection due to trauma. The blood fills the false lumen, and the true lumen is empty.

tually the sole source of energy of the mature brain, and the glycogen reserves of the CNS are meager and the oxygen reserves are nil; hence, an uninterrupted supply of oxygenated blood is essential for brain integrity. The blood supply of the brain comes via paired internal carotid and vertebral arteries. The carotids constitute the "anterior circulation" supplying the majority of the superficial and deep structures of the cerebral hemispheres; the vertebral arteries supply the "posterior circulation" which feeds the brainstem, cerebellum, and the territory of the posterior cerebral arteries. The posterior and anterior circulations anastomose via the circle of Willis. This anastomotic network at the base of the brain is quite variable, but in some fortunate individuals, the blood supply of the brain is sufficiently redundant that complete blockage of two carotids and one vertebral can be asymptomatic. Despite these elaborate hemodynamic precautions, many people experience global or focal ischemia leading to cerebral infarction.

Global ischemia leads to widespread tissue injury and the resulting condition is referred to as "ischemic encephalopathy." Global ischemia usually results from cardiopulmonary arrest or extreme hypotension in severe shock. If the perfusion failure is brief (minutes), the patient's neurological functions may quickly be restored with only transient postischemic confusion. Some patients may come back more slowly, and suffer subtle impairments of higher intellectual function that may preclude complete resumption of societal activities. More severe injury may lead to dementia and spasticity. If the ischemic period is protracted, the patient may not regain consciousness and may exhibit decorticate posturing and seizures, and may remain in a vegetative state indefinitely. Although the entire brain is inadequately perfused, there is surprising focality to the pathological alterations seen. As was mentioned earlier, certain cell populations are selectively vulnerable to ischemic injury, these include:

1. Large neurons in Sommer's sector of the hippocampus (Fig. 10-3)
2. Purkinje cells of the cerebellum
3. Neurons of layers 3 and 5 of the cerebral cortex (Fig. 10-4)

The basis of this selective vulnerability is not entirely clear but may be related to local energy metabolism requirements, hemodynamic factors, and local neurotransmitters. In particular, when ischemia leads to brain energy failure, membranes depolarize, permitting the uncontrolled release of the amino acid neurotransmitters, glutamate and aspartate. These neurotransmitters bind ligand-gated cation channels on the postsynaptic cell, opening the flood-

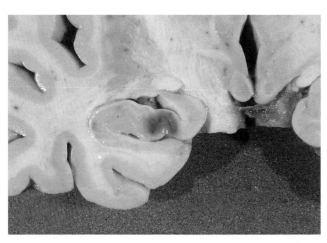

FIGURE 10-3. Selective vulnerability of the hippocampus due to ischemic injury.

gates for entry of calcium and sodium. The sodium depolarizes the cell membrane, and the calcium may activate intracellular proteases and quench mitochondrial energy production, propagating the energy failure and magnifying cellular injury. This injury done by neurotransmitters normally present, but in pathological conditions abnormally released, is "excitotoxicity." In excitotoxicity, the areas of brain injured depend on the local use of toxic neurotransmitters. For example, high levels of amino acid neurotransmitters in the mid-cortex lead to the vulnerability of specific centrally located layers of the cortex to ischemic injury resulting in a midcortical band of necrosis with relatively preserved cortex in deep and superficial layers on either side of this band. As this infarcted tissue becomes infiltrated by macrophages, it becomes grossly conspicuous and is called "laminar necrosis." The infiltration by macrophages and resorption of infarcted tissue is dependent on the re-establishment of perfusion to permit entry of these cells into the brain. If re-perfusion does not occur in global ischemia, the brain undergoes bland liquefactive necrosis devoid of macrophages or gliosis. Such a brain is referred to as a *"respirator brain"* because the patient's body may "live" on a ventilator.

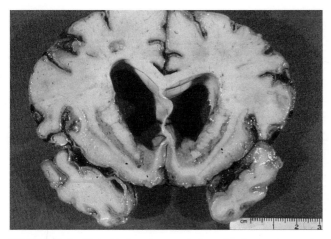

FIGURE 10-4. Global ischemic encephalopathy due to strangulation. Note the loss of cortex and basal ganglia.

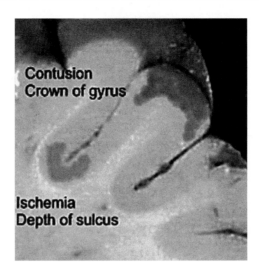

FIGURE 10-5. Infarcts involve the depths of sulci, while contusions involve the crests of gyri.

The molecular basis of selective vulnerability may depend not only on the local neurotransmitter milieu, but also on the balance of anti-apoptotic and pro-apoptotic signals in neurons undergoing damage. In the hippocampus, for example, ischemia leads to selective CA1 neuronal death while hypoglycemia results in CA3 neuronal loss. In ischemia, the surviving CA3 neurons up-regulate anti-apoptotic and stress gene proteins while the doomed CA1 neurons express pro-apoptotic genes and while they do activate stress gene responses, this is insufficient to save them. The opposite pattern of gene expression is seen in hypoglycemia. Clearly there are regional differences in apoptotic bias and cellular stress response that may be important in decreeing life or death of neurons.

Hemodynamic factors are primary in the production of *watershed or borderzone infarcts,* which occur at the junctions of major arterial supply zones. The zones exist at the precarious distal regions of arterial supply, and as perfusion pressure drops, these are the first regions to experience perfusional insufficiency. The classical borderzone is that between the anterior and middle cerebral arteries' distal territories. With global ischemia, this area in both hemispheres may undergo infarction leading to symmetrical wedge-shaped parasagittal high convexity infarcts (Fig. 10-5 and 10-6).

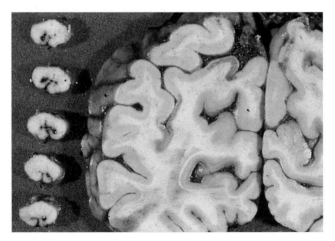

FIGURE 10-6. Infarcts at the depths of sulci lead to dusky discoloration.

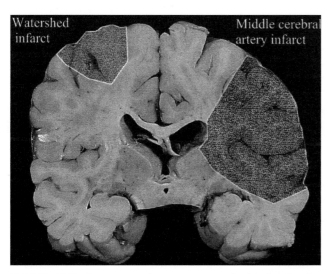

FIGURE 10-7. Compare and contrast watershed infarction between vascular territories versus large vessel occlusion within vascular territories.

Focal ischemia leads to circumscribed tissue injury or infarction; hence the term "cerebral infarction" is applied (infarcts are often easily localized by the signs and symptoms produced, allowing greater spatial precision in the diagnostic term applied; hence, "left cerebral infarct," "right cerebellar infarct," "right lateral medullary infarct," etc.). Focal ischemia may complicate global hypotension in areas supplied by stenotic vessels, or in hemodynamic border-zones as discussed above. More commonly, however, cerebral infarcts result from thrombotic or embolic obstruction of blood flow in large cerebral arteries or their branches (Fig. 10-7). During herniation, infarcts result from compression of vessels against unyielding dural structures.

Most infarcts resulting from thrombosis are anemic or bland, and are difficult to discern grossly for several hours, whereupon softening and discoloration become increasingly prominent. Swelling and liquefaction follow within the next 3–5 days, during which time the patient is in peril from the mass effect of the infarct (Fig. 10-8). The infarct then matures over weeks to

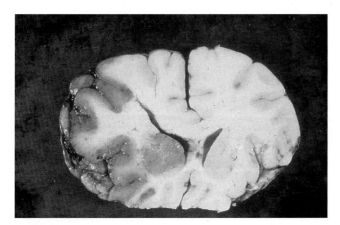

FIGURE 10-8. Acute middle cerebral artery infarction with swelling, discoloration and cingulate herniation.

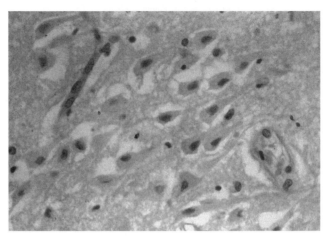

FIGURE 10-9. The shrunken red neuron is the earliest classical microscopic finding in ischemia.

months into a cystic space sometimes accompanied by compensatory ventricular enlargement. If blood flow is restored to a bland infarct (as often occurs in embolic or compressive vascular disease), then blood may seep into the softened tissues resulting in a hemorrhagic infarct, which is readily discernible grossly and radiologically.

As in other tissues, an orderly procession of gross and histopathological alterations is seen permitting estimation of the age of an infarct. If the patient survives for only minutes or even several hours, no alterations are seen. If the patient survives for 6–24 h, then shrunken eosinophilic neurons are seen in the infarct; grossly, the infarct is slightly discolored and softened with blurring of the border between gray and white matter (Fig. 10-9).

These changes become more pronounced as the infarct ages, and by 24–72 h, the tissue is infiltrated by neutrophils and the blood vessels are prominent. The tissue is soft and edematous, and may be sufficiently swollen to cause lethal mass effect.

By 72–96 h, the neutrophils are replaced by macrophages which may persist for weeks or months clearing the debris in the infarct at a rate of about 1 cc/month. The infarct is now frankly mushy. During the second week, proliferating astrocytes join the macrophages, and over the following weeks to months form a dense fibrillary glial meshwork around the dead tissue so that as the macrophages dispose of debris in the infarct, the infarct evolves into a cystic glial-lined cavity at points traversed by delicate glial sheets and small vessels, and invested with residual lipid- and hemosiderin-laden macrophages (Figs. 10-10 through 10-13).

Here is a summary of gross features of cerebral infarcts:

1. They occur in arterial distributions involving depths of sulci more than crests.
2. "Watershed" infarcts occur where arterial systems anastomose—distal tenuous "last valley" distribution—high parietal/occipital.
3. Not grossly evident for first 6–12 h, then slight discoloration/softening.
4. Within 48–72 h, gross necrosis is evident.
5. From 3–5 days, cerebral edema is maximal; herniation may occur.
6. Swelling subsides, liquefaction of necrotic tissue for days to weeks.
7. Dead tissue removed by macrophages and replaced by cystic cavity traversed by delicate glial strands and surrounded by gliotic tissue; compensatory asymmetrical ventricular enlargement may be seen.

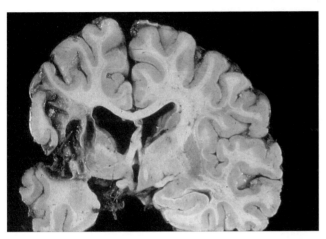

FIGURE 10-10. Remote middle cerebral artery distribution infarct is now cystic with a gliotic lining. Note the compensatory hydrocephalus ex vacuo.

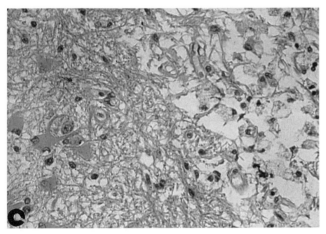

FIGURE 10-11. Wall of a remote cystic infarct with reactive astrocytes with plump cytoplasm. Macrophages with foamy cytoplasm are also present.

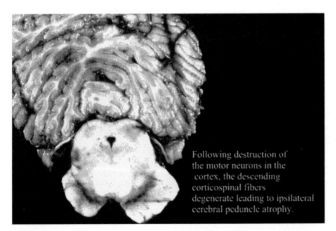

Following destruction of the motor neurons in the cortex, the descending corticospinal fibers degenerate leading to ipsilateral cerebral peduncle atrophy.

FIGURE 10-12. Destruction of motor neurons by a middle cerebral artery infarct leads to axonal degeneration and atrophy of the cerebral peduncle in the midbrain.

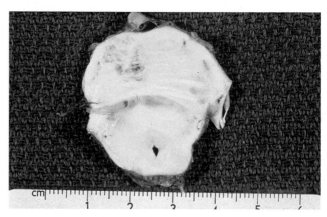

FIGURE 10-13. Infarct in the pons. Very small infarcts in the brainstem can be devastating.

This is a summary of the time sequence of neuronal ischemic death:

1. Microvacuolation (minutes to few hours) appears then regresses.
2. Neuronal shrinkage and eosinophilia (red neuron); 6–24 h; classically said to be the first sign of irreversible damage.
3. Incrustation phase—small dense fragments of neuronal cytoplasm flake from dendrites; 24–72 h.
4. Homogenizing cell change—complete loss of cytoplasmic detail, nucleus disintegrates; 24 h to days.

Here is a summary of glial, microglial, and vascular reaction to ischemic injury:

1. If the astrocytes survive, they react by swelling (12–36 h) and multiplying (gliosis 48 h to months).
2. Macrophages appear within 48 h and exhibit neuronophagy (consumption of necrotic neurons).
3. Polymorphonuclear leukocytes invade within hours, peaking at 48—72 h, being replaced by macrophages, which peak at about 14 days, but persist for months to years.
4. Small blood vessels are prominent by 48 h, and vascular proliferation ensues.

The blood-brain barrier is not intact; both vasogenic and cytotoxic cerebral edema seen, as is contrast enhancement on computed tomography. At this stage, an infarct may be mistaken radiologically and pathologically for a glioblastoma.

Thrombosis usually results from atherosclerotic disease in the common and internal carotid, vertebral, and lower basilar arteries. Arterial occlusion may result from clot formation over an ulcerated atherosclerotic plaque or from hemorrhage into a plaque. Prior to occlusion, debris from the plaque may be swept into the arterial stream leading to distal occlusive symptoms that are either transient or permanent.

Emboli tend to lodge in the distal bifurcations of the cerebral arteries, although they may come to rest as proximally as the middle cerebral artery itself. The middle cerebral artery and its branches are most commonly affected. Atherosclerotic plaques in the common and internal carotid arteries may lead to emboli, but the heart is also a rich source of emboli, spawning them from infected or defective valves, hypokinetic thrombogenic endocardial wall fol-

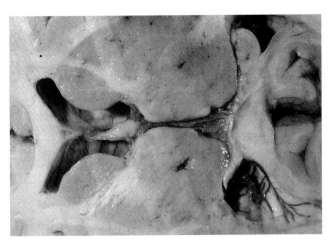

FIGURE 10-14. Multiple lacunar infarcts in the basal ganglia of a hypertensive patient.

lowing myocardial infarction, and atrial thrombi in atrial fibrillation particularly when associated with mitral insufficiency. Fat emboli and deep vein thrombi from the systemic venous circulation may find their way to the brain via a patent foramen ovale (paradoxical embolization). Rarely tumor emboli (usually from atrial myxoma) or amniotic emboli are seen. The spinal cord may experience infarction due to embolization of herniated disk material.

Lacunar infarcts ("lacunes" = small lakes) result from processes leading to narrowing of deep basal perforating arterioles rather than the large arteries and their distal branches. Lacunar infarcts range in size from a few millimeters to a maximum of 1.5 cm, and are most commonly situated in the basal ganglia and surrounding white matter, and in the pons (Fig. 10-14).

Lacunar infarcts may be asymptomatic, and it is common at autopsy to see astonishing numbers of lacunes in hypertensive patients who had no history of neurological impairment. Conversely, however, a strategically placed lacune in the internal capsule or pons may render the descending motor fibers of an entire hemisphere inoperative, resulting in profound hemiparesis. Similarly, sensory and cerebellar inflow-outflow tracts are vulnerable to lacunar infarcts. These small infarcts in the deep diencephalon, white matter, brainstem, and cerebellum result from lipohyalin change in the walls of small perforating arteries and arterioles induced by hypertension. The walls become thickened, but paradoxically weak. If the lumen is encroached upon by the thickening, ischemia ensues; if the wall weakening dominates, intracerebral hemorrhage may result.

UNUSUAL CAUSES OF ISCHEMIC CEREBROVASCULAR DISEASE

Much less commonly, arteritides or hypercoagulopathies will lead to thrombotic cerebral infarction (Fig. 10-15). Systemic lupus erythematosus (SLE), neurosyphilis, temporal arteritis (isolated granulomatous arteritis if exclusively intracranial) (Fig. 10-16 and 10-17), polyarteritis nodosa (infarcts + SAH due to aneurysmal dilations); and vasculitis of chronic and acute infections may lead to infarction. Rheumatic fever (Sydenham's chorea) and pregnancy (chorea gravidarum) can both be complicated by vasculitis leading to chorea.

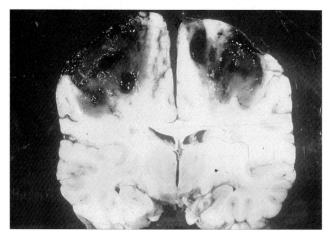

FIGURE 10-15. Bilateral venous infarcts due to superior sagittal sinus thrombosis. The blood can get in but it cannot get out leading to vascular stasis, infarction and hemorrhage

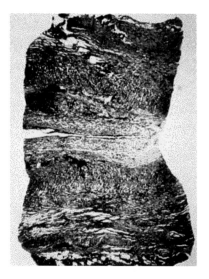

FIGURE 10-16. Temporal artery biopsy with marked narrowing of the lumen due to wall thickening in temporal arteritis.

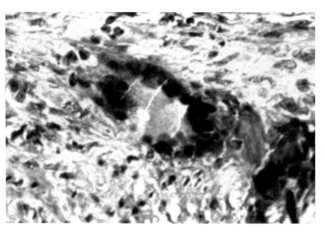

FIGURE 10-17. Multinucleated giant cell in the wall of a vessel involved in granulomatous angiitis.

Vasculitides are classified by a variety of means. One approach is to place a vasculitis into one of four categories including systemic necrotizing vasculitis, hypersensitivity vasculitis, giant cell vasculitis, or localized vasculitis. In all cases it is important to recognize that the diagnosis of vasculitis can only be confidently made on biopsy if transmural vessel wall inflammation is present. A few lymphocytes in the connective tissue around a vessel (the adventitia) is entirely normal.

The systemic necrotizing vasculitides involve small and medium sized vessels. Small artery involvement is common in polyarteritis nodosa whereas capillaries and venules can be involved in the other necrotizing vasculitides. Systemic involvement should be sought before resorting to brain biopsy.

Hypersensitivity vasculitis predominantly involves small vessels. Systemic involvement is common, and isolated nervous system damage is uncommon.

The giant cell or granulomatous vasculitides are among the more common justifications for a brain biopsy for vascular disease. Takayasu's arteritis involves the aorta and its large branches and may also produce large vessel occlusive or embolic cerebrovascular disease. Temporal arteritis involves the medium-sized vessels of the head and neck, and can usually be diagnosed with generous temporal artery biopsy.

Isolated granulomatous angiitis involves only intracranial vessels and may occur sporadically or following herpes zoster infections. Vascular narrowing and beading may be seen angiographically. The morphology of these conditions is one of giant cell infiltration of the vessels often accompanied by lymphocytes. These conditions are often responsive to high dose corticosteroids. In view of the long-term morbidity of steroid therapy, many believe that biopsy confirmation of temporal arteritis is justified. Biopsy of intracranial vessels is more problematic.

Isolated CNS angiitis includes isolated granulomatous vasculitis as its major member, but other nongranulomatous vasculitides may rarely be seen confined to the CNS. These cases are usually confirmed at autopsy, and biopsy is rarely done.

Lymphomatoid granulomatosis (LG) is occasionally encountered on brain biopsy for mass or cognitive decline and at one time was thought to be vasculitis. The condition is now regarded as a neoplastic lymphoproliferative disorder with variable malignant potential. Immunophenotyping reveals that LG is an angiocentric T-cell lymphoma in contrast to the usual B-cell primary CNS lymphoma. Distinction of LG from granulomatous angiitis or primary CNS lymphoma is impossible by simple light microscopy, but with immunohistochemical phenotyping of the lymphoid elements, the distinction becomes clearer. Antigenic monomorphism favors neoplasm, and the distinction between T and B-lymphocytes can be done using surface markers. Vasculitis has a mixture of T and B-lymphocytes as well as other constituents including giant cells, polymorphonuclear cells, and plasma cells. Often the T cells outnumber the B cell populations, but absolute monomorphism is not present. Infections can produce perivascular inflammatory infiltrates that may mimic vasculitis or neoplasm, but the infiltrate is a balanced mixture of T and B cells.

CADASIL (**C**erebral **A**utosomal **D**ominant **A**rteriopathy with **S**ubcortical **I**nfarcts and **L**eukoencephalopathy) results from a mutation of the signaling molecule Notch3 borne on chromosome 19. This disorder leads to subcortical white matter ischemic damage with myelin loss, lacunar infarcts and gliosis. There is fibrosis of small arteries and arterioles with deposition of eosinophilic, PAS positive, Congo Red positive granular material in the media. Ultrastructurally, this granular material consists of coarse irregular aggregates of electron dense material. These ultrastructural findings can be seen in vessels in skin and muscle obviating brain biopsy. CADASIL, episodic ataxia

2 and familial hemiplegic migraine all map to 19. CADASIL results from a defect of notch3 while EA2 and FHM appear to be different phenotypes resulting from damage to the same allele coding for the voltage-gated P/Q type calcium channel.

HEMORRHAGE

Hemorrhage may occur predominantly within brain parenchyma or predominantly in the subarachnoid space. The etiologies of hemorrhage in these two locations are strikingly different; hence, defining the location of a hemorrhage gives information about the probable cause of the bleeding. Bleeding may also occur in the epidural and dural cell layer spaces, and in these locations is almost always due to trauma, and will therefore be discussed in the section on neurotrauma (very rarely dural hematomas result from primary or metastatic tumor involvement).

Intracerebral hemorrhage is most commonly due to hypertensive arteriolar damage leading to rupture of these vessels. The vascular injury may take the form of transmural necrosis or microaneurysms (Charcot-Bouchard aneurysms). Such hypertensive hemorrhages characteristically occur in the basal ganglia (65%), subcortical white matter (15%), pons (10%), and cerebellar hemispheres (10%) (Figs. 10-18 and 10-19). Onset is abrupt and may be immediately lethal if massive rupture of the hematoma into the ventricular system occurs or if herniation ensues. If the patient survives the initial hemorrhage and edema, the hematoma is gradually cleared by macrophages and walled off by astrocytes leading grossly to a collapsed tan-brown cavity that microscopically possesses more hemosiderin-laden macrophages than the cystic cavity of a resolved infarct.

Intracerebral hemorrhage may less commonly occur within tumors, in patients who have a defect of coagulation, and in patients with amyloid angiopathy (Fig. 10-20). Hemorrhages in these circumstances tend to be multiple and within the white matter of the hemispheres rather than in the basal ganglia, pons, or cerebellum (Figs. 10-21 and 10-22).

Subarachnoid hemorrhage (SAH) injects blood into the cerebrospinal fluid and, to a lesser degree, into adjacent brain parenchyma. Aneurysms are the most common cause of spontaneous nontraumatic subarachnoid hemorrhage,

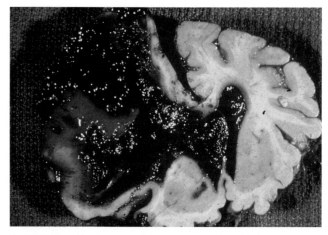

FIGURE 10-18. Catastrophic intraparenchymal hypertensive hemorrhage beginning in the basal ganglia, extending in the ventricles, and jetting to the surface.

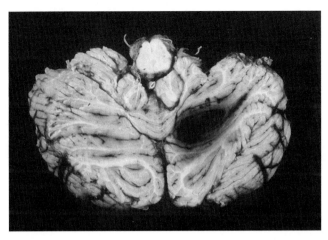

FIGURE 10-19. Cerebellar hypertensive hemorrhage is a neurosurgical emergency requiring prompt evacuation to avoid brainstem compromise.

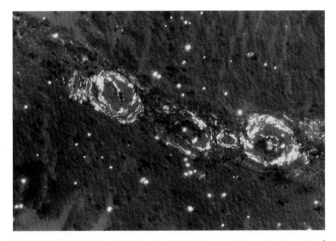

FIGURE 10-20. Amyloid angiopathy is an uncommon cause of lobar hemorrhage but should be considered whenever hemorrhage is seen in a location other than the classical sites of hypertensive hemorrhage.

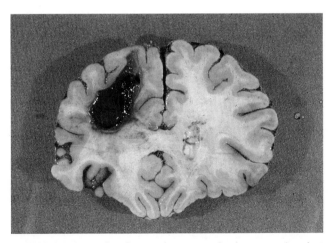

FIGURE 10-21. Lobar hemorrhage may be hypertensive, but consider amyloid angiopathy, hemorrhagic tumor, and coagulopathy.

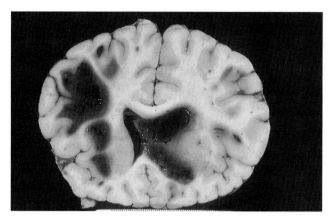

FIGURE 10-22. Multifocal intraparenchymal hemorrhage suggests coagulopathy or multifocal hemorrhagic tumor.

TABLE 10-1. SUMMARY OF ESSENTIAL FACTS ABOUT ANEURYSMS

1. Defect of arterial media with dilatation usually at proximal bifurcations.
2. Ninety percent are in the proximal carotid distribution: roughly 30% at internal carotid termination (posterior communicating artery aneurysms and carotid bifurcation aneurysms), 30% on anterior communicator (single commonest site of intracranial aneurysm) or anterior cerebral, 30% at first main branches of middle-cerebral artery.
3. Roughly 10% of aneurysms are in the vertebrobasilar distribution.
4. Multiple aneurysms in 10–20% cases.
4. Risk of rupture increases with size of aneurysm (7–8 mm critical); giant aneurysms are defined as those greater than 2.5 cm in diameter.
6. Predisposing factors: fibromuscular dysplasia, polycystic kidney disease, aortic coarctation; role of hypertension in formation disputed; 3–9% of patients with arteriovenous malformations have berry aneurysms.
7. Aneurysm may present with hemorrhage, compression of adjacent structures, or distal transient ischemic attacks (TIAs) from intraaneurysmal thrombus; following nonlethal hemorrhage, patient is at risk for rebleed, vasospasm with infarction, and hydrocephalus.
8. Mycotic aneurysms occur distally in contrast to saccular aneurysms; these aneurysms result from bacterial or fungal colonies in the walls of the vessel; often a complication of endocarditis.
9. Fusiform dilatation of the basilar or the internal carotid is seen in atherosclerosis—"dolichoectasia"; these "aneurysms" may compress local structures, but hemorrhage is uncommon.

with congenital berry or saccular aneurysms accounting for the majority of ruptured aneurysms. Berry aneurysms occur at bifurcationes of the major vessels at the base of the brain appearing as balloon-like outpouchings of the vessel wall (Figs. 10-23 through 10-25). The wall of the aneurysm thins toward its apex or dome, with fragmentation or absence of the internal elastic lamina and degeneration or absence of muscularis. Most aneurysms occur in the anterior circulation (85–90%), and are more or less equally divided among the anterior, middle, and internal carotid artery complexes. In 20% of cases the aneurysms are multiple. (For essential facts about aneurysms, see Table 10-1.)

Aneurysms usually produce symptoms by rupturing, but they may sometimes produce localizing symptoms by compressing adjacent structures (Fig. 10-26). Rupture usually occurs in early to middle adult life, and can range in severity from mild injections of blood into the subarachnoid space with resultant meningeal irritation with headache and photophobia to catastrophic hemorrhage with the patient suddenly grabbing his head complaining of the worst headache imaginable followed by coma and death. The initial hemorrhage is lethal in about 1/3 of patients, and those who survive are at risk for a subsequent repeat hemorrhage bearing a slightly higher mortality. The second hemorrhage usually follows within the first 30 days with the 10–14-day period be-

Aneurysm Formation

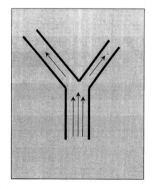
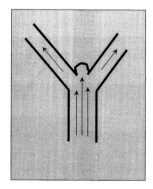

FIGURE 10-23. Aneurysms form at the bifurcations of vessels at the point of maximal rheological stress.

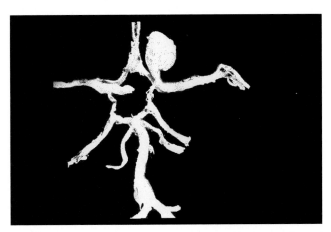

FIGURE 10-24. Berry aneurysms occur primarily proximally and on the anterior circulation near the circle of Willis.

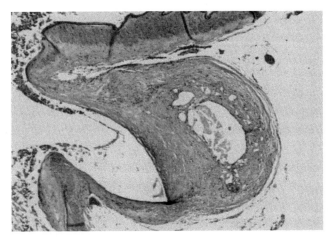

FIGURE 10-25. The loss of elastic media can be seen at the bifurcation of the vessel spawning this aneurysm.

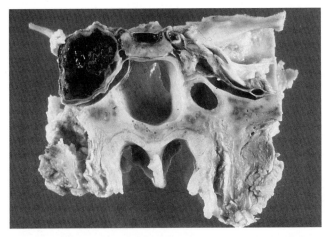

FIGURE 10-26. Cavernous sinus carotid artery aneurysm. If these rupture, there is an immediate shunting of arterial to venous circulation with a bruit and chemosis. Carotid artery aneurysms in this area may bulge into the sella, tempting the unwary to do a transphenoidal biopsy with catastrophic results.

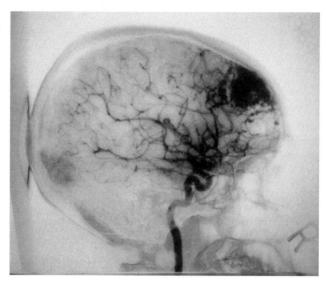

FIGURE 10-27. Arteriovenous malformation of the frontal lobe seen by angiography.

ing the time of maximal risk. Aneurysms can be prevented from hemorrhaging by the neurosurgical placement of a clip at the aneurysmal base, thus isolating the vascular defect from the circulation or by endovascular placement of thrombosis inducing coils or glue within the aneurysm. Neurosurgical management is complicated by the fact that severe cerebral arterial vasospasm often ensues in the 3–10 days following the initial hemorrhage, and neurosurgery in the face of vasospasm is often catastrophic with infarction of the brain supplied by the narrowed vessels. Even without neurosurgical intervention, the vasospasm may result in cerebral infarction that is sometimes severe enough to render issues of recurrent hemorrhage and neurosurgical intervention moot.

In addition to hypertensive intracerebral hemorrhage and SAH from aneurysms, the other significant cause of CNS hemorrhage is *vascular malformations* (Fig. 10-27). Vascular malformations are common (5–6% of all autopsies) and most are asymptomatic; those that do produce symptoms do so by hemorrhaging, by local compression or vascular steal, or by producing seizures. They come in four varieties named according to the nature of the vascular channels they contain and the intervening parenchyma between these channels (Fig. 10-28):

Arteriovenous malformations (AVMs) are large, often wedge shaped on the cortical surface, with large caliber channels having both arterial and venous features without intervening capillaries (Fig 10-29). Gliotic often hemosiderin-stained tissue resides between these channels. Importantly, this parenchyma within the AVM is nonfunctional and can be safely removed, in contrast to the parenchyma of venous angiomas and telangiectasias which is normal and may be functional.

Cavernous angiomas consist of varying caliber hyalinized vessels without intervening neural parenchyma.

Venous angiomas are made up of varying sized venous channels separated by normal neural parenchyma; a varix is a single enlarged venous channel.

Telangiectasias consist of capillary-sized vessels separated by normal neural parenchyma. They very rarely hemorrhage and are common in the pons.

It must be recognized that the vascular malformations exist on a morphological continuum and the various subtypes may blend together in indi-

Vascular Malformations

Arteriovenous Malformation

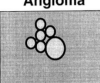

Venous Angioma

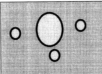

Cavernous Angioma

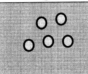

Capillary Telangiectasia

FIGURE 10-28. The classes of vascular malformations are determined by the caliber of the constituent vessels and the nature of the intervening parenchyma.

vidual cases. Vascular malformations have classically been treated by surgical excision when symptomatic, but increasingly these anomalies are being obliterated by interventional endovascular techniques or gamma-knife irradiation.

BRAIN BIOPSY IN VASCULAR DISORDERS

Ordinary large vascular territory infarcts are usually clinically and neuroradiologically conspicuous and obviously do not require biopsy. If the clinical progression is slow or sputtering rather than catastrophic, or if the imaging is done when the infarct is exerting mass effect or vascular leakiness produces contrast enhancement, an infarct may be mistaken for a tumor or rarely encephalitis or

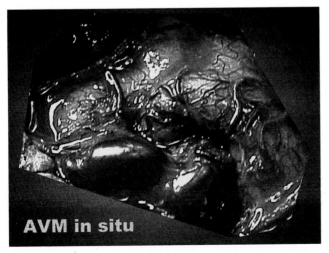

AVM in situ

FIGURE 10-29. *In situ*, an arteriovenous malformation is a fearsome sight!

cerebritis, and biopsied. Small branch occlusions or multifocal embolization may also lead to atypical presentations that may result in biopsy. Ischemic neurons, benign vascular proliferation, and macrophage infiltration will usually permit accurate diagnosis. It is wise to bear in mind, however, that ischemic changes can be seen adjacent to neoplasms and other masses.

Brain biopsy is an appropriate consideration if vasculitis is considered likely on clinical or radiological grounds. As discussed above, the vasculitides involve different types and sizes of vessels, and it is important to select the appropriate vessel for biopsy. A biopsy directed by radiological or clinical abnormalities is always preferable to one done blindly. If the patient has a systemic disorder producing vasculitis, then biopsy of a less critical organ—skin, kidney, nasal mucosa—should be considered prior to brain biopsy. Depending on the type and extent of vascular involvement, patients with vasculitis may present with large vessel occlusion, multifocal infarcts, or progressive cognitive decline.

Biopsy of aneurysms is best avoided. Aneurysms may mimic tumors if they burrow into the parenchyma and are particularly tempting if they impinge upon the pituitary gland where they may be mistaken for pituitary adenomas or sellar meningiomas. Magnetic resonance imaging will usually show a flow void or luminal enhancement, but a partially thrombosed aneurysm remains a snare for the unwary.

Intraparenchymal hemorrhages are most commonly due to hypertension and do not require biopsy. If the hemorrhage is lobar or has an area of enhancement, it may be the result of hemorrhage within a neoplasm, and should be considered for biopsy. Open biopsy is always preferable to stereotactic biopsy under these circumstances so that feeding vessels of a vascular malformation or tumor can be discerned.

11

CENTRAL NERVOUS SYSTEM TOXIC AND METABOLIC DISORDERS

PERSPECTIVE

1. The brain is a biochemically intricate organ that is exquisitely sensitive to metabolic derangement arising from deficiency of essential vitamins or metabolites, alteration of internal milieu, or exposure to toxins.
2. In most instances, neurometabolic derangements result in brain dysfunction (metabolic encephalopathy) without gross or microscopic abnormalities; however, there are several toxic and metabolic disorders associated with relatively specific gross or microscopic neuropathologic alterations.
3. Neurometabolic conditions are superimposed upon individuals with widely differing genetically determined phenotypes; hence, there is some genetically determined differential susceptibility.
4. Neurotoxicology is a major area of concern in medical practice; the clinical and neuropathological aspects of ethanol, methanol, ethylene glycol, and carbon monoxide (CO) intoxication are particularly important.

OBJECTIVES

1. Understand the neurological manifestations of vitamin deficiencies, including thiamine and B_{12} deficiency.
2. Understand the importance of the rare but treatable copper metabolism disorder, Wilson's disease.
3. Appreciate the broad range of neuropathological manifestations of ethanol use.
4. Be able to recognize the gross neuropathological features of methanol and CO intoxication.

The brain is a soggy computer: it is a biochemically intricate organ evolved for information processing. It accounts for only about 2% of body weight yet consumes 20% of glucose (77 mg/min for the average 1,400-g brain—about 100 g/day) and oxygen used by the body under resting conditions (it's finicky, too; essentially only glucose will do for energy production). Additionally, it has quite an appetite for amino acids and other metabolic morsels for the maintenance of structure, axonal transport, and neurotransmitter manufacture. It should not be shocking, therefore, that the brain is subject to malfunction due to lack or malutilization of essential substances, intoxication, and hereditary metabolic disorders. These disorders are of particular medical relevance because correction of the underlying metabolic derangement restores function. In most instances, these disturbances, while functionally profound, have no morphological correlate; however, in some cases, diagnostic gross and microscopic alterations are seen.

VITAMIN-RESPONSIVE DISORDERS

Classically, this category was reserved for vitamin deficiency disorders but in recent years a number of hereditary disorders of vitamin utilization or malabsorption have been detected (Table 11-1). While these conditions are uncommon, recognition and treatment are lifesaving since the defects can be corrected by administering large doses of the appropriate vitamin.

B₁₂ Deficiency

These patients present with progressive spastic paraparesis, sensory ataxia and paresthesiae, and if they remain untreated become demented. These symptoms may occur in the absence of megaloblastic anemia. Degeneration of the posterior and lateral white matter columns of the spinal cord with demyelination, macrophage infiltration, and axonal loss are the cardinal features and give rise to the name "subacute combined degeneration" of the spinal cord (the "subacute" refers to the indolent tempo of the disorder; "combined" refers to the combination of motor and sensory system involvement)(Fig. 11-1). In advanced disease, white matter destruction may be seen in the brain and optic nerves. The peripheral nerves may be damaged as well, a process that may obscure the spasticity seen in this condition.

Thiamine Deficiency

Thiamine (vitamin B₁) deficiency may lead to a peripheral neuropathy. More serious, however, is involvement of the CNS to produce characteristic clinical

TABLE 11-1. CLINICAL FEATURES OF VITAMIN DEFICIENCY DISORDERS THAT IMPACT ON THE NERVOUS SYSTEM

Disease	Vitamin	Clinical Features
Alcoholism	Thiamine/lipoate	Wernicke-Korsakoff syndrome
Combined system disease	B₁₂	Neuropathy, sensory loss, ataxia, anemia
Methylmalonic aciduria	B₁₂	Recurrent lethargy, Reye's-like disease, aciduria
Recurrent Reye's-like disease	Biotin	Alopecia, thrush, recurrent encephalopathy
Multiple carboxylase deficiency	Biotin	Recurrent encephalopathy with acidosis
Pellegra	Niacin	Dermatitis, diarrhea, neuropathy, dementia
Hartnup's disease	Niacin	Recurrent ataxia and amino aciduria
Lactic acidosis	Thiamine/lipoate	Recurrent ataxia, lethargy, acidosis
Mitochondrinopathies	Riboflavin	Recurrent encephalopathy, muscle disease
Bassen-Kornzweig disease	Vitamine E	Neuropathy, ataxia, acanthocytosis
Cholestatic liver disease	Vitamin E	Neuropathy, ataxia
Friedreich-like ataxia	Vitamin E	Ataxia, sensory neuropathy

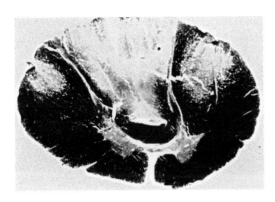

FIGURE 11-1. Cross section of the spinal cord of an individual with vitamin B$_{12}$ deficiency. Degeneration of the dorsal columns and lateral corticospinal tracts has resulted in secondary loss of myelin.

and pathological features of the Wernicke–Korsakoff syndrome. The early, reversible portion of the syndrome is known as Wernicke's encephalopathy and is characterized by abrupt onset of confusion, nystagmus, extraocular palsies, and ataxia. Grossly, brown soft hemorrhagic foci are seen in the mammillary bodies, the walls of the 3rd ventricle, around in the aqueduct of Sylvius, and in the floor of the 4th ventricle (Fig. 11-2). The nuclei of 3, 4, 6, and 10 may be involved. Microscopically, intense vascular proliferation, dilatation, and leakage accompanied by brisk gliosis and macrophage infiltration is seen. Importantly, neurons and their axons are relatively spared. Timely administration of thiamine at this point may completely reverse the condition.

If thiamine is not given in time or in adequate quantity, irreversible damage may lead immediately to death or if the patient survives, he is left with a profound disturbance of recent memory and he may confabulate vividly. The lesions are in the same distribution as those in Wernicke's encephalopathy although there is a greater tendency for thalamic involvement, and the lesions microscopically are characterized by intense gliosis, neuronal loss, and hemosiderin-laden macrophages.

Leigh's Disease (Subacute Necrotizing Encephalomyopathy)

This shares with Wernicke's syndrome the tendency for deep, periventricular, gray matter hemorrhagic necrosis with, the important exception that the

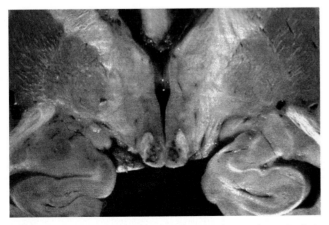

FIGURE 11-2. Mammillary bodies showing hemorrhage and atrophy in thiamine deficiency. Similar changes are seen in the periventricular and periaqueductal gray matter.

mammillary bodies are spared and involvement of medulla and cord is common. Onset is in infancy and the outlook is dismal. The underlying biochemical defect is variable and in some cases unknown, but these children may have elevated plasma pyruvate and lactate levels suggesting a defect in entry into the tricarboxylic cycle or subsequent electron transport. In some cases, defects of pyruvate dehydrogenase, cytochrome c oxidase, mitochondrial DNA deletion, or point mutations of mitochondrial DNA (NARP: neuropathy, ataxia, retinitis pigmentosa) are seen. Despite the morphological similarity to Wernicke's encephalopathy, response to thiamine is disappointing.

Niacin Deficiency

Pellagra is the clinical triad of dermatitis, diarrhea, and dementia; central chromatolysis is present in neurons.

Pyridoxine Responsive Seizures

Rarely neonatal seizures result from a disorder of pyridoxine utilization (if you can't use pyridoxine, you can't make GABA, which is a major inhibitory neurotransmitter implicated in seizure suppression). Neonates with seizures should receive a 50-mg dose of pyridoxine; if they have this condition, the seizures generally stop within minutes.

TREATABLE HEREDITARY METABOLIC DISORDERS

Increasingly, the metabolic disorders which have an impact on the CNS are being diagnosed early enough that genetic counseling, pregnancy termination, or in some instances therapy can be instituted. The sphingolipidoses, neuronal storage disorders, mucopolysaccharidoses, glycogen storage diseases, and leukodystrophies are diagnosable early enough that counseling can be offered, but therapy in these disorders has been disappointing. Several of the aminoacidopathies and organic acidopathies can, however, be diagnosed early and treated with dietary manipulation so that neurological complications can be minimized. Early recognition of these conditions is essential, and state-mandated newborn screening for some of these disorders has averted tragedy for a number of families. Individually, most of these disorders are very rare, but in aggregate they constitute a significant cause of human misery. The morphological neuropathology of these disorders is quite nonspecific, although, in some, the staining and fluorescent qualities of the storage product within neurons may provide diagnostic insight. Early in the storage diseases, the brain may be heavy and large due to storage product accumulation; however, as normal constituents are lost, the brain weight declines. The only treatable hereditary metabolic disorder to be considered in detail here is Wilson's disease.

Wilson's Disease

This is an uncommon autosomal recessive disorder of copper metabolism characterized by the intraparenchymal accumulation of copper in the liver, brain, and cornea leading to cirrhosis, neurological manifestations, and Kayser-Fleischer rings. Hepatic and neurological symptoms may occur synchronously, sequentially, or in isolation. The neurological features generally include extrapyramidal movement disorders, spasticity, coarse tremor, dysarthria, and dementia. Most have reduced serum ceruloplasmin, elevated urinary copper excretion, and aminoaciduria. Gross examination of the brain discloses shrinkage (sometimes cavitation) of the putamen, accompanied by brown discoloration. Microscopic changes are widespread and consist of neuronal loss and proliferation of large astrocytes with watery nuclei (Alzheimer type II astrocytes). Such astrocytes are not specific for Wilson's disease; they may be seen in a variety of acquired metabolic disorders, especially hepatic encephalopathy (which may, of course, occur in Wilson's disease). Wilson's disease must be considered in every case of hepatitis, cirrhosis, movement disorder, and dementia because it is treatable with penicillamine.

ACQUIRED METABOLIC DISORDERS

Metabolic Encephalopathy

The brain malfunctions in the face of systemic metabolic derangements due to cardiopulmonary, renal, hepatic, or endocrine diseases occurring singly or in combination. Such disturbance of cerebral function is referred to rather nonspecifically as "metabolic encephalopathy." Clinically, the patient has a decline in level of consciousness starting with inattentiveness sometimes accompanied by rowdiness, progressing to lethargy, and finally to states of unarousability regardless of level of stimulation. The change in consciousness may be accompanied by tremor, asterixis, and changing multifocal neurological signs. The computed tomography shows no structural abnormality, and the electroencephalogram demonstrates a progressive slowing of the rhythmic cortical activity sometimes accompanied by periodic high amplitude discharges known as triphasic waves (triphasic waves are seen most commonly in hepatic encephalopathy but they are not specific for this condition). Biochemically, metabolic encephalopathy is characterized by diminished cerebral glucose and oxygen utilization regardless of the inciting derangement. No specific morphological features are seen in metabolic encephalopathy although the presence of Alzheimer type II astrocytes is suggestive but not diagnostic of hepatic encephalopathy. Hepatic encephalopathy may also trigger transformation of astrocytes into Opalski cells—astrocytes with fluffy abundant cytoplasm.

INTOXICATION

Neurotoxicology is a major aspect of contemporary neuropathology. The breadth of this area far exceeds the scope of this review so we will concentrate on the more common and better-understood toxic injuries to the brain.

Ethanol

This toxin has widespread detrimental effects acutely and chronically in an individual, and more widespread societal repercussions due to its behavioral effects (Fig. 11-3). Lethal intoxication usually occurs when drinking takes on a competitive quality as in "chugging" contests and other rituals of youth (Table 11-2).

Chronic alcohol use is associated with a number of neurological complications arising from nutritional deficiency (Wernicke–Korsakoff syndrome and possibly peripheral neuropathy), hepatic failure (hepatic encephalopathy and non-Wilsonian hepatocerebral degeneration), and metabolic derangement (central pontine myelinolysis from rapid correction of hyponatremia). Less well understood is anterior superior vermal cerebellar degeneration which occurs predominantly in alcoholic men and presents with truncal ataxia, and is grossly evident as atrophy of the vermis. Also seen in alcoholics is central

TABLE 11-2. ETHANOL EFFECTS ON BEHAVIOR ACCORDING TO BLOOD LEVEL IN A NOVICE DRINKER

Ethanol (mg/dL)	Clinical features
0.05–0.1	Disinhibition (rowdy)
0.1–0.3	Inebriated/ataxic (obnoxious)
0.3–0.35	Very intoxicated
>0.35	Potentially lethal

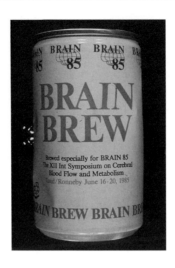

FIGURE 11-3. The behavioral effects of ethanol intoxication are well known and widely appreciated. Structural neuropathological consequences can also be seen.

necrosis of the corpus callosum (Marchiafava-Bignami disease—initially thought to occur only in Italian drinkers of red wine; now known to have a more cosmopolitan distribution) (Figs. 11-4 through 11-6).

Methanol

In their quest for bottled hope, alcoholics will from time to time consume methanol, which is oxidized by the liver to damaging formaldehyde and formic acid. This toxin is sometimes an adulterant of alcoholic drinks introduced either accidentally by poor manufacturing practices or occasionally intentionally to increase the volume of the liquid sold (methanol is less expensive than ethanol). Since both ethanol and methanol are metabolized by the same alcohol dehydrogenase system in the liver, ethanol will compete with methanol for the enzyme and will slow the production of formaldehyde and formic acid to potentially tolerable levels. Ethanol is the medical treatment for methanol intoxication, and when methanol is an adulterant, the ratio of ethanol to methanol in the drink is critical in determining if the patient experiences methanol toxicity. Patients dying of methanol intoxication have severe cerebral edema with hemorrhagic necrosis of the lateral putamen (Fig. 11-7). The retina is also a very sensitive target of the damaging effect

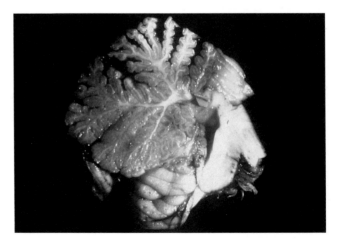

FIGURE 11-4. Cerebellar vermis atrophy due to chronic ethanol use.

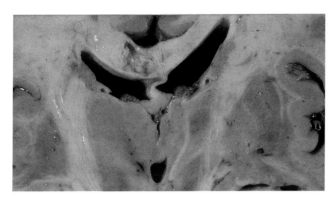

FIGURE 11-5. Marchiavava-Bignami syndrome of necrosis of the corpus callosum may be a pathophysiological cousin to central pontine myelinolysis. This lesion can be seen in experimental hyponatremia just as one can see central pontine myelinolysis.

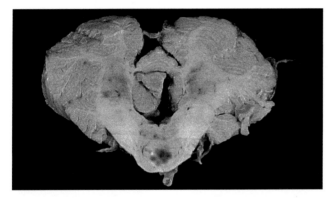

FIGURE 11-6. Central pontine myelinolysis resulting from too rapid correction of hyponatremia. The condition is commonly seen in alcoholics but can be seen in other hyponatremic individuals.

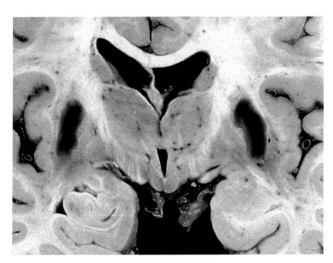

FIGURE 11-7. Methanol ingestion results in bilateral hemorrhagic necrosis of the putamen.

of methanol. Retinal edema and ganglion cell degeneration is observed, and accounts for the blindness that afflicts these patients. Blindness may result from the ingestion of as little as 4 mL, whereas a lethal dose is in the range of 8–10 mL of pure methanol, although usually 70–100 mL is consumed in fatal cases.

Ethylene Glycol

Like methanol, ethylene glycol (automotive antifreeze) is sometimes consumed by desperate individuals as an alternative to ethanol. In addition, due to its beguilingly sweet taste, children or animals may ingest ethylene glycol. Oxalic acid is the primary degradation product, and the resulting severe organic acidosis may lead to coma and renal failure, and survivors may have residual neurological deficits.

Carbon Monoxide

This colorless, odorless, tasteless gas is formed by incomplete combustion. Carbon monoxide (CO) binds avidly to hemoglobin forming carboxyhemoglobin reducing the oxygen carrying capacity of blood. Carboxyhemoglobin is red and imparts a "cherry-red" hue to victims of this poison. Severe intoxication results in striking bilateral liquefactive necrosis of the dorsolateral globus pallidus (Figs. 11-8 and 11-9). Other areas of CNS ischemic injury may be seen particularly in the cerebellum, cerebral cortex and hippocampus. Also a patchy loss of white matter myelin presumably due to oligodendroglial ischemia can be seen in long-term survivors. The mechanism of the selective globus pallidus injury is unclear, but the recent discovery that CO may function as a neurotransmitter analogous to nitric oxide (NO), raises the possibility that areas rich in heme-iron (such as the basal ganglia) may use this compound under physiological conditions for cell-to-cell signaling. Analogous to the amino acid excitotoxicity story, in excess a neurotransmitter such as CO might inflict injury in the very areas where it normally plays a physiological role. Some believe that the pallidal necrosis results from vascular compromise due to brain swelling with compression of the anterior choroidal arteries.

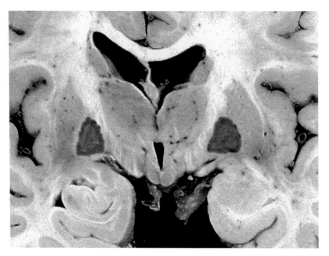

FIGURE 11-8. Carbon monoxide intoxication produces bilateral liquefactive necrosis of the globus pallidus.

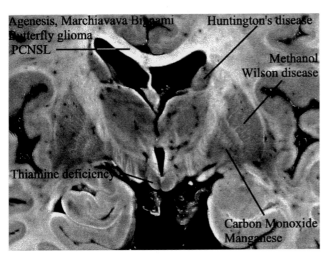

FIGURE 11-9. Composite image of disorders affecting the periventricular region.

Metal Intoxication

A number of metals employed in industry and medicine can result in neurological disease; additionally, the biocidal properties of some of these substances such as arsenic and thallium have made them favorite tools of murderers, suicidal individuals, and pesticide users. Lead and mercury are, however, the most common metal intoxicants.

Lead

Lead intoxication produces an edema-based encephalopathy in acute poisoning especially in childhood; microscopically, amorphous exudate is seen around microvessels, and some vascular proliferation may be seen (Figs. 11-10 and 11-11). Children may acquire lead intoxication by ingesting lead-based paint, fishing sinkers, and other lead weights. Chronic lead exposure in childhood may result in learning and behavior disturbances, but this issue is very complex and thus far largely lacks neuropathological illumination. In adults,

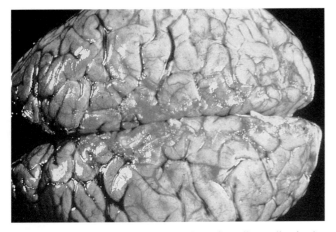

FIGURE 11-10. Lead intoxication with profoundly swollen brain. This is most commonly seen in children while adults tend to have peripheral neuropathy.

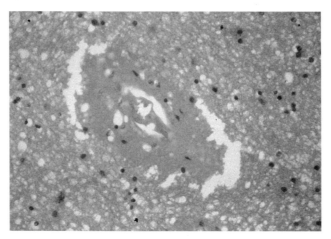

FIGURE 11-11. Lead intoxication leads to disruption of endothelium with leakage of fluid into the neuropil and resultant edema. Here is the necrotic remains of a brain capillary in lead intoxication.

lead intoxication more commonly presents as a neuropathy rather than as an encephalopathy.

Mercury

Chronic inorganic mercury compound intoxication may present with dementia, delirium, tremor, irritability, and insomnia. Intoxication of this type is currently rare, but in the 19th century, mercury intoxication decimated workers in cinnabar mines, hat manufacturing ("mad as a hatter" possibly derives from the psychic state of felt hat factory workers exposed to mercury in the processing of felt), mirror silvering plants, and manufacturers of scientific instruments. Cerebellar atrophy with loss of Purkinje cells was seen. In the modern world, organomercurial poisoning is more prevalent, with industrial disasters occurring in Japan (Minamata bay disease: mercuric chloride in the manufacture of vinyl chloride was dumped into the bay, the marine food chain obligingly concentrated the Hg, and fishermen and local inhabitants then ate contaminated seafood: 1,500 people damaged or dead) and Iraq (grain intended for planting only was dusted with the fungicide methylmercury, was poorly labeled and given to illiterate farmers, the grain was converted by the hungry populace into flour; in 1972, 459 deaths and 6,530 hospitalizations occurred in a single outbreak in Iraq). Cerebellar and cerebrocortical atrophy is seen with some cortical damage elsewhere; these patients are afflicted with ataxia and blindness. Congenital methylmercury neurotoxicity resulting from *in utero* exposure results in severe mental retardation, athetosis, ataxia, and spastic quadriparesis. Severe atrophy of the cerebrum with milder cerebellar atrophy is evident, with loss of the cortical lamellar organization perhaps indicating a defect in neuronal migration and organization in development.

Arsenic

Arsenical intoxication manifests with gastrointestinal complaints (nausea, vomiting, diarrhea), cutaneous features (hyperkeratosis and increased pigmentation of the soles and palms, and Mees' lines on the nails), and a severe axonal neuropathy. In the brain, swelling and petechiae may be present.

Thallium

Like arsenic, gastrointestinal disturbances are prominent, the major cutaneous manifestations consist of late alopecia and Mees' lines occasionally, and severe axonal neuropathy.

Manganese

Basal ganglionic damage produced by manganese is classically seen in manganese miners. The globus pallidus takes the brunt of the damage, while the substantia nigra is spared.

Tin

Triethyltin exposure acutely results in white matter vacuolation, and with chronic exposure, demyelination and gliosis are seen.

ASSORTED METABOLIC NIGHTMARES

Metabolic neuropathology provides abundant fodder for clinical rounds and examinations. We provide the following compilations for those anticipating interrogation about these disorders.

It is sometimes handy to have a handful of genetic disorders in mind arranged according to mode of inheritance when rounding with the Marquis de Sade (Tables 11-3 and Table 11-4).

TABLE 11-3. GENETIC DISORDERS ARRANGED ACCORDING TO MODE OF INHERITANCE

Autosomal dominant disorders
  Huntington's chorea, neurofibromatosis, myotonic dystrophy, von Hippel–Lindau's disease, OPCA in many cases
Autosomal recessive disorders
  Most inborn errors of metabolism are autosomal recessive—phenylketonuria, Pomp's disease, homocystinuria, maple syrup urine disease, Wilson's disease, alipoproteinemias, Refsum's disease . . . if you don't know the inheritance pattern of a disease, assume it's autosomal recessive.
X-linked recessive
  Duchenne dystrophy, Becker dystrophy, adrenoleukodystrophy, Fragile X syndrome, Lesch–Nyhan syndrome, Fabry's disease.
Mitochondrial genetic disorders
  Kearns–Sayre syndrome—large deletions in mitochondrial genome
  MERRF—defect in mt-tRNA (Lys)
  MELAS—defect in mt-tRNA (Leu)
  Leber's hereditary optic atrophy—mutation at 11778

TABLE 11-4. APPROACH INBORN ERRORS OF METABOLISM WITH TREPIDATION, BUT AN APPROACH ORGANIZED AROUND DISEASE PHENOTYPE IS OFTEN MORE USEFUL THAN AN APPROACH BASED ON DIMLY REMEMBERED BIOCHEMICAL PATHWAYS

Symptom	Disease
Cataract	Galactosemia, Lowe's syndrome, cerebrotendinous xanthomatosis, Cockayne's syndrome, Zellweger's syndrome
Corneal clouding	Hurler's disease (MP1) and Fabry's disease
Retinitis pigmentosa	Cockayne's syndrome, abetalipoproteinemia, Refsum's disease, Spielmeyer–Vogt, progressive external ophthalmoplegia (Kearns–Sayre)
Cherry red spot	Tay-Sachs, Sandoffs, infantile Niemann-Pick, Infantile GM1 gangliosidosis, Mucolipidosis II (I–cell disease)
Glaucoma	Lowe's syndrome, Zellwegers, Sturge–Weber
Lens dislocation	Homocystinuria and Marfan's
Red eyes	Ataxia-telangiectasia
Pendular nystagmus	Pelizaeus–Merzbacher leukodystrophy
Opsoclonus	Neuroblastoma
Deafness	Cockayne's syndrome, Refsum's disease, Mannosidosis
Renal disease	Fabry's disease, Wilson's, Hartnup, Lowe's, Zellwegers, and Lesch–Nyhan (urate stones)
Ichthyosis	Refsum's disease and Austin's variant of MLD; not to be confused with the eczema of PKU
Yellow tonsils	Tangier disease (A-alpha-lipoproteinemia, familial high density lipoprotein deficiency)
Acanthocytosis	Abetalipoproteinemia (Bassen–Kornzweig) and some forms of familial chorea
Photosensitivity	Cockayne's syndrome, xeroderma pigmentosa, porphyria
Angiokeratoma	Fabry's disease and fucosidosis
Fair complexion	PKU, spongy degeneration of the CNS (i.e., Canavan's)
Pellagra-like rash	Hartnup's disease

MLD, metachromatic leukodystrophy; PKU, phenylketonuria.

How Are Gangliosides Named?

One of the most frustrating and confusing aspects of inborn errors of metabolism is the incorporation of arcane biochemical nomenclature into the clinical literature. A prime example is the naming of the disorders of gangliosides. The gangliosides are named according to the Svennerholm code system. G stands for ganglioside. The next letter is the index standing for asialyic (A), monosialyic (M), disialyic (D), or trisialyic (T) units. Most gangliosides of concern to us are monsialyic, hence GM. Gangliosides are made up of ceramide as the basic molecule with 2, 3, or 4 carbohydrate molecules linked to it forming an oligosaccharide chain. Each carbohydrate molecule has a number—and here is the problem—gangliosides with four carbohydrate chains are designated 1, with three unit chains are designated 2, and with two unit chains are designated 3. Therefore, GM1 indicates a ganglioside in which the ceramide has 4 carbohydrates with the final one being sialyated.

12

NEURODEGENERATIVE DISORDERS

PERSPECTIVE

1. The neurodegenerative disorders are characterized by loss of functionally related groups of neurons. The cause of the neuronal loss is unknown but is clearly multifactorial. The clinical symptoms produced depend on which neuronal populations are lost (Fig. 12-1).

2. In some instances, the etiologies of diseases that were previously classified as neurodegenerative disorders are now known, and these diseases have been reclassified into more appropriate etiological categories (Fig. 12-2).

3. Increasing attention is being directed at chronic cellular injury and stress from excitotoxic and free radical mechanisms as potentially causative in the neurodegenerative disorders.

OBJECTIVES

1. Three major causes of dementia are Alzheimer's disease (AD), Pick's disease, and Lewy body dementia (LBD). Learn the clinical manifestations, and gross and microscopic features of each of these.

2. Learn the clinical features, gross and microscopy pathology, genetics, and neurochemistry of Huntington's disease and Parkinson's disease. Understand the differences and similarities between Parkinson's disease, progressive supranuclear palsy, and postencephalitic Parkinson's disease.

3. Understand the two most common degenerative disorders associated with ataxia—multiple system atrophy and Friedreich's ataxia.

4. Understand amyotrophic lateral sclerosis, familial amyotrophic lateral sclerosis, and infantile spinal muscular atrophy.

The neurodegenerative disorders are among the most common and devastating neurological diseases. For organizational purposes, we will discuss these conditions in turn according to the primary target—cerebral cortex, basal ganglia, brainstem and cerebellum, and spinal cord. These conditions are beginning to yield their secrets thanks to a full frontal assault from investigators using modern molecular and morphological techniques (Figs. 12-1 and 12-2). A theme of cellular stress with abnormal protein polymerization (fibrillization) is emerging and provides a molecular underpinning for the many classical observations of intracellular inclusions in these diseases (Fig. 12-3).

Neurodegenerative Diseases

- **Loss of functionally related neurons**
- **Many causes for neuronal loss**
- **Symptoms depend on specific neuronal populations lost**
  - Cortical neurons: Dementia
  - Basal ganglia neurons: Movement disorder
  - Cerebellar neurons: Ataxia
  - Motor neurons: Weakness

FIGURE 12-1. The clinical manifestations of neurodegeneration depend on the affected system.

Neurodegenerative Diseases

As causes of specific disorders are elucidated, the causes of other disorders may become clear

- **Prions (infectious entities without nucleic acid)**
- **Toxins (MPTP)**
- **Trinucleotide repeat amplification**
- **Oxidative stress**

FIGURE 12-2. Neurodegenerative diseases may arise due to a variety of pathophysiological mechanisms. Elucidation of one disease may clarify others.

INTRACELLULAR INCLUSIONS: ORIGIN, SIGNIFICANCE, AND SPECIFICITY

Intracellular, and in particular, intracytoplasmic inclusions have a history that is inextricably linked to the neurodegenerative disorders, and since these engaging features of diseased cells were among the first histological abnormalities of the nervous system recognized, inordinate significance is often bestowed upon them. Modern techniques have largely dispelled the romance of the inclusions, and show them to be markers of cellular stress. They are cytoplasmic landfills comprised of deranged cytoskeletal proteins and heat shock proteins.

The cellular cytoskeleton is an intricate cytoplasmic organelle linking the cellular membrane with the nuclear envelope. Beyond its obvious structural function, the cytoskeleton may play a role in transcellular signaling. It is composed of three major classes of proteins forming filaments of increasing diameter: the microfilaments (5 nm), the intermediate filaments (10 nm), and the microtubules (22 nm). Microfilaments are composed of actin. The intermediate filaments are made up of relatively tissue-specific proteins. In the nervous system, neurofilament (NF) is the neuronal intermediate filament and glial fibrillary acidic protein (GFAP) is the glial intermediate filament. Multiple forms of these proteins are present in the normal brain, and posttranslational modifications (in particular, phosphorylation) can modify their functional characteristics. The microtubules consist of cylindrical aggregates of globular tubulin molecules. In addition to tubulin, microtubules contain a variety of microtubule-associated proteins (MAPs). The most important of these is tau which exists in multiple isoform and phosphorylation states. The normal cytoskeleton is formed from the complex interdigitation of these three classes of proteins to form a visually delicate cytoplasmic web.

When the cell is stressed by a wide variety of physiological perturbations, the intermediate filament network immediately collapses to form perinuclear bundles or clumps. This molecular response may reflect increased phosphorylation or proteolysis of these proteins due to the influx of calcium into the

Fibrillization and Inclusions

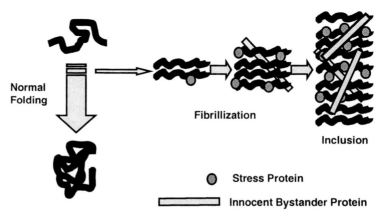

Normal Folding

Fibrillization

Inclusion

- Stress Protein
- Innocent Bystander Protein

FIGURE 12-3. Fibrillogenesis results from the polymerization of cellular proteins and an increased propensity to this biophysical process appears to underlie many neurodegeneration conditions. During fibrillization, abnormal protein polymerizes, induces stress protein conjugation, and may entrap innocent bystander proteins.

Neurodegenerative Buzzword: Fibrillogenesis

- Alzheimer's disease
- Parkinson's disease
- Pick's disease (FTD)
- CJD
- Huntington's disease and other CAG repeat disorders
- Familial ALS

- A-beta amyloid
- Alpha-synuclein
- Tau
- Prion protein
- Huntingtin, ataxin etc. form fibrillar aggregates as intranuclear inclusions
- Superoxide dismutase

FIGURE 12-4. Specific proteins are involved in fibrillogenesis in a variety of disorders spanning the entire spectrum of neurodegeneration.

stressed cell. If the stress experienced by the cell is not lethal, the cell deploys an adaptive response called the "heat shock response" since it was first recognized in cells exposed to thermal stress. The cell manufactures several proteins that may restore functional activity of partially denatured proteins, or if the denaturing is too severe to permit restoration, the proteins are marked for proteolysis. Proteins designated for destruction are conjugated with the stress protein ubiquitin. Other stress proteins may be invoked including crystallin and a family of heat shock proteins (hsp's). If the proteins conjugated to these stress proteins are not degraded, these conjugated complexes aggregate to form intracellular inclusions.

The inclusions in neurodegenerative disorders are examples of such aggregates. They can now be described in terms of the damaged native cytoskeletal protein and the stress response conjugates (Figs. 12-4 and 12-5). The stress response is evoked anytime the cell is damaged; therefore, the presence of stress response inclusions gives no insight regarding the inciting insult. The neuropathological inclusions are made from a relatively limited number of permutations of cytoskeletal proteins and stress proteins (Fig. 12-6). Indeed, this number of permutations is substantially smaller than the number of

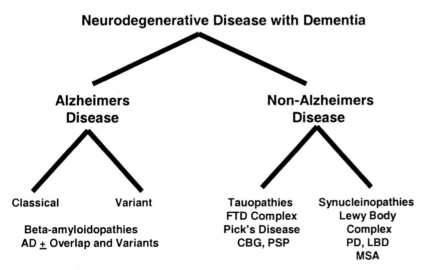

FIGURE 12-5. A synthesis of the cortical dementias based on the polymerizing proteins may be fruitful and bring order out of chaos.

Cytoplasmic Inclusions

Cytoplasmic Landfills

Structural Protein	Stress Protein
Neurofilament Tau Synuclein	Ubiquitin Crystalline Heat Shock Proteins

FIGURE 12-6. Cytoplasmic inclusions are simply cytoplasmic landfills.

apparently discrete types of inclusions described. The observation that several of the inclusions are biochemically identical calls into question their diagnostic specificity. Ubiquitin immunoreactivity is seen in many intracellular inclusions and in and of itself is not "diagnostic" of any particular disease, but the morphology, cellular distribution, and clinical context of ubiquitin positive inclusions may be very important diagnostically. Ubiquitin-immunoreactivity is much more sensitive than classical staining methods, and is therefore increasingly the method of choice in the detection of cellular protein inclusions. Antibodies are now commercially available that allow identification of the proteins conjugated with ubiquitin. Hence, neurofilament, tau, and synuclein can all be discerned. In summary, inclusions give no data about the precise stress damaging the cell, their biochemical composition overlaps in many cases, and final diagnostic categorization often is dependent on clinical data. A number of abnormal proteins associated with neurodegenerative diseases tend to polymerize more readily than their normal counterparts. This polymerization leads to linear fibrils seen ultrastructurally; therefore, the polymerization process is called "fibrillogenesis" (see Figs. 12-3 through 12-6). Once arrays of fibrils begin to condense in the cell, other proteins may be caught up in the process. The cellular stress response is activated and the fibril aggregates and their constituents are ubiquinated. Much remains to be learned about how these fibril accumulations may exert pathogenic effects, and it remains to be seen if pharmacological intervention to prevent polymerization will be beneficial.

Common Cortical Dementias

- Senile dementia of the Alzheimer's type
- Pick's disease
- Dementia with Lewy bodies

FIGURE 12-7. The common cortical dementias.

CORTICAL DEGENERATIONS

The major diseases in this category are AD, LBD, and Pick's disease (Fig. 12-7). They share the clinical manifestation dementia—loss of previously acquired intellectual skills and information. Previously, this loss of intellect was incorrectly regarded as a normal part of aging; hence, dementia was divided into senile dementia for those over age 65 years and presenile dementia when it occurred in those under 65 years of age. It is recognized that dementia is a manifestation of neurological disease regardless of the age of onset.

The neuropathological diagnosis of the "classical" forms of these diseases is straightforward, but there remains considerable controversy about the precise criteria for diagnosis of more subtle, atypical or overlapping forms. As in other areas of clinical neuroscience, there is considerable tension between "lumpers" and "splitters" in this area.

The range of non-Alzheimer dementias has increased in recent years, and many "new" syndromes have been described. There has been a confusing proliferation of imposing names applied to these syndromes, and it appears likely that there are, in fact, only a limited number of clinically or pathologically unique conditions among all of these. The myriad of aliases, however, exaggerates the number of these atypical dementias and obstructs synthesis of concepts about them. "Frontal lobe dementia" (FLD), "nonspecific degeneration," "progressive subcortical gliosis," "progressive aphasia," and "dementia lacking distinctive histological features" (DLDH) belong to this poorly defined and controversial set of dementias. Furthermore, there has been an almost absurd proliferation of Pick's disease variants. These include Pick's disease without Pick bodies, hereditary Pick's disease (hereditary dysphasic dementia), Pick's disease with parkinsonism (Akelaitis variant of Pick disease), and amyotrophy with Pick's disease. The very existence of Pick's disease as a unique entity is in doubt, and there is sufficient neuropathological and clinical overlap of classic Pick's disease, the Pick variants, and other rare and poorly characterized non-Alzheimer dementias that a unifying concept of dementia with lobar atrophy (hence relative focality) has emerged under the name of "frontotemporal dementia" (FTD). Molecular subclassification of these disorders may be possible based on the substances exhibiting fibrillogenesis with the triad of beta-amyloidopathies, tauopathies, and synucleinopathies providing a conceptual framework.

ALZHEIMER'S DISEASE

AD is the single most common cause of dementia. The decline in intellectual ability generally commences between 50 and 65 years, although onset in the 30's and 40's may occur. Women are affected two to three times more commonly than men, and in about 15% of cases a positive family history is evident. In probands with AD, there is an increased incidence of chromosomal abnormalities including trisomy 21 (Down's syndrome); conversely, almost all patients with Down's syndrome develop AD if they live to be older than 30 years. The amyloid precursor protein gene resides on chromosome 21, and mutations of this gene account for about 10% of autosomal dominant AD. Two forms of autosomal dominant familial AD are linked to chromosomes 14 and 1, and result from missense mutations of integral membrane proteins (presenillin 1 and presenillin 2) which may be receptors, membrane channels or proteins involved in docking and fusion of membrane-bound vesicles. There is evidence that the presenillins may be involved in proteolytic processing at the cell surface required to release Notch and APP fragments into the extracellular space. The presenillin mutations may result in increased APP production. These familial forms of AD tend to have earlier onset and a more aggressive course than sporadic or apolipoprotein E4 linked AD. Homozygosity for the E4 allele of apolipoprotein E has been shown to confer increased risk for AD. ApoE is involved in lipid transport, but the precise molecular basis of the AD connection is unclear. The liver is the primary producer of ApoE, but the brain is a close second, and it is possible that brain-derived ApoE may modulate the CNS stress response to injury. Interestingly, ApoE4 is associated with poor outcome from traumatic head injury lending support to this notion.

Clinically, patients undergo steadily progressive intellectual deterioration without remissions or plateau periods, and death generally occurs in 3 to 12 years at which time the individual is generally bedridden and unable to attend to even the most fundamental bodily processes.

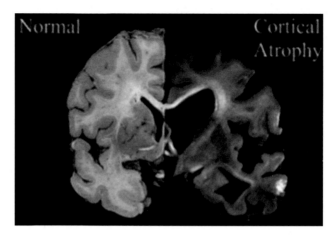

FIGURE 12-8. Cortical atrophy leads to widened sulci and hydrocephalus ex vacuo.

Alzheimer's Disease

• **Senile plaques**

• **Neurofibrillary tangles**

• **Granulovacuolar degeneration**

• **Amyloid angiopathy**

FIGURE 12-9. Histopathology of Alzheimer's disease.

Examination of the brain discloses cortical atrophy with thinning of the cortex and widening of the sulci, the ventricles are enlarged (compensatory hydrocephalus or hydrocephalus *ex vacuo*), and the brain weight is decreased (Fig. 12-8). Microscopically, one sees neurofibrillary tangles, senile plaques, and granulovacuolar degeneration. Additionally, amyloid angiopathy is sometimes seen (Fig. 12-9).

Tangles are intraneuronal cytoplasmic collections of poorly soluble 7–9-nm paired helically wound filaments with a periodicity of 80 nm. These filaments share some antigenic sites with neuronal intermediate filaments, and are best stained with classical silver methods or thioflavin S. Tangles are found predominantly in projection neurons. Hyperphosphorylated tau protein is a major component of tangles although neurofilament protein and ubiquitin are also present in significant amounts.

Plaques are extracellular 20–150-μm structures consisting of a central pink amyloid core surrounded by blunt swollen neuritic processes; like tangles, they stain well with silver stains and have the appearance of burnt out campfires against the delicate background of the neuropil (Fig. 12-10).

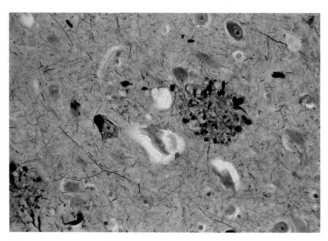

FIGURE 12-10. Senile plaque and neurofibrillary tangle in Alzheimer's disease.

The third microscopic hallmark is granulovacuolar degeneration that appears as small (5 μm), clear, intraneuronal cytoplasmic vacuolation with each vacuole containing a single argyrophilic granule (Fig. 12-11).

Some believe that the severity of dementia correlates well with the number of mature or neuritic plaques per unit area in the brain, while others hold that the neurofibrillary tangles correlate better with dementia. All agree that diffuse plaques, which are large diffuse areas of staining devoid of central cores or swollen neuritic processes, do not correlate with the severity of dementia. The diffuse plaque may be a precursor of the neuritic plaque, but the correlation with severity of dementia and the specificity of the diffuse plaque is much weaker than the mature form. Many neuropathologists eschew counting diffuse plaques in the assessment of dementia brains, but these structures contribute substantially to interobserver variability in the evaluation of brains at autopsy.

Plaques contain beta-amyloid protein, a peptide having 28 to 43 amino acids. This small amyloidogenic peptide is derived from proteolytic cleavage of a large transmembrane glycoprotein, amyloid precursor protein (APP). This precursor protein is synthesized in three major forms (695, 751, and 770 amino acid residues) by differential mRNA splicing. The two larger forms have regions that have homology with serine protease inhibitors. Beta-amyloid is toxic to mature neurons; this peptide may bind protease inhibitor receptors on cell surfaces permitting the accumulation of extracellular proteases leading to membrane and eventually cytoskeletal damage

In terms of neurotransmitter alterations, AD is characterized by a striking reduction in cortical acetylcholine as reflected in the amount of choline acetyl transferase (CAT) in the cortex. This biochemical information led to the observation that the basal forebrain nucleus responsible for the majority of cortical cholinergic projections, the basal nucleus of Meynert, is depleted of cells in AD. Other neurochemical abnormalities have been described in AD, but cholinergic reduction remains the major alteration and development and moderately successful clinical application of multiple central choline esterase inhibitors validates the importance of this biochemical alteration.

The neuropathological diagnosis of AD has been the topic of heated discussion for several years, but a consensus is beginning to emerge from these discussions. The guidelines developed by the multicenter AD project CERAD (Consortium to Establish a Registry for AD) probably represent the most widely used diagnostic criteria. The CERAD protocol employs a semi-quantitative evaluation of neuritic plaques coupled with the patient's age to reach an age-related plaque score. Three sections of neocortex including superior and middle temporal gyrus, middle frontal gyrus, and inferior parietal lobule are examined at 100x using either the Bielschowsky silver technique or the more sensitive thioflavin S staining technique. The thioflavin S technique requires access to fluorescence microscopy, and is not as widely available as silver staining. The number of plaques is designated as none, sparse, moderate, and frequent. CERAD provides images illustrative of these plaque (and tangle) frequencies to help neuropathologists calibrate their estimates. Fewer plaques are tolerated in young (age less than 50 years) than in the elderly (age greater than 75 years), and the presence or absence of a history of dementia is taken into account. Recent CERAD studies have disclosed substantial variability in stain selection, staining technique, and plaque estimation between 18 centers and 24 neuropathologists in the United States and Canada. In this study, unstained sections from 10 cases (eight AD and two control cases) were sent to the 18 CERAD participating centers, and stained and examined. There was 75% interobserver agreement regarding the semiquantitative assessment of the sections for neuritic plaques. Diffuse plaques were over-counted by some neu-

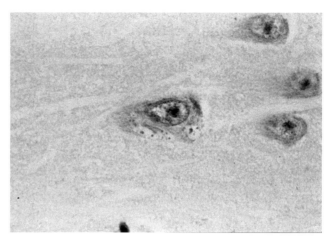

FIGURE 12-11. Granulovacuolar degeneration in Alzheimer's disease.

ropathologists contributing to the variability. The two control cases were very consistently ranked as having few plaques Braak and Braak redirected attention to the neurofibrillary tangles and described spread of tangles from the transentorhinal cortex and hippocampus (stage 1 and 2) to limbic system (stage 3 and 4) to isocortex including frontal, temporal, parietal and occipital neocortex (stage 5 and 6) as AD progresses. They have provided compelling evidence that description of the distribution of NFTs is important in the neuropathological assessment of AD. Individuals in stage 1 and 2 are generally asymptomatic, those in stage 3 and 4 have incipient or mild AD, and those in stage 5 and 6 have symptomatic AD. The Braak and Braak classification can be simplified to three tiers: transentorhinal cortex, limbic, and isocortex involvement.

A National Institutes of Health National Institute on Aging sponsored consensus conference on the neuropathological diagnosis of AD was convened in 1998, and while diagnostic consensus was not even remotely approached, it was agreed that future research programs funded by the NIA should include assessment of both plaques and tangles. This requirement is referred to as the NIA Reagan consensus and basically requires that neuropathological assessment include a CERAD designation as well as Braak and Braak staging (Figs. 12-11 through 12-13).

Recent Evolution of AD Diagnosis

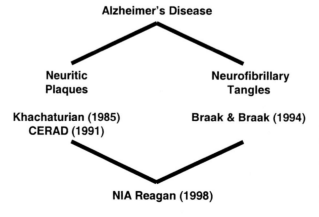

FIGURE 12-12. The diagnostic classification of Alzheimer's disease should take both plaques and neurofibrillary tangles into account.

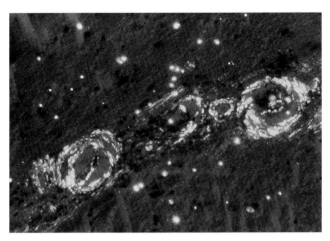

FIGURE 12-13. Amyloid angiopathy is common in Alzheimer's disease and may result in lobar hemorrhage.

PICK'S DISEASE

Much less common and sometimes clinically indistinguishable from AD, this condition is characterized pathologically by severe ("knife-edge") cortical atrophy involving predominantly the frontal and temporal regions with relative sparing of the posterior two-thirds of the superior temporal gyrus and the parietal and occipital lobes (Fig. 12-14). Loss of frontal inhibition of socially unacceptable and previously suppressed behavior may emerge early in the disease often eclipsing the memory disturbance. Microscopically, severe cortical neuronal loss with gliosis is seen as are intraneuronal cytoplasmic oval silver-loving filamentous inclusions (Pick bodies)(Fig. 12-15). In addition to classic Pick bodies, ballooned neurons with achromatic cytoplasmic inclusions are commonly seen (Fig. 12-16). These ballooned neurons overlap with the neuronal changes seen in corticobasal ganglionic degeneration (CBGD). Plaques, tangles and granulovacuolar degeneration are not seen, clearly distinguishing this condition from AD. Biochemical studies and examinations of the basal nucleus of Meynert have yielded inconsistent results. Pick's disease is now classified as one of several FTDs, which share

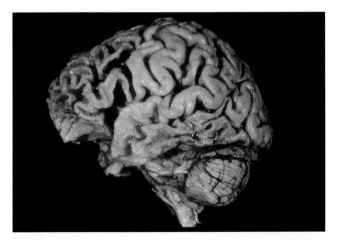

FIGURE 12-14. Frontotemporal dementia (Pick's disease) with marked atrophy of frontal and temporal lobes with less involvement of the parietal and occipital regions.

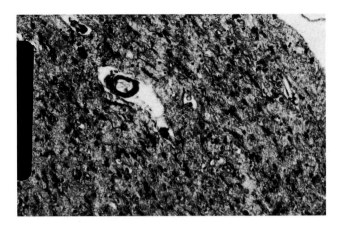

FIGURE 12-15. Gliosis, vacuolation, and neuronal loss in frontotemporal dementia.

cortical neuronal loss and gliosis preferentially affecting the frontal and temporal lobes. FTD may be associated with motor neuron disease. Chromosome 17 linked familial FTD results from intronic tau gene mutation leading to abnormal splicing and overexpression of selected tau isoforms that have a propensity to be hyperphosphorylated. This principle may generalize to other FTDs, including Pick's disease, leading to the concept that they are "tauopathies." In addition, progressive supranuclear palsy and corticobasalganglionic degeneration show a tau isoform imbalance.

LEWY BODY DEMENTIA (LBD)

This disorder exhibits highly variable clinical and neuropathological overlap between AD and Parkinson's disease. Some regard LBD as a variant of the above diseases but most regard it as a separate disease. Classic early onset cases are characterized by parkinsonism unresponsive to standard medications, whereas later onset cases are dominated by cognitive decline. Fluctuating deterioration of cognition characterized by "good days" with relatively intact function separated by "bad days" with confusion and visual hallucina-

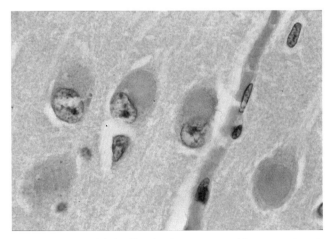

FIGURE 12-16. Pick bodies are intraneuronal intracytoplasmic tau-positive inclusions.

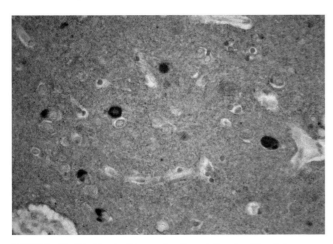

FIGURE 12-17. Cortical Lewy bodies stained with alpha-synuclein immunohistochemistry.

tions are particularly useful in distinguishing this condition from AD. In some recent autopsy series, DLBD is second only to AD as a cause of dementia (7–30% of all dementia cases). Pathologically, there are neuronal cytoplasmic inclusions having structural and antigenic features similar to classical Lewy bodies in Parkinson's disease. Cortical Lewy bodies are not as distinctive as those in the substantia nigra and may be difficult to discern without immunohistochemical staining. Neurofilament, ubiquitin, and crystallin are all present in these bodies, but alpha-synuclein immunoreactivity is the most specific feature (Fig. 12-17). Relatively few cortical Lewy bodies seen in the neocortex (particularly cingulate cortex) are required for a neuropathological diagnosis of this condition. In addition, there is loss of neurons in the substantia nigra similar to that seen in Parkinson's disease, and loss of basal nucleus of Meynert neurons similar to AD. In the hippocampus, there are neurofibrillary tangles and senile plaques as well as granulovacuolar degeneration similar to AD. Cortical microvacuolation is also common and may lead to diagnostic consideration of a prion encephalopathy! LBD is the great mimicker of other neurodegenerative disorders; neuropathologists who believe in the disease probably overdiagnosis it, and nonbelievers clearly under diagnose the condition. Use of alpha-synuclein immunohistochemistry will lead us out of this morass.

CORTICOBASAL GANGLIONIC DEGENERATION

This disorder is characterized by striking asymmetrical gait and speech apraxia, "alien hand syndrome," rigidity, myoclonus, and cortical sensory loss. Dementia usually is a late manifestation of the disease. Pathologically, there is pre- and postcentral cortical neuronal degeneration with achromatic intracytoplasmic neuronal inclusions. These inclusions are also in the thalamus, subthalamic nucleus, red nucleus, and substantia nigra. On hematoxylin and eosin-stained sections, the achromatic inclusions are very similar to Pick bodies, and immunohistochemical studies reveal that these inclusions share neurofilament, ubiquitin, crystallin and tau immunoreactivity seen in Pick bodies. This immunohistochemical similarity leads to corticobasal ganglionic degeneration (CBGD) being classified as a tauopathy.

RECENTLY CHARACTERIZED NON-ALZHEIMER DEMENTIAS: FRONTOTEMPORAL DEMENTIA

This set of disorders exists in a perpetual state of flux, and has spawned a bewildering number of diagnostic terms. One unifying thread which runs through this morass is the prominence of non-amnestic focal cortical clinical signs and symptoms. Hence, these disorders bear names reflecting their relentless progressive initially focal clinical manifestations as well as their lobar pathology. The cellular neuropathology is variable. In some instances these conditions appear to be focal variants of Pick's disease, AD, or LBD. In others the histopathology is not congruent with these disorders, raising the possibility that some of the non-Alzheimer dementias represent unique new diseases. Some use the term *frontotemporal dementia* to encompass these disorders, and these have been the focus of several international meetings and conferences attempting to reach diagnostic consensus. Genetic studies of familial FTD with extrapyramidal symptoms linked to chromosome 17 have demonstrated splicing defects of tau.

Frontal lobe dementia is a syndrome characterized by prominent frontal lobe symptoms in contrast to the more pronounced amnestic symptoms seen in classic AD. These patients have reduced frontal cerebral blood flow. Grossly, there is slight symmetrical frontal and anterior temporal atrophy with frontal ventricular enlargement. The atrophy is usually not as severe as in classic Pick's disease. No striatal, amygdala, or hippocampal atrophy is seen. Microscopically there is microvacuolation and gliosis predominantly of the outer 3 laminae of cerebral cortex. Neurons are lost in laminae 2 and 3, but lamina 4 is relatively spared. No classic Pick bodies, ballooned neurons, or Lewy bodies are seen. No neuronal inclusions immunoreactive to tau or ubiquitin are seen. The microscopic alterations are most marked in the frontal cortex. In some cases there is mild to moderate loss of pigmented neurons of the substantia nigra. Patients exhibiting frontal lobe dementia plus these neuropathological findings are now classified as having *frontotemporal dementia of the frontal lobe degeneration type (FTDFLD)*.

Some patients have the clinical features of frontal lobe dementia but have much more pronounced frontal lobe atrophy, and in addition to microvacuolation, gliosis, and neuronal loss, they have ballooned or inflated neurons and Pick bodies. The gliosis may extend throughout the cortex and into the white matter. Such patients are classified as having *frontotemporal dementia of the Pick-type (FTDPT)*. This semantic maneuver leaves open the possibility that these patients have Pick's disease while maintaining sufficient flexibility to encompass atypical cases.

Finally, there is *frontotemporal dementia of the motor neuron type (FTDMNT)* in which the previously described clinical and neuropathological findings are coupled with spinal motor neuron degeneration. The motor neuron loss is usually most severe in the cervical and thoracic segments. In Japan and more recently in Western countries, sporadic cases of ALS plus dementia have been described and designated *amyotrophy-dementia complex (ADC)* that appear to be identical to *FTDMNT*.

Importantly, the presence of histopathological features of AD, including senile plaques, diffuse amyloid plaques, amyloid angiopathy, or neuropil threads serve as exclusionary diagnostic features of FTD as does the presence of prion protein detected by immunohistochemistry.

In 1990, Knopman et al. described 14 patients out of 460 demented patients whose brains were contained in a regional brain bank as *dementia lacking distinctive histology (DLDH)*. These patients had gliosis and neuronal loss in multiple sites including frontoparietal cortex, striatum, thalamus, substantia nigra, and hypoglossal nucleus. No senile plaques or neuronal inclusions were seen. There was more atrophy of the amygdala and hippocampus than is generally expected with FTD of the frontal lobe degeneration type, but the neuropathological features are otherwise very similar. Lumpers are inclined to place DLDH into the same diagnostic bin as FTD of the frontal lobe degeneration type, whereas splitters celebrate the birth of yet another diagnostic category!

Progressive aphasia, a linguistic syndrome of progressive aphasia FTD of the frontal lobe degeneration type except that the speech areas are more heavily involved. Progressive aphasia has also been described in the context of AD, CJD, CBGD, and classic Pick's disease (Fig. 12-18).

Progressive Aphasia
- **Frontotemporal dementia**
- **Alzheimer's disease**
- **CBGD**
- **CJD**

FIGURE 12-18. Progressive aphasia can result from a variety of disorders and is not a specific diagnosis.

A LUMPER'S VIEW OF AD, PICK'S DISEASE, CBGD, AND NON-ALZHEIMER DEMENTIAS

The following is our rather irreverent view of the dementias we have covered so far. We are confessed and unrepentant lumpers, but we recognize that in our broad sweep toward synthesis we may overlook some important subdivisions of diseases. Listed in *italics* are the diagnostic terms we prefer to use, and listed with these preferred terms are their numerous aliases. The aliases should be used sparingly, if at all, so that they may undergo linguistic atrophy.

Alzheimer's disease: Clinical features of dementia, CERAD plaque quantification, and Braak and Braak staging, in other words, the Reagan consensus on neuropathological features are required for the definitive diagnosis, and recognize that focal and overlap forms may occur. Focality may be acknowledged in the diagnosis, i.e., "AD with progressive aphasia" or "AD with disproportionate visuospatial dysfunction." Overlap can be denoted by AD with Parkinson's disease, or AD with diffuse Lewy body disease. Eschew progressive aphasia or dementia with disproportionate visuospatial dysfunction used alone as diagnostic terms. Eschew use of the term Lewy body variant of AD.

Pick's disease: Dementia plus classic Pick bodies on histopathology are required for a firm diagnosis. Recognize that focal and overlap forms may occur. Focality and overlap can be handled the same as with AD, i.e. hereditary Pick's disease (hereditary dysphasic dementia), Pick's disease with parkinsonism (Akelaitis variant of Pick disease), and amyotrophy with Pick's disease. *Frontotemporal dementia, Pick type* is an acceptable alternative term since it acknowledges Arnold Pick's contribution while attempting synthesis with the other FTDs. Aliases to be eschewed, in our opinion, include Pick's disease type A (which is classic Pick's disease as we use the term here), Pick's disease type B which is really CBGD, Pick's disease type C, which is FTD of the frontal degeneration type, and Pick's disease without Pick bodies, which is also FTD of the frontal degeneration type.

CBGD: Appropriate clinical features and achromatic neuronal inclusions but no classic Pick bodies are required for the diagnosis. Eschew dementia with swollen chromatolytic neurons, corticodentatonigral degeneration, and corticobasal degeneration.

Lewy body dementia (LBD): Appropriate clinical features plus Lewy bodies in neocortex (particularly demonstrated by alpha-synuclein immunohistochemistry) are required for the diagnosis.

Frontotemporal dementia of the frontal degeneration type (FTDFDT): Appropriate clinical features, gliosis, microvacuolation and neuronal loss are required. Recognize focal forms such as FTDFDT with progressive aphasia. Eschew use of the terms dementia lacking distinct histopathology (DLDH), progressive subcortical gliosis, Pick's disease without Pick bodies, and nonspecific degeneration.

Frontotemporal dementia of the Pick type: see *Pick's disease.*

Frontotemporal dementia of the motor neuron type: Dementia plus motor neuron disease required with neuropathological features of FTD and ALS. Eschew ALS with dementia, Pick's disease with amyotrophy, amyotrophy-dementia complex.

BASAL GANGLIA DEGENERATIONS

Disorders impacting on this area often produce movement disorders, but varying degrees of intellectual impairment may be seen as well. Overlap syndromes can also be seen. For example, concurrent Huntington's disease and AD have been described, and more commonly one can see AD with Parkinson's disease.

HUNTINGTON'S DISEASE

This autosomal dominant disorder carried on chromosome 4 combines dementia with choreiform movements having their onset in the 20's to 40's well after affected individuals have had time to reproduce. The disease may begin with psychiatric symptoms or abnormal movements, and progresses relentlessly to death in 10 to 15 years (Fig. 12-19).

The brain is atrophic, and striking atrophy of the caudate nucleus and, to a lesser degree, the putamen is seen. Compensatory hydrocephalus is evident (Fig. 12-20). Microscopically, preferential loss of the small spiny striatal neurons accompanied by gliosis is seen. Biochemically, there is diminished gamma-aminobutyric acid (GABA), encephalins, and substance P.

The genetic basis of seven neurodegenerative disorders—Huntington's disease, hereditary spinocerebellar atrophy type 1, myotonic dystrophy, spinobulbar atrophy and fragile-X mental retardation, dentatorubro-pallidoluyseal degeneration, and Machado-Joseph disease—is trinucleotide repeat amplification. This novel mechanism of genetic disease may underlie other disorders, and may explain the previously mysterious phenomenon of "anticipation" in which these disorders had earlier onset in succeeding generations.

Huntington's Disease

- **Autosomal dominant**
- **Chromosome 4**
- **Trinucleotide repeat in "huntingtin" gene**
- **Caudate atrophy**
- **Loss of spiny GABA neurons**
- **Chorea**
- **Dementia or psychosis**
- **Rigid variant in the young**

FIGURE 12-19. Features of Huntington's disease.

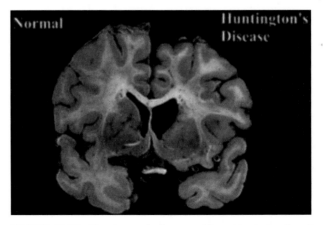

FIGURE 12-20. Huntington's disease with marked atrophy of the caudate nucleus.

We all normally have a number of trinucleotide repeats but when instability of the DNA leads to increased numbers of repeats in a given sequence, disease may result. The severity of the disease and age of onset increases with increased trinucleotide repeat numbers, and since repeats may amplify between generations "anticipation" may be seen (Figs. 12-21 and 12-22).

The CAG trinucleotide repeat disorders possess polyglutamate sequences within the proteins produced by the mutated genes. The molecular basis of pathogenesis in these disorders remains obscure, but it is possible that this change in the primary structure of the protein may lead to abnormal interactions with other proteins or may alter the functional characteristics of the proteins. Huntington's disease and SCA1 both have intranuclear neuronal inclusions resulting from precipitation of nuclear proteins. Recent studies suggest that abnormally long polyglutamine stretches coded by CAG repeats result in intranuclear inclusions and neurodegeneration regardless of the location of the repeats in the genome. This means that the pathological effect of CAG repeats is independent of genomic context.

IDIOPATHIC PARKINSONISM (PARKINSON'S DISEASE, PARALYSIS AGITANS)

This common disease was first described by James Parkinson in 1817 and is dominated by disturbances of motor function including reduced facial expression (reptilian faces), stooped posture, slowness in initiating and executing voluntary movements, rigidity, pill rolling tremor, and festinating gait (Fig. 12-23). This disease usually appears between ages 50 and 80 years, and is characterized pathologically by loss of pigmentation of the substantia nigra and locus ceruleus with decreased neuromelanin-containing neurons in these structures (Fig. 12-24). Affected neurons contain large homogenous eosinophilic cytoplasmic inclusions called "Lewy bodies" that possess neurofilament, ubiquitin, and crystallin immunoreactivity (Fig. 12-25). Importantly, however, Lewy bodies also contain alpha-synuclein which is relatively specific for both classical Lewy bodies and cortical Lewy bodies of LBD.

The molecular basis of Parkinson's disease is incompletely understood, but neurotoxicologic models have focused attention on impaired free-radical handling as mechanistically important (Fig. 12-26). The exceptionally high

---

Trinucleotide Repeat Syndromes

- Trinucleotide DNA repeats are part of normal genetic polymorphism
- Excessive amplification at some sites produces disease
- Severity and age of onset of disease correlate with degree of amplification
- Amplification may increase in successive generations leading to "anticipation"

FIGURE 12-21. Mechanism of trinucleotide repeat amplification in neurological disorders.

Trinucleotide Repeat Syndromes

- Huntington's disease
- Myotonic dystrophy
- Fragile X syndrome
- Friedreich's ataxia
- Spinocerebellar ataxia
- Spinobulbar atrophy
- Dentatorubroluyseal degeneration
- Machado-Joseph disease

FIGURE 12-22. Neurodegenerative diseases with trinucleotide repeat amplification.

Parkinson's Disease

- Sporadic
- Common in older persons
- Atrophy of substantia nigra
- Loss of dopaminergic neurons projecting to striatum; Lewy bodies
- Rigidity
- Tremor
- Bradykinesis

FIGURE 12-23. Features of Parkinson's disease.

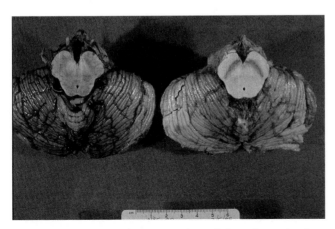

FIGURE 12-24. Loss of pigmentation of the substantia nigra (*left*) compared to normal (*right*)

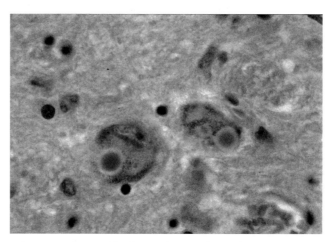

FIGURE 12-25. Lewy bodies in the cytoplasm of pigmented neurons of the substantia nigra in Parkinson's disease.

MPTP Parkinsonism Directed Attention to Free Radicals

- **MPTP is converted to toxic MPP+ by monoamine oxidase B**
- **Toxicity can be prevented by MAO-B inhibitors**
- **Selegiline is a MAO-B inhibitor that may slow the progression of idiopathic Parkinson's disease**

FIGURE 12-26. MPTP-induced Parkinsonism refocused attention on free radical mechanisms in neurodegeneration.

Other Causes of Parkinsonism

- **Post-encephalitic parkinsonism**
- **Progressive supranuclear palsy**
- **Manganese intoxication**
- **Dopamine antagonist medications**

FIGURE 12-27. Parkinsonism can result from a variety of conditions.

---

iron content of the basal ganglia, and the substantia nigra, in particular, portends vulnerability to oxidative damage. A very rare form of familial Parkinson's disease results from an alpha-synuclein mutation (chromosome 4). This rare mutation led to the observation that synuclein immunohistochemistry is a very sensitive and specific method for detecting Lewy bodies.

Parkinson's disease was until the mid-1960's a disease with almost as dismal an outlook as AD today. Recognition of the biochemical defect—relative dopaminergic insufficiency—led to the therapeutic triumph of levodopa therapy (administration of neurotransmitter precursor). Rather than a bedridden death, these patients are able to function for years to decades after onset of symptoms. In addition, pharmacological measures designed to reduce free-radical damage appear to retard the progression of the disease. Many researchers hope that the Parkinson's disease paradigm of therapeutics can be applied to other neurodegenerative disorders.

POSTENCEPHALITIC PARKINSONISM

This disease is now an almost nonexistent but nevertheless extremely important disease which followed the 1914–1918 influenza pandemics (Fig. 12-27). Some individuals developed encephalitis, and in the months to years following recovery from the acute illness, they developed parkinsonism attended by prominent oculogyric symptoms. The condition was nonprogressive. Pathologically, depigmentation of the substantia nigra and locus ceruleus is seen, but no classic Lewy bodies are present and neurofibrillary tangles are evident.

MPTP PARKINSONISM

This condition occurred as an epidemic in drug abusers unfortunate enough to have used "synthetic heroin" (MPPP: 1-methyl-4-phenyl-4-propionoxy-piperidine; a Demerol analogue) contaminated by MPTP (1-methyl-4-phenyl-1,2,5,6-tetrahydropyridine) which is converted by MAO-B to MPP+, which is selectively toxic to dopaminergic neurons. Cell loss is seen in the pars compacta of the substantia nigra; no true Lewy bodies are present although smaller eosinophilic cytoplasmic inclusions with antigenic features identical to Lewy bodies have been seen. This neurotoxicological model is used to produce

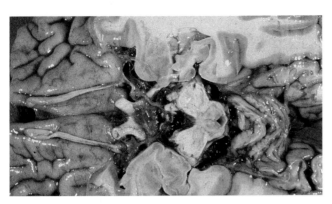

FIGURE 12-28. Progressive supranuclear palsy showing the characteristic "Mickey Mouse" midbrain.

experimental Parkinson's disease in animals, and has focused much attention on toxins as potential mediators of neurodegenerative disorders.

PROGRESSIVE SUPRANUCLEAR PALSY

In progressive supranuclear palsy (PSP; Steele-Richardson-Olszewski syndrome), an uncommon disorder, supranuclear ophthalmoparesis (down gaze in particular), rigidity, and gait disturbance dominate the clinical presentation. 60–80% of PSP patients may exhibit subcortical dementia. There is widespread diencephalic, mesencephalic (grossly leading to "Mickey Mouse" midbrain), brainstem and cerebellar nuclear neuronal loss (Fig. 12-28). Globose neurofibrillary tangles are seen. These tangles exhibit paired helical filament, tau protein and ubiquitin immunoreactivity.

SPINOCEREBELLAR DEGENERATIONS

Multiple System Atrophy

This group of disorders is characterized by extreme clinical variability and nosological chaos (Fig. 12-29). They tend to be familial but may be transmitted either dominantly or recessively, and sporadic cases are common. Neuronal atrophy is seen to a variable degree in the brainstem, cerebellum, spinal cord, and peripheral nerves, usually associated with mild gliosis.

Olivopontocerebellar atrophy (OPCA) is one of the most common and most variable of these conditions. Neuronal loss with gross atrophy is concentrated in the pons, medullary olives, and cerebellum, but other areas may be involved (Fig. 12-30). Ataxia, rigidity, spasticity, and oculomotor movement disturbances are present to variable degrees in combination. OPCA is currently classified as one of the multiple system atrophies (MSAs) that include OPCA, striatonigral atrophy, and the Shy-Drager syndrome (marked atrophy of the lateral horns). There is considerable clinical and pathological overlap among these syndromes, and recently glial cytoplasmic inclusions (GCIs) have been recognized as apparently unique cellular pathological markers of MSA (Fig. 12-31). These are intracytoplasmic predominantly oligodendroglial argyrophilic inclusions that exhibit modest tau and strong alpha-synuclein immunoreactivity.

Multiple System Atrophy

- Olivopontocerebellar degeneration
- Striatonigral degeneration
- Dysautonomia

FIGURE 12-29. Multiple system atrophy is one disease where once there were three.

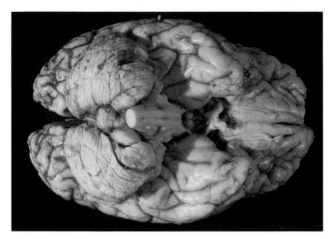

FIGURE 12-30. Olivopontocerebellar atrophy in multiple system atrophy.

Friedreich's Ataxia

Friedreich's Ataxia

- Most common hereditary ataxia
- Autosomal recessive
- GAA triplet repeat expansion
  - Both alleles with expansion
  - One allele with expansion + other with mutation
- Frataxin
- CNS, cardiac, pancreas

FIGURE 12-32. Features of Friedreich's ataxia.

Friedreich's ataxia is more clearly defined than MSA, and is autosomal recessive (Fig. 12-32). Ataxia, clumsiness, dysarthria, loss of tendon reflexes, and impaired sensation may all occur and are accompanied by interstitial myocarditis. The spinal cord is small with loss of axons and gliosis of the posterior columns, corticospinal tracts, and spinocerebellar tracts. Neuronal loss is seen in Clark's column, the lower cranial nuclei, and the dentate nucleus as well as the Purkinje cell layer and the dorsal root ganglia (Fig. 12-33 and 12-34).

This disease is a triple repeat amplification disorder, and is unique among the triplet repeat disorders in that it is recessive; both alleles of the frataxin gene have abnormal triplet repeat amplification, or one allele has a triplet repeat amplification and the other allele has another kind of mutation. Evidence is accumulating that frataxin is involved in mitochondrial iron regulation, and that a defect in this protein leads to excessive mitochondrial iron content with attendant excess free radical production. The affected protein, frataxin, is homologous to Yfh1p in yeast, a protein that regulates mitochondrial iron homeostasis.

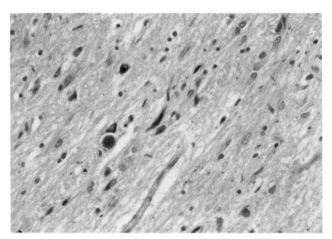

FIGURE 12-31. Glial intracytoplasmic inclusion in multiple system atrophy.

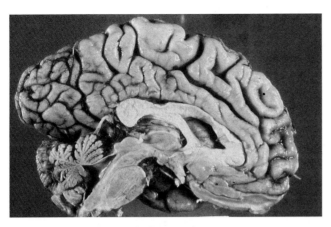

FIGURE 12-33. Spinocerebellar atrophy.

Understanding of the hereditary ataxias has undergone a remarkable transformation with the elucidation of the genetic mechanisms of these disorders. The following is a partial listing of the major hereditary ataxias.

Motor Neuron Disease

In contrast to the spinocerebellar degenerations, the motor neuron degenerative disorders are remarkably homogenous (Fig. 12-35). In these conditions, the upper motor neuron (soma in the motor cortex—axon in corticospinal tracts), the lower motor neuron (cranial nerve motor nuclei and anterior horn cells of the spinal cord), or both atrophy over a period of months to years (Figs. 12-36 through 12-38).

Amyotrophic lateral sclerosis is the term applied when the degeneration involves both upper and lower motor neurons. The patients present with weakness that is often initially asymmetrical. The lower motor neuron involvement will be evidenced by muscle atrophy, weakness, and fasciculations (spontaneous grossly visible twitching of muscle fiber groups). The upper motor neuron involvement is manifested by weakness and spasticity. Progression is relentless with eventual loss of all voluntary movement with the exception

---

Motor Neuron Disease

- **Amyotrophic lateral sclerosis**
- **Familial ALS - Superoxide dismutase mutation**
- **Spinal muscular atrophy**
- **Wernig-Hoffman disease**

FIGURE 12-35. Variety of motor neuron disease.

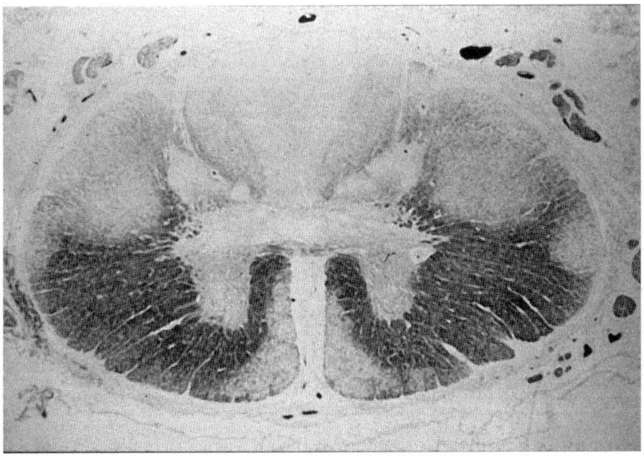

FIGURE 12-34. Spinal cord in Friedreich's ataxia showing degeneration of spinocerebellar, lateral corticospinal, and dorsal column tracts.

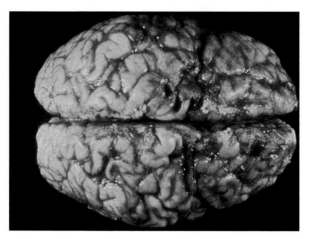

FIGURE 12-36. Upper motor neuron loss in amyotrophic lateral sclerosis manifested as atrophy of the motor strip.

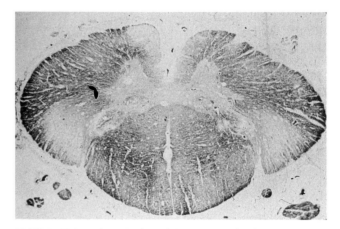

FIGURE 12-37. The spinal cord in amyotrophic lateral sclerosis showing loss of the lateral and anterior corticospinal tracts.

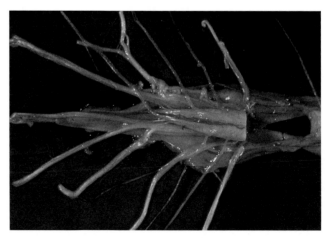

FIGURE 12-38. Anterior (motor) spinal root atrophy in ALS. The intact posterior sensory roots are white due to myelin and thick due to intact axons.

generally of extraocular motility. Death results from respiratory insufficiency or bedsores with sepsis. The patient's intellect is unimpaired. The anterior roots of the spinal cord are of diminished caliber reflecting the anterior horn cell loss that is evident microscopically. The degenerating lateral corticospinal tracts are gliotic and therefore firm and white (hence "lateral sclerosis"). Skeletal muscle is atrophic (hence "amyotrophic"), and exhibits fiber-type grouping indicative of denervation. Recently, autoantibodies to muscle voltage-gated calcium channels have been reported to be elevated in ALS patients, raising the possibility that autoimmunity may play a role in some patients with this disease. Familial ALS in some instances results from mutations of superoxide dismutase, which was initially thought to result in impaired handling of free radicals. No abnormalities in free-radical handling have yet been convincingly demonstrated in either hereditary or sporadic ALS, and it is now believed that the superoxide dismutase mutations result in a gain of function by fibrillization. Finally, there is considerable interest in the potential role of excitotoxicity in ALS with excess glutamate activity being posited as the operative mechanism.

If the degeneration involves predominantly the cranial nerve nuclei with resulting dysarthria, dysphagia, and respiratory embarrassment, the term *progressive bulbar palsy* is applied. If spinal cord anterior horn cell involvement predominates, the term *progressive muscular atrophy* is used. If involvement is confined largely to the lateral corticospinal tracts, the term *primary lateral sclerosis* applies.

Infantile progressive spinal muscular atrophy (Werdnig-Hoffman disease) is a horrifyingly common autosomal recessive condition presenting in infancy with extreme muscle weakness and atrophy due to severe loss of the anterior horn cells; it is clinically and pathologically analogous to progressive muscular atrophy of adulthood. Death ensues from respiratory failure or aspiration pneumonia usually within a few months of diagnosis. Accurate diagnosis is critical for genetic risk management.

OVERLAP SYNDROMES

As was discussed under the cortical dementias, amyotrophy may accompany variants of AD, Pick's disease, and is part of FTD of the motor neuron type.

ALS–Parkinsonism–Dementia of Guam

The ultimate overlap syndrome is ALS–parkinsonism–dementia of Guam, which exhibits gross atrophy of the frontotemporal regions, depigmentation of the substantia nigra, and loss of anterior roots. Histologically, there are neurofibrillary tangles in the cortical neurons, loss of pigmented neurons in the substantia nigra without Lewy body formation, and loss of anterior horn cells with neurofibrillary tangles.

BIBLIOGRAPHY

Consensus Recommendations for the Postmortem Diagnosis of Alzheimer's Disease. *Neurobiol Aging* 1997;18:S4.

Dickson DW, Yen SHC. In: Mayer J, Brown I, eds. *Heat shock in the nervous system.* New York: Academic Press, 1994.

Mirra S, et al. *Arch Pathol Lab Med* 1993;17:132–144.

Mirra S, et al. *J Neuropathol Exp Neurol* 1994;53:303–315.

13

TRAUMA

PERSPECTIVE

1. Physical injury of the brain, spinal cord, and peripheral nervous system constitutes a major cause of loss of life and productivity. Populations at highest risk for such injuries include children, men in late adolescence and early adult life, and the elderly.
2. Injury results from the transfer of energy to the tissues. The severity of injury depends on the magnitude and time course of energy transfer to the brain or spinal cord.

OBJECTIVES

1. Compare and contrast the cause, clinical course, and pathology of epidural hematoma versus subdural hematoma.
2. Describe where cerebral contusions are most commonly seen. Compare and contrast coup and contra-coup contusions.
3. Comprehend that kinetic energy is the primary physical determinant of the severity of injury from a bullet. You can tell the trajectory of the bullet by examining the skull for beveling.
4. Understand that diffuse axonal injury (DAI) is found in the white matter and develops over a period of hours to days.

The brain and spinal cord are enclosed in protective bony cases which serve to dissipate forces delivered to these delicate nervous system structures; however, evolutionary selection has not yet adequately responded to the need to survive vehicular crashes, personal assaults with small arms, or dives into shallow pools. Events like these and others that injure the nervous system share the common principle of transfer of energy to the neural tissues: the degree of injury often correlates with the quantity of energy delivered and the time over which it was delivered (Fig. 13-1). This energy transfer may directly disrupt tissues leading to penetrating injuries, or the energy may be translated into movement and compression of neural structures within the confines of the skull or spinal canal in a closed injury. It is important to realize that extreme injury of the brain and cord is possible with little or no disruption of the overlying tissues. Conversely, very dramatic injury of the superficial tissues can occur with no damage to the underlying nervous system.

HEAD INJURY

Injuries to the head will be considered first. These most commonly result from assaults, vehicular accidents, and falls. Injuries will be considered from the outside going inward.

Scalp

The scalp is well vascularized and, when lacerated, bleeds copiously and sufficiently to lead to shock. Blows to the head often lead to jagged stellate lacerations of the scalp, whereas bullet wounds tend to be discrete rounded defects. Thorough descriptions (or better yet, photographs) of scalp injuries are important pieces of forensic evidence, and should not be neglected during the pandemonium of treating these patients. Fortunately, the scalp is very resilient, and only the most severe avulsing injuries lead to permanent damage (these avulsion injuries usually result from entanglement of hair in machinery or in vehicular accidents in which the head is dragged on the pavement).

Skull

The skull is the major protector of the brain. Its function is to soften blows, and when the forces are intense enough, to fracture, dissipating the energy of the blow. The relationship of the skull and the brain is analogous to that of an eggshell and the yolk, and if you've cracked enough eggs you already have an intuitive understanding of skull fractures. Fractures tend to radiate from the point of impact, and if they communicate with the surface they are said to be open; if not, they are closed. The most common boney defect is a linear skull fracture, so named because they appear on skull x-rays as radiolucent lines, which may run considerable distances from their origins. If the bone is splintered, then the fracture is called "comminuted." Usually, the edges of a skull fracture line up at the same level, but if one edge is forced deeper into the head than the other then a depressed skull fracture is present. Blood and cerebrospinal fluid (CSF) may seep through skull fractures and drain through the nose and ears. Also seepage of blood into the soft tissues of the head can lead to black eyes and blood in the middle ear. Fractures of the base of the skull are sometimes difficult to detect on x-rays, but they bespeak major impact energy and are apt to lead to CSF or blood leaks. CSF leaks can be troublesome sources of recurrent meningitis.

Dural Injuries

Lacerations of vessels of the dura lead to life-threatening accumulations of blood within the cranial vault.

Epidural hematomas are accumulations of blood between the inner table of the skull and the outer surface of the dura mater. They usually occur in the context of a skull fracture involving the groove of the middle meningeal artery in which that artery is lacerated by the jagged edges of bone. This arterial bleeding leads to rapid accumulation of blood in the epidural space with concomitant increased intracranial pressure. The patient may be deceptively lucid in the early phases of hematoma accumulation, but within minutes to hours, progressive mental status deterioration will occur, and only timely surgical evacuation of the hematoma will save the patient. Less commonly, venous epidural hematomas are seen, and while they may pursue a more leisurely course, they are nevertheless dangerous. Epidural collections of blood have a characteristic computed tomography (CT) scan appearance; they do not cross suture lines of the skull (Fig. 13-2).

Subdural hematomas are blood accumulations classically regarded as occurring between the inner aspect of the dura mater and the arachnoid; with the demise of the subdural space, they are more correctly thought of as hematomas within the dural border cell layer. They usually occur over the cerebral convexities, are bilateral in 15% of cases, and, in contrast to the epidu-

Head Injury is a Process NOT an Event

Primary injury sets into motion a neurochemical cascade of secondary injury

FIGURE 13-1. Head injury is a process not an event.

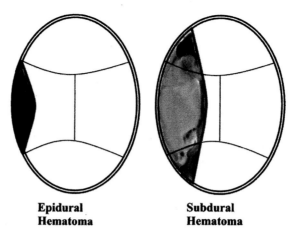

FIGURE 13-2. Epidural hematoma strips the dura away from the skull until it reaches the coronal and occipital sutures. Acute subdural hematoma does not respect the coronal and occipital sutures.

Epidural Hematoma

Subdural Hematoma

ral, they cross suture lines. Acute subdural hematomas are similar to epidural hematomas in that they occur immediately in the context of severe head injury usually with open fractures of the skull, and laceration of the underlying dura and brain. Acute subdural hematomas may pursue a more indolent course than epidural hematomas since they are often the result of venous bleeding. Chronic subdural hematomas are deceptively lethal, slowly progressive accumulations of blood which result from tearing of bridging veins which normally connect venous sinuses and the cortical surface; these veins traverse a longer more tightly tethered course as the brain atrophies with aging or abuse, hence the high risk populations are comprised of elderly or alcoholic persons. "Subdural" hematomas begin as simple accumulations of blood, but soon the overlying dura thickens with granulation tissue and the inner surface of the hematoma is covered by a thinner layer of fibroblasts and granulation tissue (Fig. 13-3). These inner and outer membranes encase a core of degenerating blood, which is gradually encroached upon by the expanding membranes. Since these membranes possess numerous delicate blood vessels, recurrent hemorrhage occurs leading to gradual expansion of the lesion. Surgical drainage of the hematoma and removal of the membranes is necessary for definitive treatment.

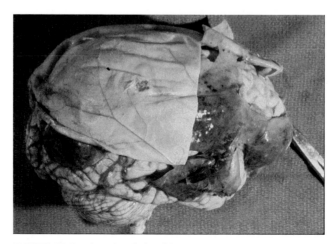

FIGURE 13-3. Chronic subdural hematoma.

Brain Injury

Injury to the brain ranges in severity from transient physiological disturbances to gross disruption of parenchyma, and any of these may result without major damage to overlying structures.

Concussion is a transient alteration of consciousness following a nonpenetrating blow to the head. The structural and physiological basis of this phenomenon is unclear, though it may involve transient torsion with malfunction of the reticular activating system. The autopsy in the rare death that occurs in this setting may disclose no structural abnormalities or minimal swelling.

A *contusion* consists of an area of hemorrhagic necrosis (a brain bruise, in essence) usually occurring on the crests of gyri (in contrast to watershed infarcts which occur in the depths of sulci). These injuries result from the brain being jostled against intracranial boney and dural surfaces. The irregular boney contours of the floor of the anterior and middle cranial fossae are particularly prone to inflict injury; hence, contusions are frequently seen on the subfrontal and anterior temporal cortical surfaces. The severity and distribution of cerebral contusions is determined in part by the mobility of the head at impact (Figs. 13-4 and 13-5). If the head is struck while immobilized, the focus of the injury will be at the impact site—a so-called "coup" injury. If the head is not immobilized when struck, the majority of the injury may be to the brain on the opposite side of the head from impact—a "contra-coup" injury. Contra-coup injuries are thought to result from acceleration or deceleration (in the case of falls) imparted to the brain by the impact. Contra-coup injuries are particularly notable in the occipital region. Acutely, these contusions may be associated with increased intracranial pressure. Histologically, acute contusions consist of hemorrhagic

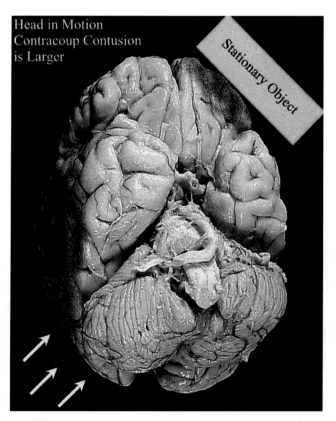

FIGURE 13-4. Contra-coup contusion—head in motion with deceleration.

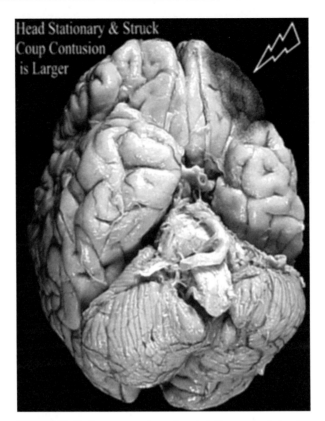

FIGURE 13-5. Coup contusion—head stationary and struck.

necrosis; later the dead tissue is removed by macrophages leaving an irregular tan defect with a glial floor on the cortical surface. The yellow-tan color of remote contusions lead to the designation "plaques jaunes."

Brain *lacerations* are tears in the brain parenchyma with necrosis and hemorrhage. These result from penetration by a foreign body or skull fragments, or may occur in extremely high-energy vehicular accidents. Like the contusion, the laceration resolves via macrophage infiltration and gliosis, but instead of being confined to the cortical surface, a laceration may extend deep into the brain, or even be a perforating (that is, through and through) injury. Lacerations often result from bullets passing through the brain (Fig. 13-6). The ex-

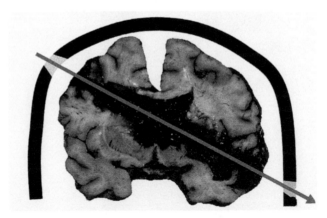

FIGURE 13-6. Perforating brain laceration due to gunshot. The beveling of the skull is the most reliable indicator of the trajectory of the missile.

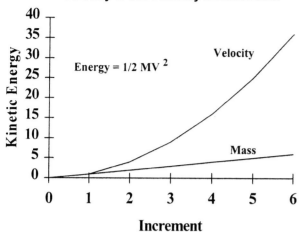

Kinetic Energy of a Projectile
Velocity is the Primary Determinant

FIGURE 13-7. Kinetic energy in relationship to velocity and mass.

tent of injury by a bullet is related to the amount of kinetic energy possessed by the bullet that is transferred to the tissue during transit. Elementary mechanics taught us that kinetic energy $= 1/2\ mv^2$; therefore, the velocity of a projectile determines the kinetic energy to a large extent (Fig. 13-7).

The amount of energy possessed by a bullet increases much more rapidly as a function of velocity than mass. Injury is related more to missile velocity than mass (obviously supersonic bowling balls would be missiles to be contended with, but in the real world of Houston, Texas, a .357 Magnum will inflict more damage than a standard load .38 due largely to differences in muzzle velocity) (Fig. 13-8). Missile passage through the soft compliant brain is associated with cavitation lasting several milliseconds with subsequent collapse of the cavity to form the bullet track within the tissue. Bullet injuries can be amplified by bullet fragmentation and ricochet as well as formation of secondary missiles from fragmented skull. The cranial vault can be penetrated by objects other than bullets by sufficiently determined or creative assailants (Fig. 13-9)!

Intraparenchymal hemorrhages may occur within the brain in both closed and penetrating head injury. They tend to occur in the corpus callosum, quadrigeminal plate, and diencephalon are common sites of these hemorrhages. Their origin is unclear, although some may result from impact against relatively unyielding falcine or tentorial dura. In any case, they bespeak a high-energy injury.

1 inch		VELOCITY	ENERGY
22		1200	90
25		835	70
32		900	110
	380	1000	190
357	38	1100	250
	357	1450	735
45		1025	466

FIGURE 13-8. Kinetic energy of common civilian handguns in the United States.

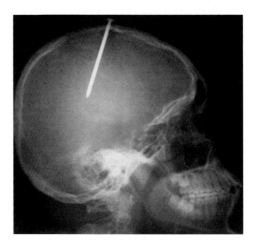

FIGURE 13-9. Projectiles can reflect creative mayhem as in this nail gun projectile.

DIFFUSE AXONAL INJURY

Some patients who are head injured are severely impaired in the absence of gross lacerations or hematomas. These patients are generally comatose from the instant of injury, and subsequently have only limited recovery. They have sustained widespread microscopic axonal injury evidenced by the presence of ruptured axons that retract to form spheroids (Fig. 13-10). This syndrome is called "diffuse axonal injury" (DAI) and is believed to result from shearing forces that damage axons during acceleration or deceleration. There is strong evidence that this axonal alteration matures over a period of hours to days and may therefore be amenable to therapeutic intervention (Fig. 13-11). Initially, the axons appear normal, but soon there is focal accumulation of axoplasmic cytoskeletal components and organelles indicating a malfunction of axonal transport. After several hours of increasing focal swelling, the axon splits and the severed ends retract. Study of DAI is providing insight into the brain's acute stress response which may in turn give us clues about the cellular stress response in other neurological disorders. DAI, for example, results in a rapid up-regulation of APP expression and formation of diffuse neuritic plaques. The parallels with Alzheimer's disease are made even stronger by the observation that head-injured patients bearing even a single ApoE4 allele fare considerably worse that those devoid of this hateful gene!

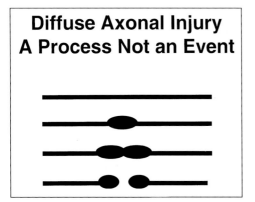

Diffuse Axonal Injury
A Process Not an Event

FIGURE 13-11. Diffuse axonal injury is a process that evolves over time, not an event.

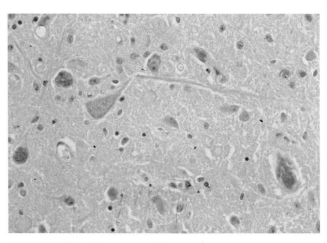

FIGURE 13-10. Diffuse axonal injury.

Trends in Neurotraumatology

- Detection and reduction of secondary injury
- On-line neurometabolic monitoring to complement physiological monitoring
- Reduction of excitotoxic injury
- Augment NO production to increase CBF
- Reduction of inflammatory component of secondary injury
- Arrest evolution of diffuse axonal injury
- Optimize gene expression in injured tissue
- Examine stem cell-driven repopulation of damaged cerebral tissue

FIGURE 13-13. Contemporary neurotraumatology is focusing on molecular, cellular and physiological derangements in head injury.

SECONDARY INJURY MECHANISMS

The mechanisms of traumatic brain injury include primary injury consisting of the initial transfer of kinetic energy to the neural tissues, and secondary injury from neurochemical and vascular perturbations (Fig. 13-12 through 13-15). Primary injury is best approached by primary prevention while secondary injury may be favorably influenced by critical care management and is the subject of intense scientific scrutiny. Many mechanistic overlaps exist between acute ischemic injury and trauma, and both invoke excitotoxicity and free radical damage as major elements.

SPINAL CORD INJURY

Like the brain, the spinal cord is heavily protected by surrounding soft tissue and bone. Injury results from penetrating wounds in stabbings or shootings with laceration of the cord. Spinal column damage with subluxation, dislocation, or fracture of the vertebrae may lead to compression with contusion, lac-

Secondary Injury Mechanisms in Head Trauma

- Ischemia
- Excitotoxicity
- Free radical generation
- Nitric oxide disturbances
- Acidosis
- Cerebral acute phase response
- Inflammatory response

FIGURE 13-12. Contributing to the evolution of traumatic brain injury are secondary injury mechanisms.

Neuromonitoring 10-15 years ago

Pressure	Ventriculostomy
Flow	CPP global CBF Kety-Schmidt ^{133}Xe CBF
Oxygenation-metabolism	SjvO$_2$ CVP catheter fiberoptic catheter CSF

FIGURE 13-14. Greater understanding of the mechanisms underlying head injury are reflected in the monitoring techniques used in the past.

Neuromonitoring Present Day

Pressure	Ventriculostomy, miniature transducer-tipped catheters		
Flow	CPP transcranial Doppler global CBF Kety-Schmidt ^{133}Xe CBF	regional CBF stable Xe CBF SPECT PET	continuous local CBF TD-CBF laser Doppler
Oxygenation-metabolism	global O$_2$ SjvO$_2$	regional O$_2$ NIRSO$_2$	local O$_2$ PbtO$_2$
	global CSF CMRO$_2$,-G,-L	regional PET	local metabolism microdialysis pCO$_2$, pH

FIGURE 13-15. Neuromonitoring in the present day reflects increased understanding of the underlying mechanisms of tissue injury.

eration, or even transection of the spinal cord; these injuries are most common in vehicular and diving accidents with the majority affecting the cervical and lumbar spine. Transient malfunction analogous to cerebral concussion sometimes occurs in the spinal cord, but caution is warranted since unstable spinal column injury may result in transient symptoms which if ignored may be followed by devastating permanent injury.

Vascular injury may complicate spinal trauma leading to epidural hematomas or spinal cord infarction. The latter may also complicate injury of the aorta and its branches as well as surgical correction of aortic disorders.

Depending on the tempo of spinal cord compression, two major myelopathic syndromes are seen:

1. Acute myelopathy with initial spinal shock with flaccidity, anesthesia below the level of injury, and full atonic bladder. Spinal shock is a poorly understood pathophysiological state in which intact cord deprived of descending pathways ceases to function. With the passage of time, some functional autonomy is seen is the disconnected cord leading to spasticity of the extremities, bowel and bladder, and autonomic nervous system.
2. Subacute myelopathy occurs with more slowly progressive compression of the spinal cord such as occurs in masses of the spine or epidural space. Spinal shock is not seen; instead, the patient develops spasticity and anesthesia below the level of the lesion. Local pain is often present.

Evaluation of myelopathies in the past relied on myelography in which contrast material was placed in the CSF outlining the spinal cord and its roots. Today, however, CT and magnetic resonance imaging (MRI) produce excellent images of the spinal cord.

PERIPHERAL NERVOUS SYSTEM INJURY

The brachial and lumbosacral plexuses and the peripheral nerves may suffer traumatic injury. Peripheral nerves are most commonly compressed leading to sensory and motor disturbances in the territory of the damaged nerve that are usually colloquially referred to as "falling asleep." Such injuries may occur if a person maintains a particular position for a period of time. Persons with impairment of consciousness (alcoholic stupor, for example) or impaired mobility due to orthopedic injuries may sustain serious compression injuries of peripheral nerves (the ulnar, radial, and peroneal nerves are most commonly

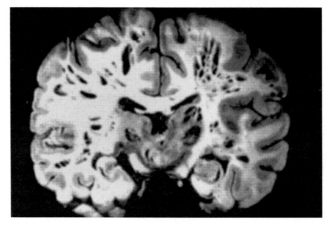

FIGURE 13-16. Swiss cheese artifact.

affected). Peripheral nerves may also be lacerated during assaults and accidents; immediate expert medical care is essential in such cases if permanent damage is to be avoided—if the nerve is anastomosed in a timely and skillful manner, good recovery can be anticipated. High energy injuries may lead to devastating spinal root avulsion with the characteristic radiological finding of extravasation of myelographic contrast material through the dural sleeve of the avulsed root.

POSTMORTEM ARTIFACT

And finally, an appropriate place to end this section on destruction and mayhem is one of the most distinctive gross brain images extant—*swiss cheese brain*—a postmortem artifact resulting from gas pocket formation due to the metabolic activity of gas-forming microbes in the decaying corpse (Fig. 13-16)!

14

NEUROMUSCULAR DISEASES

PERSPECTIVE

1. Neuromuscular disorders affect components of the motor unit—the motor neuron and its myelinating Schwann cells, the neuromuscular junction, and skeletal muscle.
2. Disorders of the motor neuron or its myelinating Schwann cells produce neuropathies. Neuropathies are subdivided into axonal or demyelinating depending on whether the motor neuron axon or the Schwann cells are most affected. These changes can be seen on nerve biopsy and with electrophysiological studies.
3. Biochemical and physiological features of muscle fibers are controlled by the motor neurons innervating those fibers. Diseases of the motor neurons can, therefore, change the histochemical appearance of muscle fibers seen on biopsy.
4. There is a set of disorders in which signal transmission across the neuromuscular junction is impaired. Myasthenia gravis is the prototype disease in this category.
5. Non-neoplastic muscle disorders are called "myopathies" and are usually degenerative—dystrophies—or inflammatory—myositis. There are many kinds of dystrophies, and some of these can be distinguished on muscle biopsy alone, but usually integration of the clinical history, family history, and genetic studies is required.

OBJECTIVES

1. Understand the components of the motor unit and the clinical and pathological manifestations of disorders of each component (Table 14-1).
2. Be able to distinguish between an axonal versus demyelinating neuropathy.
3. Understand the clinical features and pathophysiology of neuromuscular junction disorders.
4. Learn the primary manifestations of myopathies and be able to discuss the differences between dystrophic myopathies, congenital myopathies and inflammatory myopathies.

The corticospinal pathways, extrapyramidal circuits and the cerebellum work together to control motor activity. The final common pathway of movement is the lower motor neuron and the muscle it innervates (Fig. 14-1). The dendrites and cell bodies of the lower motor neurons reside within the spinal cord and brainstem and are therefore within the CNS. The axons of the lower

TABLE 14-1. FEATURES OF THE MOTOR UNIT IN HEALTH AND DISEASE

Motor unit—motor neuron plus the muscle fibers it innervates
1. Neuron 30–100 μ diameter at cell body, axon up to 14 μ diameter and 1 m long
2. Slow postural versus fight-or-flight; oxidative versus ATPase enzymes; red versus white; the fiber type differentiation is specified by the innervating neuron
3. Branch to innervate scattered fibers of single histochemical type
4. Number of fibers/neuron varies inversely with skill (eye 10, gastrocnemius 2,000)

Muscle fiber diameter
1. Increases with age and use, from 10 to 60 μ
2. Inversely proportioned to skill (eye 10 μ, gastrocnemius 60 μ)
3. Varies by sex and type
   a. Female—type I 58 μ, type II 50 μ
   b. Male—type I 62 μ, type II 70 μ

Criteria for disease
1. Loss of power or abnormal contracture; myopathy usually produces proximal weakness and neuropathy distal weakness
2. Elevation of serum muscle enzyme markers; may normalize in advanced disease; highest values seen in rhabdomyolysis and Duchenne's dystrophy
3. Histological alterations:
   a. Muscle—size, shape, nucleus, fibril changes, vacuoles, necrosis, inclusions
   b. Inflammation—vascular, myofiber, fibrous
   c. Fatty change—end stage alteration
   d. Enzyme alterations—size, grouping, target fibers, deficiencies
4. Characteristics of neurogenic disease
   a. Type grouping
   b. Group atrophy
   c. Atrophic angular fibers of both type 1 and 2
   d. Target fibers
5. Characteristics of myopathic disease
   a. Fiber degeneration-regeneration
   b. Myophagocytosis
   c. Fiber splitting
   d. Fibrosis
   e. Increased internal nuclei (>3%) Increased internal nuclei normally seen near tendon insertions—don't biopsy here
   f. Rounded atrophic fibers

motor neurons leave the CNS and constitute the motor fibers of the peripheral nerves. These axons branch repeatedly and eventually come into contact with skeletal muscle at the neuromuscular junction. The motor fibers activate the skeletal muscle by releasing acetylcholine which diffuses across the neuromuscular junction synaptic space to bind to nicotinic cholinergic acetylcholine receptors on the muscle. The muscle membrane is depolarized leading to contraction. Schwann cells surround the axons and encircle them with concentric sheets of myelin which makes rapid conduction of axonal impulses possible (saltatory conduction).

There are diseases in which damage occurs to the lower motor neuron cell body, its axon, the Schwann cell, the neuromuscular junction, or the skeletal

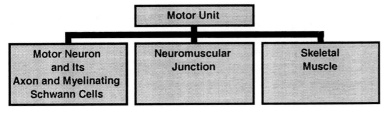

FIGURE 14-1. The motor unit.

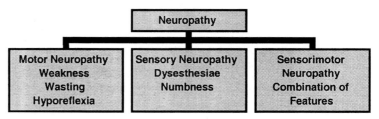

FIGURE 14-2. Types of neuropathy.

muscle. If the cell body is damaged, the condition is called "lower motor neuron disease" or "neuronopathy."

If the axon or its surrounding Schwann cells are damaged, the condition is a neuropathy (Figs. 14-2 through 14-8).

An axonal neuropathy results if the axon is damaged while a demyelinating neuropathy results if the Schwann cell is damaged. Diseases of the neuromuscular junction are known rather unimaginatively as neuromuscular junction disorders (Fig. 14-9). Disorders of muscle are known as myopathies (Figs. 14-10 through 14-19).

PERIPHERAL NEUROPATHY: SIGNS AND SYMPTOMS

Peripheral nerves may be motor, sensory or sensorimotor. Most have combined sensory and motor functions; therefore, disturbances of the peripheral nerve will lead to weakness and numbness in the anatomic distribution of that nerve. The weakness will be in muscles innervated by the nerve, and if the damage to the nerve is long-standing, the muscle innervated by the nerve will waste away (denervation atrophy). Any muscle stretch reflexes mediated by the nerve will be diminished or lost. The sensory distribution of the nerve will be described by the patient as numb (diminished sensation: hypesthesia) or more commonly as "asleep" with a disagreeable "pins and needles" sensation (dysesthesia). If you've ever had your hand or foot "go to sleep," you have experienced a temporary neuropathy due to pressure on the nerve.

If a single nerve is damaged, then the process is called a "mononeuropathy." If multiple nerves are damaged, then the process is called a "polyneuropathy." In some diseases, individual nerves are picked off one after the other, a condition called "mononeuropathy multiplex." Obviously, if enough nerves are destroyed in this fashion, a polyneuropathy will eventually result.

Sensory or motor axons may be selectively damaged by certain diseases so that even though sensorimotor nerves may be damaged, either sensory symptoms or motor symptoms may predominate. Even within sensory axons, in some diseases the small unmyelinated pain-carrying axons are spared while the myelinated faster-conducting larger axons are destroyed. The converse may

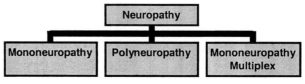

FIGURE 14-3. Types of neuropathy according to distribution of disease.

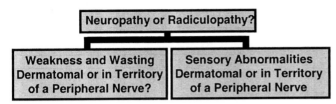

FIGURE 14-4. It is essential to distinguish a neuropathy from a radiculopathy.

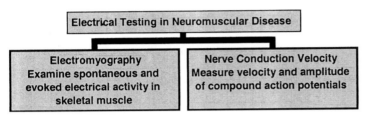

FIGURE 14-5. Electrical testing plays an important role in the evaluation of neuromuscular disease.

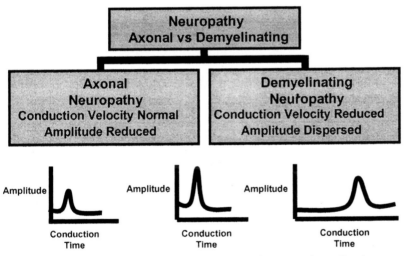

FIGURE 14-6. Electrical differentiation of axonopathy versus demyelinating neuropathy.

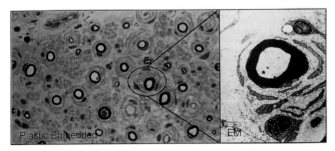

FIGURE 14-7. Onion bulbing in chronic demyelination with remyelination in a demyelinating neuropathy.

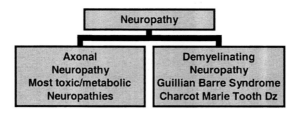

FIGURE 14-8. Neuropathies are either axonal or demyelinating.

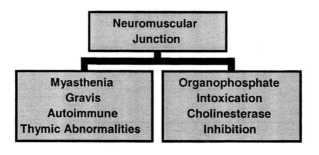

FIGURE 14-9. The neuromuscular junction can also be the locus of disease and this results in weakness and fatigue.

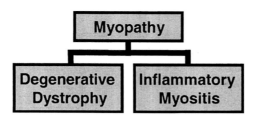

FIGURE 14-10. Primary diseases of muscle are either degenerative or inflammatory.

Neuropathy vs Myopathy

- Distal weakness
- Reduced reflexes
- Sensory loss
- Dysesthesiae
- Muscle wasting
- Fasiculations

- Proximal weakness
- Reflexes preserved
- No sensory loss
- Muscle pain +
- Wasting uncommon
- No fasiculations
- May have myotonia

FIGURE 14-11. Neuropathy and myopathy can sometimes be distinguished by clinical findings.

Muscle Biopsy Findings

Neurogenic
- Type grouping
- Group atrophy
- Angular fibers
- Target fibers

Myopathic
- Fiber size variability
- Basophilia
- Central nuclei
- Splitting
- Macrophages
- Fibrosis

FIGURE 14-12. Often the primary distinction made on muscle biopsy is neurogenic versus myopathic disease.

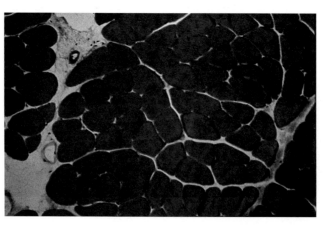

FIGURE 14-13. Normal skeletal muscle shows uniform polygonal fibers with subsarcolemmal nuclei and minimal connective tissue.

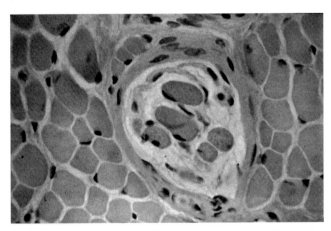

FIGURE 14-14. Muscle spindle may be mistaken by the novice for a parasite.

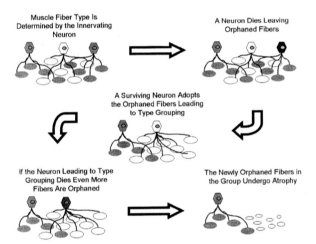

Muscle Fiber Type Is Determined by the Innervating Neuron

A Neuron Dies Leaving Orphaned Fibers

A Surviving Neuron Adopts the Orphaned Fibers Leading to Type Grouping

If the Neuron Leading to Type Grouping Dies Even More Fibers Are Orphaned

The Newly Orphaned Fibers in the Group Undergo Atrophy

FIGURE 14-15. The muscle biopsy shows distinct differences between neuropathic and myopathic processes. The fiber type composition of skeletal muscle is determined by the neurons innervating the muscle. There are characteristic alterations seen on skeletal muscle biopsy in neurogenic disorders.

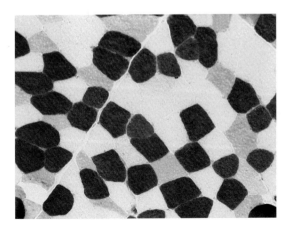

FIGURE 14-16. Normal fiber type mosaic seen on enzyme histochemistry.

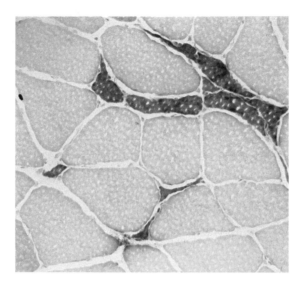

FIGURE 14-17. Angular atrophic fibers rich in esterase are seen in denervation. (Courtesy of Dr. Hannes Vogel, Baylor College of Medicine, Houston, Texas.)

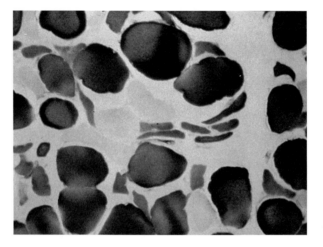

FIGURE 14-18. Individual atrophic muscle fibers of both types are seen in denervation. (Courtesy of Dr. Hannes Vogel, Baylor College of Medicine, Houston, Texas.)

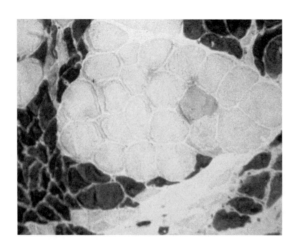

FIGURE 14-19. Fiber type grouping of both fiber types indicates denervation with reinnervation. (Courtesy of Dr. Hannes Vogel, Baylor College of Medicine, Houston, Texas.)

also occur. For example, there is a rare genetic neuropathy in which the pain fibers are lost so that the patient has normal fine touch but cannot appreciate painful injuries. Conversely, and unfortunately more commonly, the larger fibers are lost leading to loss of motor function and loss of fine touch, while painful sensations are conducted properly or may be amplified leading to dysesthesia.

PERIPHERAL NEUROPATHY: EVALUATION

The physical examination of muscle strength, muscle stretch reflexes, and the sensory examination encompassing fine touch as well as thermal and pain sensation usually allow you to diagnose a peripheral neuropathy. The distinction between mononeuropathy and polyneuropathy is made by examining multiple areas of the body to see if single nerves or multiple nerves are involved.

A specialized test called an "electromyogram" (EMG) is sometimes used in the evaluation of neuromuscular disorders. This test complements the physical examination, and permits ascertainment of the distribution and electrophysiological severity of peripheral nerve problems. The test has two phases—both of them quite unpleasant—the nerve conduction velocity (NCV) and the actual electromyogram (EMG) itself. For the NCV, selected peripheral nerves are shocked using a stimulating electrode. Detecting electrodes are placed over the distal portions of the stimulated nerve or over its innervated muscles. By knowing the distance between the site of stimulation and the site of detection, the conduction velocity of the nerve can be calculated. The speed of conduction of the signal depends on the integrity of myelinated fibers, whereas the amplitude of the signal depends on the number of axons carrying the signal. The NCV allows distinction between an axonal neuropathy and a demyelinating neuropathy—a distinction of considerable differential diagnostic importance. The second part of the EMG involves sticking needle electrodes into the muscles and observing the electrical activity of the muscle at rest and when volitionally activated. (Yes, you are asked to contract the muscle while the needle is in the muscle—ouch!) The electrical activity of the muscle measured by EMG allows the distinction between a neuropathic process versus a myopathic process, and permits some determination of how widespread a process might be.

PERIPHERAL NEUROPATHY: AXONAL VERSUS DEMYELINATING

Axonal neuropathy results in a reduced number of axons in nerve fibers conducting action potentials. Those impulses which are conducted, however, are conducted at normal velocities; nerve conduction electrophysiological studies show normal conduction velocities but reduced response amplitude.

Demyelinating neuropathy has preserved axons devoid of myelin; the conduction velocity is reduced, but response amplitude is normal or only slightly diminished. Biopsy of axonal neuropathy shows reduced numbers of axons sometimes with enlarged axons. Demyelinating neuropathy shows preservation of axons, but loss of myelin—if repeated demyelination and remyelination occurs, then "onion-bulbing" is seen. Most toxic, metabolic, and many hereditary neuropathies are axonal. Lead neuropathy, Guillain–Barré syndrome, diphtheria neuropathy, and leukodystrophies produce demyelinating neuropathy.

NEUROMUSCULAR JUNCTION DISORDERS

Myasthenia gravis is the prototype for neuromuscular junction disorders. Myasthenia gravis is an autoimmune disorder of the neuromuscular junction in which acetylcholine receptors are destroyed leading to impaired transmission of signals across the neuromuscular junction. This leads to weakness especially conspicuous in muscles depending strongly on numerous rapid high fidelity neuromuscular transmissions. Muscles of this type include the muscles responsible for moving the eyes, so eye muscle weakness with resultant diplopia (double vision) is common, and may be the sole manifestation of myasthenia gravis. More severe disease involves other muscles leading to weakness sometimes sufficiently severe to embarrass respiration. Myasthenia gravis is associated with a thymoma in 25% of cases and thymic hyperplasia in 50% of cases. This condition may be associated with hyperthyroidism in 5% of cases. Histopathology shows only scattered collections of lymphocytes ("lymphorrhages") and electron microscopy shows simplification of myoneural junction folds.

MUSCULAR DYSTROPHIES

Dystrophinopathies: Duchenne's and Becker's Muscular Dystrophy

The most common muscular dystrophies of childhood are dystrophinopathies (Figs. 14-20 through 14-22). Dystrophin is a muscle structural protein coded by an extremely large and complex gene on chromosome X. Mutations of this gene are numerous, but they have the common phenotypic presentation of an X-linked muscular dystrophy. The age of onset, severity, and rate of progression of the dystrophy depend on the site of the mutation and the impact of the mutation on the functional integrity of dystrophin. Duchenne muscular dystrophy involves larger or functionally more significant mutations, and hence is a more severe, earlier onset disorder. Becker's dystrophy also involves mutations of the dystrophic gene, but these are of lesser functional significance, and the disorder has a later onset, milder symptoms, and slower progression. These disorders are known referred to as "dystrophinopathies."

There are dystrophies which phenotypically are similar to Duchenne's and Becker's dystrophy, but that are autosomal recessive and thus are called "autosomal recessive muscular dystrophy" (ARMD). These result from mutations of dystrophin-related proteins in the dystrophin–glycoprotein complex

---

Dystrophinopathies

Duchenne's	Becker's
• Severe	• Milder
• Early onset	• Later onset
• Rapid progression	• Slower progression

Dystrophin: subsarcolemmal structural protein

Gene: X chromosome

X-linked recessive muscular dystrophy

FIGURE 14-20. The most common dystrophic myopathies are dystrophinopathies.

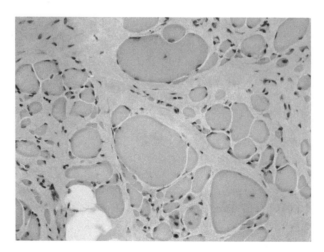

FIGURE 14-21. The muscle biopsy in a dystrophic myopathy shows fiber size variability, fibrosis, fiber necrosis, increased connective tissue and basophilic fibers.

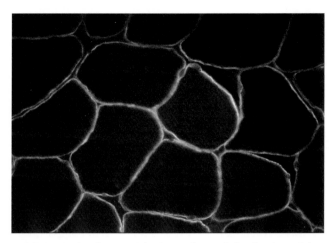

FIGURE 14-22. The normal subsarcolemmal distribution of dystrophin. In the dystrophinopathies this pattern is missing.

at the sarcolemma. Proteins in this complex include α-sarcoglycan (adhalin), β, γ, δ-sarcoglycan, (-sarcoglycan, merosin and calpain-3. Other mutations of this complex may lead to late onset limb-girdle muscular dystrophy (LGMD).

Myotonic Dystrophy

Myotonic dystrophy is an autosomal dominant multisystem disorder characterized by variable age of onset, predominantly distal weakness, and the presence of myotonia—slow relaxation of muscles after contraction and spontaneous sustained muscle contractions (Fig. 14-23). Adult onset disease is usually fairly mild and slowly progressive whereas infantile myotonic dystrophy results in severe weakness sometimes leading to respiratory failure. Myotonia has a characteristic repetitive discharge detectable on electromyography which has been likened to the sound of a dive bomber. Muscle biopsy shows frequent internal nuclei and "ringbinden"—arrays of contractile elements occurring circumferentially in fibers rather than the normal arrangement along the long axis of the fibers (Fig. 14-24 through 14-26). Severe dystrophic features are uncommon. Myotonic dystrophy results from a trinucleotide repeat amplification mutation of the myotonin gene on chromosome 19. Normal

---

Myotonic Dystrophy

- **Autosomal dominant**
- **Trinucleotide repeat amplification**
- **"Myotonin"**
- **Myotonia: impaired muscle relaxation**
- **Distal wasting**
- **Frontal balding**
- **Endocrine abnormalities**

FIGURE 14-23. Clinical features of myotonic dystrophy.

Myotonic Dystrophy

- **Internal nuclei**
- **Abnormal arrangement of contractile elements**
- **Myopathic changes**

FIGURE 14-24. Histopathologic features of myotonic dystrophy.

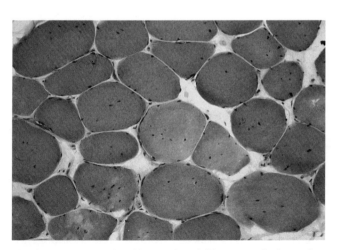

FIGURE 14-25. Increased internal nuclei in myotonic dystrophy.

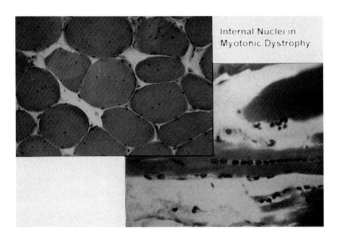

FIGURE 14-26. Myotonic dystrophy is characterized by more internal nuclei than any other neuromuscular disorder.

people have 0–20 trinucleotide repeats in the gene and suffer no effects, but affected individuals have 30–60 trinucleotide repeats. The severity and age of onset depend on the number of trinucleotide repeats present. Children of affected individuals may have amplification of the defect leading to early onset severe disease. This occurrence of more severe disease earlier in successive generations is known as "anticipation."

Other Dystrophic Myopathies

Facioscapulohumeral muscular dystrophy (FSH) is an autosomal dominant (4q35) disorder with onset in childhood but associated with a normal lifespan. Slowly progressive facial, proximal shoulder, and scapular weakness are the primary manifestation; and cardiac involvement or mental retardation is rare. Histopathology is similar to Duchenne's but not as severe. FSH is also notorious for the presence of inflammatory cells on muscle biopsy sufficient to lead to a misdiagnosis of inflammatory myopathy. Despite these enigmatic inflammatory features, FSH does not respond to immunosuppressive therapy.

Limb-girdle muscular dystrophy (LGMD) is not a single disease, but rather is a heterogeneous collection of muscular dystrophies that involve predominantly the proximal muscles. The diagnosis is one of exclusion after dystrophinopathies, myotonic dystrophy and FSH have been eliminated. Some cases of pediatric onset LGMD result from mutations of skeletal muscle cytoskeletal proteins. Particularly interesting is the fact that the sarcoglycans (alpha, beta, delta and gamma) involved in anchoring dystrophin to the skeletal muscle membrane are involved in the LGMDs.

CONGENITAL MYOPATHIES

Central Core Disease

Central core disease is a familial disorder usually presenting as a floppy infant with proximal non-progressive weakness. Laboratory studies show normal enzymes. Enzyme histochemistry shows that most if not all type I fibers have central pallor leading to the disorder's name—central core disease (Fig. 14-27). Electron microscopy of a central core shows myofibrillar disarray and ab-

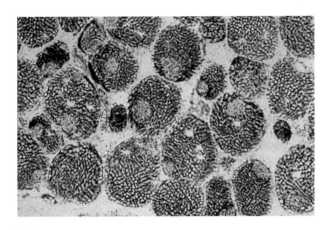

FIGURE 14-27. Central core disease microscopic features.

sence of mitochondria. In some cases of central core disease, there is a mutation of the ryanodine receptor. This finding is of additional interest because mutations of this gene are involved in some cases of familial malignant hyperthermia, and individuals with central core disease are at increased risk for malignant hyperthermia.

Nemaline Myopathy

Nemaline myopathy usually manifests as a floppy infant with nonprogressive weakness and normal serum muscle enzymes. These patients may have peculiar facies with high arched palate, small jaw, and a thin face. Enzyme histochemistry shows type I fiber predominance with multiple dense rods ("threads," from which this disorder gets its name) associated with the Z lines. The nemaline rods can be seen very well on plastic embedded sections and on electron microscopic examination are seen to protrude from the Z lines (Fig. 14-28 and 14-29). The autosomal recessive form of nemaline myopathy results from a mutation of slow tropomyosin while the autosomal dominant form, in some but not all pedigrees, results from a mutation of alpha-tropomyosin.

Centronuclear or Myotubular Myopathy

Centronuclear myopathy has its onset between ages 5–30 years with variable progression and clinically emphasizes the oculofacial and distal muscles.

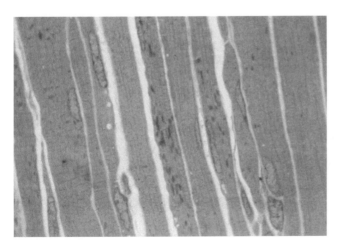

FIGURE 14-28. Light microscopy of nemaline myopathy showing small dark "threads" of Z-disc material.

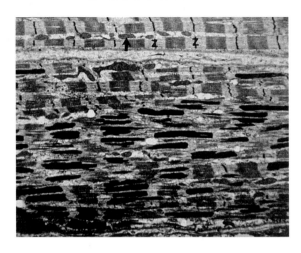

FIGURE 14-29. Electron microscopy of nemaline myopathy showing Z-line streaming.

Serum enzymes are slightly elevated or normal. Histopathological evaluation shows central nuclei with halos and type I atrophy. The fibers with central nuclei resemble primitive myotubes during skeletal muscle development hence the disorder is sometimes called "myotubular myopathy."

The X-linked myotubular myopathy results from a mutation of the gene encoding for myotubularin, a protein tyrosine phosphatase.

Inflammatory Myopathies: Polymyositis and Inclusion Body Myositis

Polymyositis produces predominantly proximal muscle weakness and may be associated with muscle pain (Fig. 14-30). The condition is sporadic, has a variable age of onset, and may be associated with muscle pain and tenderness, dysphagia, elevated serum creatine kinase and erythrocyte sedimentation rate (ESR). Histopathological examination shows lymphocytic infiltration and muscle fiber destruction (Fig. 14-31). Histopathology may show vasculitis (15–20%), type II atrophy (90%), type grouping (60%), perifascicular atrophy (50%), IgG on sarcolemma (60–80%), degeneration with necrosis and phagocytosis (5–10%), fibrosis (5%), regeneration of isolated fibers. This form of inflammatory muscle disease in its most common form is usually responsive to corticosteroid therapy and spontaneous remissions may occur. Polymyositis may be associated with collagen vascular diseases such as systemic lupus erythematosus (SLE), periarteritis nodosa, rheumatoid arthritis, systemic sclerosis, Sjögren's disease, or polymyalgia rheumatica. If muscle pain

Inflammatory Myopathy

Polymyositis	Inclusion Body Myositis
• Lymphocytic infiltration	• Lymphocytic infiltration
• Muscle fiber destruction	• Muscle fiber destruction
• Pain and weakness	• Rimmed vacuoles
• Rx: immunosuppression	• Painless weakness
	• Immunosuppression not effective

FIGURE 14-30. Inflammatory myopathies.

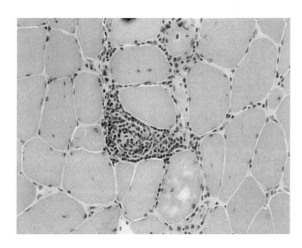

FIGURE 14-31. Microscopy of inflammatory myopathy.

and weakness are associated with a rash (particularly in sun exposed regions of the face) then the condition is more likely to be dermatomyositis which is more a disease of small blood vessels than a primary inflammatory myopathy. The purported association of polymyositis with occult neoplasm in older persons remains controversial. There is a malignant variant of polymyositis called the "anti-tRNA synthetase syndrome," consisting of polymyositis plus arthritis and pulmonary fibrosis. Serum anti-tRNA synthetase antibodies are present and this condition has a very poor response to therapy.

Inclusion body myositis afflicts older individuals and presents as distal weakness. An inflammatory infiltrate is present as in polymyositis, but additionally, there are rimmed vacuoles within the myocytes. Inclusion body myositis does not respond well to immunosuppression.

OTHER INFLAMMATORY MYOPATHIES

Myoinflammation can occur locally or globally in a variety of systemic inflammatory conditions. Trichinosis from ingestion of inadequately cooked pork infested with the pig tapeworm was once common (5–10% of all autopsies up to 1950) but fortunately is now rare. There may be systemic eosinophilia as well as infiltration of skeletal muscle with eosinophils. The parasite itself may be seen on microscopic examination of the skeletal muscle. Heavy infestations can produce massive calcification of the muscle visible on x-rays. Toxoplasmosis is now more common than trichinosis and causes fever with myositis and lymphadenopathy. Cysticercosis myositis is common in Mexico, Central, and South America producing eosinophilia and calcified ovoids in muscle. Idiopathic inflammation of sarcoidosis may involve skeletal muscle and under these conditions the muscle biopsy may help in the diagnosis of the systemic disease. When giant cells are seen out of the appropriate clinical context, care must be taken to consider the possibility of foreign body giant cell reaction to exogenous material either factiously injected or embolic from intravenous administration.

Infections can produce myositis. Mycobacterial myositis may selectively involve single muscles producing granulomata mimicking soft tissue tumors. Gas gangrene occurs when Gram-positive Clostridial organisms thrive in necrotic muscle; the biopsy shows intense acute inflammation, edema, and separation of fibers by gas and fluid. Staphylococcus may cause myoabscess formation with intense local pain and swelling; examination shows acute polymorphonuclear cell infiltration. Viral myositis is very common; anyone who has experienced muscle aches and pains during a viral infection such as influenza probably has some degree of skeletal muscle inflammation. Coxsackie B viral infections are the most frequent cause of life-threatening generalized myositis with myoglobinuria; involvement of the heart (myocarditis) and the CNS (encephalitis or aseptic meningitis) may occur simultaneously. The myocarditis may be sufficiently severe as to necessitate cardiac transplantation. Neuronotropic viruses including polio and rabies replicate in skeletal muscle and are then transported by retrograde axonal flow to the CNS. While in residence in the muscle, these infections may produce muscle pain and tenderness. Inflammatory myopathy can complicate HIV infection, and in addition, treatment with AZT leads to a mitochondrial myopathy that can be distinguished from the inflammatory myopathy by the presence of ragged red fibers and abnormal mitochondria. Other drug-induced myopathies include those produced by the cholesterol lowering drugs. Epidemic eosinophilic myositis has been seen in patients consuming large amounts of L-tryptophan for its purported sleep-inducing properties; this epidemic was apparently due to small quantities of a microbial byproduct.

METABOLIC MYOPATHIES

Thyrotoxic myopathy results in proximal weakness with myopathic EMG abnormality in 90% of cases. Percussion may lead to fasciculations suggesting terminal branch hyperirritability. Due to the association of other neuromuscular disorders with hyperthyroidism there may be coexisting myasthenia gravis or periodic paralysis.

Hypothyroidism can produce a myopathy characterized by weakness, stiffness, cramps, and pseudomyotonia that may precede the diagnosis of hypothyroidism. Percussion provokes prolonged contraction with slow release and laboratory evaluation shows increased serum enzymes.

Periodic paralysis occurs in hypokalemic, hyperkalemic, and eukalemic forms usually occurring as autosomal dominant conditions with male predominance and onset usually in childhood. These individuals experience abrupt onset profound flaccid paralysis in episodes lasting for several hours. The weakness only rarely leads to respiratory compromise but is otherwise very severe. Between attacks muscle strength is normal but the patient may develop a persistent weakness between attacks. Attacks may be triggered by carbohydrate load, exercise, or exposure to cold. If a muscle biopsy is obtained during an attack, fibers show PAS-positive vacuoles that appear as clear holes on light and electron microscopy. Between attacks the muscle biopsy is normal. Molecular mechanisms include mutations of the voltage-gated sodium and calcium channels.

Glycogen storage disorders can result in metabolic myopathies with a broad range of clinical and pathological features. Type II glycogen storage disease (Pompe's disease) results from autosomal recessive acid maltase deficiency (1,4 glucosidase) and most commonly presents in the infantile form with profound floppiness at age 1–2 months, congestive heart failure at 3 months, and death by 6 months. This severe condition has concurrent macroglossia and hepatomegaly. Milder juvenile and adult forms are less common. Microscopic examination shows severe vacuolation with PAS+ glycogen deposits in skeletal and cardiac muscle. Type III glycogen storage disease, Forbes-Cori disease, caused by debrancher deficiency (1,6 glucosidase) results in childhood hypotonia and hypoglycemia with hepatocardiomegaly. The prognosis is variable with occasional adult onset. Type V glycogen storage disease, McArdle's disease, is caused by myophosphorylase

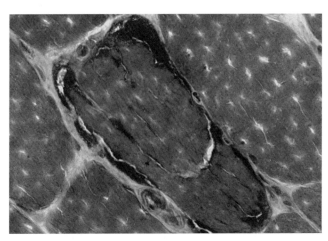

FIGURE 14-32. Ragged red fiber on Gomori methenamine silver–stained section in a mitochondrial myopathy.

deficiency and is an autosomal recessive disease with onset in childhood or adulthood. McArdle's disease is characterized by exercise-induced pain, cramps, stiffness, weakness, and myoglobinuria that may be severe enough to induce renal shutdown. An ischemic exercise test demonstrates failure of lactate to go up and EMG silence. Histopathology shows absence of myophosphorylase and PAS+ glycogen crescents in fibers.

Alcoholic myopathy may mimic McArdle's disease by showing low myophosphorylase and impaired lactate production with ischemic exercise, however, the clinical progression is insidious with proximal muscle weakness with unimpressive biopsy and limited serum enzyme elevation. Acute rhabdomyolysis with generalized weakness, cramping, edema, renal failure may complicate binge drinking. Myoglobinuria is seen with massive muscle lysis seen in crushing trauma, burns, snake bites, drugs, infections, acute polymyositis, infarction, or excessive exercise. Serum creatinine kinase is dramatically elevated and acute tubular necrosis may supervene. Hyperkalemia due to release of intracellular potassium may trigger cardiac arrhythmias.

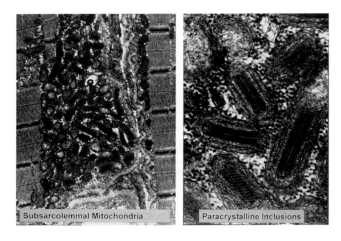

Subsarcolemmal Mitochondria

Paracrystalline Inclusions

FIGURE 14-33. Electron microscopy in a mitochondrial myopathy shows paracrystalline mitochondrial matrix inclusions.

Mitochondrial myopathies are maternally inherited disorders of energy metabolism characterized by lactic acidosis and weakness. Ophthalmoplegia may also be present. These disorders may be accompanied by CNS, cardiac, hepatic, or renal involvement since these organs are also prodigious consumers of energy. On the muscle biopsy there are subsarcolemmal accumulations of mitochondria visible by light microscopy using the modified Gomori trichrome stain and on electron microscopy. The mitochondria impart a subsarcolemmal red hue to the otherwise green muscle fiber and these are called "ragged red fibers." On electron microscopy, excessive numbers of abnormally shaped mitochondria may be seen, and particularly indicative of mitochondrial disease is the presence of paracrystalline arrays within the mitochondrial matrix (Figs. 14-32 and 14-33).

15

DEVELOPMENTAL DISORDERS

PERSPECTIVE

1. In the United States, some experts believe that 3% of neonates have major systemic or CNS malformations, and 75% of fetal deaths and 40% of deaths within the first year of life are associated with CNS malformations. Up to 15% of pediatric neurology hospital admissions are related to malformations.
2. Neurodevelopmental abnormalities result from teratogenic events in any one of three major periods of nervous system development: neural tube formation (neurulation), segmentation and cleavage, and proliferation and migration.
3. The most common CNS malformations involve defects in neural tube closure (neurulation). Neural tube closure is complete by day 28 of embryogenesis; therefore, the neural tube defects occur before the mother even knows she is pregnant. Therefore, women of child-bearing age (10–50 years) should be carefully treated by their physicians in order to avoid exposure to teratogenic drugs.
4. Defects occurring during segmentation and telencephalic cleavage lead to the Arnold-Chiari malformation and the holoprosencephaly series of defects.
5. Defects of cellular proliferation and migration result in cerebral cortical malformations ranging from absence of sulci (lissencephaly) to malformed gyri (polymicrogyria). Focal lesions such as schizencephaly may also occur as a result of germinal matrix disruption.
6. The perinatal period is not immune from pathological processes interrupting or destroying neurodevelopmental activities.

OBJECTIVES

1. Understand the timing and consequences of failure of neural tube closure. Failure of anterior neuropore closure leads to anencephaly when severe and encephaloceles when milder. Failure of posterior neuropore closure leads to spina bifida ranging in severity from spina bifida occulta to meningocele to meningomyelocele. Folate supplementation reduces the frequency of these malformations.
2. Learn about the timing during embryogenesis of prosencephalon cleavage into the two cerebral hemispheres, and how failure of this process leads to the holoprosencephaly series of malformations.
3. Learn how disorders of cellular migration and proliferation at 1–7 months of gestation lead to lissencephaly, schizencephaly, and polymicrogyria.
4. Understand the pathological events associated with acquired intrauterine and perinatal congenital defects.

DEVELOPMENTAL NEUROPATHOLOGY

There is a cruel hoax perpetrated on virtually every serious student of biological sciences at some point in their career. The setup consists of the following statement made in deeply reverent tones, "In order for you to truly understand gross anatomy of the mature organism, you must first understand embryology!" The student is then assaulted with a bewildering array of sheets folding, hollow spheres developing, layers emerging, clefts and arches emerging and regressing, gills and tails emerging and regressing, structures coming, going, rotating, twisting, and involuting. More often than not this experience does not contribute one iota to the student's understanding of adult anatomy and it completely poisons any interest in embryology. That's a pity because developmental biology (an alias for this dark art adopted by those who wish to interest bright minds rather than repel them), and in particular, developmental neurobiology, is one of the most vibrant and exciting areas of modern neuroscience.

In developmental neuropathology, timing is everything. The type of developmental abnormality seen depends largely on when during embryogenesis a pathogenic event occurs. Limited knowledge of the three essential steps in normal brain development is necessary in order to understand abnormalities in development (Fig. 15-1). Those steps are neurulation (formation of the neural tube), segmentation and cleavage (formation of the major subdivisions of the CNS), and proliferation and migration of the cellular constituents that eventually populate the nervous system.

Critical Events in Neurodevelopment

- Neurulation
  - Complete by 4 weeks
- Segmentation and telencephalic cleavage
  - Complete by 8 weeks
- Proliferation and migration
  - Most occur between 8 weeks gestation and birth but some continue after birth

FIGURE 15-1. Critical events during neurodevelopment.

DEFECTS IN NEURULATION

The nervous system begins as an area of specialization in the ectodermal layer when the embryo is composed of the three primeval layers—ectoderm, mesoderm, and endoderm. The neuroectoderm is oriented along the anterior to posterior axis of the developing organism in the form of the neural groove; indeed, the establishment of this axis is one of the signal events in early development. Few would dispute the importance of discerning one's head from one's ass, and now the molecular basis of this important axis is beginning to be understood. Emergence of the neuroectoderm results from signaling from mesodermal notochord primordia that suppresses the expression of bone morphogenetic proteins (BMPs), a family of proteins that are constitutively expressed in ectoderm. The primary mesodermal signaling molecule that forces the emergence of neuroectodermal specialization is sonic hedgehog, a ubiquitous signaling molecule named whimsically after the computer game which delighted the child of the discoverer of this molecule. Exposure of ectoderm to sonic hedgehog (SHH) from the notochord results in suppression of BMP and specialization of the neuroectoderm. The anterior to posterior axis is defined by the presence of other molecules such as noggin in the cephalic region, that works in concert with SHH to permit emergence of the neuroectodermal phenotype. The neural groove sinks into the mesoderm and the lips of the groove approximate to form the neural tube that seals shut bidirectionally in a salutatory fashion from the midsection of the emerging tube. Eventually a neural tube is formed with two openings—the anterior (cephalad) and posterior (caudal) neuropores (Fig. 15-2).

Even as the neural tube descends into the mesoderm as if drawn by the notochord, there is also differentiation of the dorsal portion toward the sensory phenotype and the ventral portion toward the motor phenotype. In the spinal cord, this dorsal—sensory and ventral—motor distinction is main-

---

Neural Tube Defects

- Anterior neuropore
  - Anencephaly
  - Encephalocoele
- Posterior neuropore
  - Meningomyelocoele
  - Meningocoele
  - Spina bifida occulta

FIGURE 15-2. Neural tube defects result from failures of neurulation.

tained with stark clarity throughout development. In the brainstem and cerebral hemispheres, the distinction is blurred to some extent, but if one views the frontal lobes (executive, motoric higher functions) as being ventral and the parietal and occipital lobes (complex visual and polymodality sensory functions) as being dorsal, this early differentiation of function is preserved. The molecular basis of the ventral to dorsal differentiation is the establishment of a gradient of retinoic acid concentration directed by the interplay of BMPs and HSS. Hence an emerging cell "knows" whether to express the sensory or motor phenotype based on its local retinoic acid concentration. This subtle shading of retinoic acid concentration can be hopelessly washed out by the systemic administration of retinoic acid homologues such as 13-cis-retinoic acid (Accutane), a widely prescribed medication for severe acne—a malady of great importance to young women entering the child bearing years. Without the retinoic acid gradient to provide a gentle sculpting influence, the neural tube fails to develop. Hence, an otherwise innocuous compound given at the wrong time results in a catastrophic impact on the emerging nervous system. In teratogenesis, timing is everything.

Failure of the anterior neuropore to close leads to the most severe, common, lethal CNS malformation—anencephaly. The brain and calvarium are absent, and are replaced by a tangle of glial and connective tissue known as cerebrovasculosum (Fig. 15-3). Remnants of the brainstem and pituitary may be present, and the brainstem may be sufficient to support vegetative functions so that anencephalics may be born "alive." There is no prospect for meaningful neurological existence, and these newborns invariably die. There is considerable geographic variability in the frequency of anencephaly with high frequencies being seen in Ireland, intermediate levels in the United States, and low levels in Japan. There is considerable evidence that folate supplementation of women of child-bearing age reduces the risk of anencephaly; therefore, women of child-bearing age should receive supplemental folate (325 μg/day) and any that have previously had pregnancies with neural tube defects should receive 4000 μg/day.

Less severe defects of anterior neuropore closure lead to boney defects in the midline through which brain tissue may protrude. These defects are called "encephaloceles" and are most commonly located in the occipital region (Fig. 15-4). The prognosis depends on the quantity of cerebral tissue that herniates into the defect.

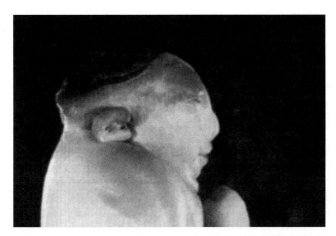

FIGURE 15-3. Anencephaly is the most severe form of neural tube defect. The brain is missing and is replaced by a tangle of soft tissue and vessels.

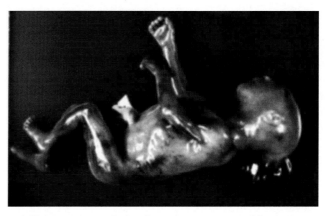

FIGURE 15-4. Encephalocele with protrusion of brain into a fluid-filled sac. (Courtesy of Dr. S.Z. Powell, Baylor College of Medicine.)

Defects of posterior neuropore closure lead to defects in the lumbosacral region. The least severe defect is one in which the posterior arches of the vertebrae in this region fail to fuse; this is called "spina bifida occulta." More severe defects allow the herniation of meninges filled with cerebrospinal fluid to thin atrophic skin. This form of spina bifida is called "meningocele," and if the skin erodes, the CSF may become infected. If elements of spinal roots or cord accompany the CSF and meninges in herniating, then the defect is called "meningomyelocele" (Fig. 15-5). In addition to having the risk of infection as in the meningocele, these individuals have neurological defects—leg weakness, and bowel and bladder control abnormalities.

The third major class of dysraphic defects are the Chiari malformations. Originally, four subtypes of the Chiari (also known as Arnold–Chiari) malformations were described, but only the type 1 and type 2 forms are clinically significant. These complex malformations involve defects at the anterior and posterior neuropores. The type 1 malformation consists of downward herniation of cerebellar tonsilar tissue sometimes associated with arachnoid adhesions at the foramen magnum. There are no associated brainstem malformations, and the condition presents in adult life with headache due to impaired CSF flow and sometimes medullary signs and symptoms. The lesion is corrected by simple occipital craniectomy and high cervical decompressive laminectomy. The type 1 malformation is associated with coexisting syringomyelia in up to 50% of cases. The manifestations of the anterior neuro-

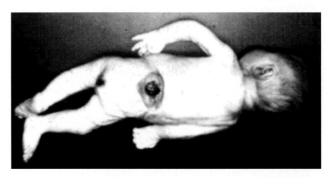

FIGURE 15-5. Meningomyelocele reflects a posterior neuropore failure. (Courtesy of Dr. S.Z. Powell, Baylor College of Medicine.)

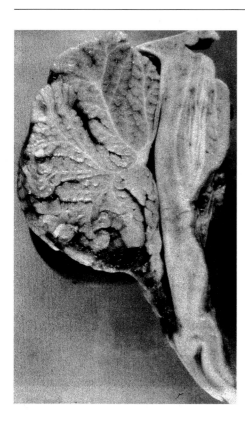

FIGURE 15-6. The Chiari type 2 malformation showing quadrigeminal plate beaking, aqueductal atresia, and protrusion of heterotopic cerebellar tissue through the foramen magnum. (Courtesy of Dr. S.Z. Powell, Baylor College of Medicine.)

pore abnormalities in the Chiari type 2 malformation include brainstem elongation and kinking, cerebellar tonsillar dysmorphic tissue displaced downward, beak-shaped mesencephalic tectum, and atretic aqueduct (Fig. 15-6). Obstructive hydrocephalus may complicate the aqueductal atresia. The cerebellum is small, the posterior fossa small, and foramen magnum big. There is often an associated lumbosacral meningomyelocele. Indeed, any infant with a lumbar neural tube defect requires imaging of the brain to evaluate for coexisting Chiari type 2 malformation so that progressive hydrocephalus can be averted. The pathogenesis of the brainstem and cerebellar abnormalities in Chiari type 2 remains obscure, but it is possible that this developmental abnormality resides at the cross roads of neurulation and segmentation, the next major neurodevelopmental process to be considered.

DEFECTS IN SEGMENTATION AND PROSENCEPHALIC CLEAVAGE

Once neurulation is complete, the neural tube has been formed, the cephalad to caudal axis has been established, and the ventral dorsal functional bifurcation into motor and sensory functions of the nervous has occurred (Fig. 15-7). The cephalad portion of the neural tube is more elaborate and bulbous, and then like a child's balloon toy, the cephalad or anterior end undergoes a series of expansions and segmentation to form the components of the supratentorial nervous system as we know it. The spinal cord maintains its fundamental structure and busies itself with forming connections with the periphery and the more central ever developing portions of the CNS.

The first phase of segmentation is the formation of three primitive vesicles or bulbous expansions of the anterior neural tube—the hindbrain (rhombencephalon), midbrain (mesencephalon) and forebrain (prosen-

---

Defects of Segmentation and Cleavage

- **Midline defects**
  - **Arrhinencephaly**
  - **Agenesis of the corpus callosum**
- **Telencephalic cleavage defects**
  - **Lobar holoprosencephaly**
  - **Alobar holoprosencephaly**

FIGURE 15-7. Defects of segmentation and cleavage occur between weeks 4 and 8 gestation.

cephalon). The mesencephalon does not segment further, but the rhombencephalon and the prosencephalon each divide to form two vesicles. The rhombencephalon segments to form the myelencephalon (medulla) and the mestencephalon (pons) while the prosencephalon segments into the diencephalon (thalamus and basal ganglia) and telencephalon—end brain (cerebral hemispheres). Hence the cephalad neural tube goes from one bulbous expansion to three and thence to five—odd numbers all—structurally and functionally distinct regions. The telencephalon is not content to leave well enough alone, however, and it divides into two functionally and structurally similar-paired vesicles to form the cerebral hemispheres in a process called "cleavage." Thus, by day 35 of development, the basic subdivisions of the CNS are in place and are basically ready to be populated.

Segmentation of the hindbrain is regulated by a family of genes called "Hox"—an ancient evolutionarily conserved family involved in the segmentation of annelids and flies. Expression of specific hox genes restricts the migration of cells within a spatial domain—in essence, a molecular fence is erected so that cells in a given neighborhood as well as the progeny of those cells will stay in the neighborhood. Disruption of Hox genes leads to abnormal hindbrain development. The genes controlling segmentation of the proencephalon and spinal cord is imperfectly defined, however, several genes included in the Emx family are emerging as candidates. Interestingly, these genes are also involved in facial and oropharyngeal development thus solidifying the relationship of the developing brain with facial features.

Between gestational days 33 and 35, the prosencephalon cleaves to form paired telencephalic vesicles (cerebral hemispheres). Failure of cleavage leads to holoprosencephaly (one cerebrum—one ventricle) in which the brain consists of a single sphere surrounding a single gaping ventricle. When viewed from below, the holoprosencephalic brain is not terribly striking; there is a well-formed brainstem and cerebellum and a cerebral enlargement is readily apparent replete with sulci and gyri. Closer inspection, however, discloses no medial fissure separating the left and right cerebri, and the olfactory nerves and bulbs are absent (Fig. 15-8). Inspection of the brain from above discloses the full extent of the malformation, the cerebral cortex extends in a continuous

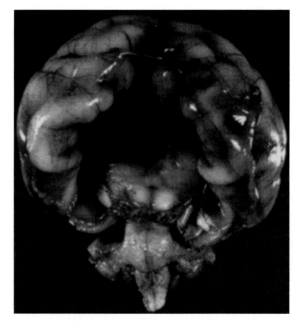

FIGURE 15-8. Holoprosencephaly is failure of telencephalic cleavage with a resultant single ventricled sphere rather than the paired cerebral hemispheres.

perverse band from the left to the right, and posteriorly, a single ventricle gapes forlornly where there should have been corpus callosum and parietal and occipital lobes. This form of holoprosencephaly is called "alobar holoprosencephaly" and is the most extreme form of this disorder. Sometimes incomplete prosencephalic cleavage occurs leading to partial formation of cerebral hemispheres, and this defect is called "lobar holoprosencephaly." The least severe form of the holoprosencephaly series is one in which the olfactory system fails to properly cleave, lead to absence of the olfactory bulbs and nerves—a condition known as arhinencephaly (*a*—without, *rhine*—nose, *encephaly*—brain: without nose brain). Holoprosencephaly may be sporadic or occur in association with trisomy 13. The hereditary form of holoprosencephaly is associated with defects in the sonic hedgehog signaling pathway.

Alobar holoprosencephaly is associated with severe abnormalities of facial development including formation of a single eye often replete with four eyelids and a primitive nose with a solitary opening located above the eye. With decreasing severity of brain abnormalities, correspondingly less profound defects of facial development are observed. With lobar holoprosencephaly and arhinencephaly, there may be hypertelorism and variable placement and maturity of the nose. Alobar holoprosencephaly is usually lethal but if the afflicted individual survives there is severe mental retardation, individuals with alobar holoprosencephaly may have moderate to severe mental retardation and variable degrees of hypertelorism, and those with arhinencephaly may have mild mental retardation, mildly abnormal facies, and anosmia due to lack of the olfactory nerves.

DEFECTS OF NEURONAL PROLIFERATION AND MIGRATION

After 2 months gestation, the major inductive processes are complete and a period of furious cellular proliferation and migration ensues lasting until birth and beyond (Fig. 15-9). The hollow core of the developing nervous system is lined by a layer of cells that spawn all of the endogenous denizens of the brain and spinal cord. This layer, the germinal matrix, is composed of pluripotential cells which divide to form progeny that can differentiate along glial or neuronal lines. During the process of cell division, the nuclei of the precursor cells conduct an oscillatory dance in which cells in the G1 phase of the cell cycle reside immediately adjacent to the ventricular surface. A cell in this state will execute the preflight checklist of cell division: is my DNA sufficiently intact to permit high fidelity replication, is there adequate synthetic precursors, are my synthetic enzymes functional. And if all is well, the cell enters S-phase, the DNA biosynthetic phase of the cell cycle. During S-phase the nucleus migrates away from the ventricle and attains its zenith when DNA synthesis is reaching completion. The cell enters the G2 phase of the cell cycle in which it once again checks to see if all is in readiness to divide: was the DNA copied with excellent fidelity, are there adequate supplies of energy and proteins to carry out mitosis? If problems are detected, the cell will attempt DNA repair and if that is unsuccessful, apoptosis will be triggered. If the checklist of G2 is satisfactory, mitosis ensues. During the G2 phase, the nucleus descends to the ventricular area and mitosis commences at this site. Following division, the daughter cell may migrate out of the germinal matrix to populate the cerebral cortex or will itself become a precursor cell. Students often envision this cell division as being a solitary and indolent act, but during the frenzied periods of cellular proliferation in brain development up to 250,000 daughter cells are being created every minute! After all, there is an entire nervous system to be

Defects of Proliferation and Migration

- **Global**
  - **Micrencephaly**
  - **Megalencephaly**
- **Gyral pattern formation**
  - **Lissencephaly**
  - **Pachygyria**
  - **Polymicrogyria**
- **Cortical organization**
  - **Band heterotopia (collections of neurons in white matter)**
  - **Double cortex**
  - **Focal cortical neuronal heterotopia**

FIGURE 15-9. Defects of proliferation and migration.

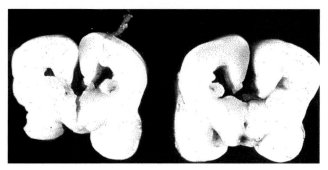

FIGURE 15-10. Agenesis of corpus callosum with characteristic bat-wing ventricles. (Courtesy of Dr. S.Z. Powell, Baylor College of Medicine.)

populated. One can well imagine, however, the adverse consequences on the ultimate cellular population of the nervous system of even brief exposure to situations that impair cellular proliferation. Conditions that may impair cellular proliferation include irradiation, many forms of chemotherapy, and hyperthermia among others. If there is a global impairment of cellular proliferation, there will be a global defect in cortical development, but it is important to recognize that specific areas of the germinal matrix produce cells destined for specific final locations. If a patch of germinal matrix is damaged, then the preordained destination of the cells arising in this patch will be depleted of cellular populations ranging from complete absence to simple numerical reduction. The defects occurring during this period in development lead to agenesis of the corpus callosum, lissencephaly, schizencephaly, double cortex syndrome and polymicrogyria.

Agenesis of the corpus callosum consists of partial or complete absence of the corpus callosum. The fibers that would have crossed between the cerebral hemispheres in the corpus callosum run beside the lateral ventricles and are called "Probst bundles" (Fig. 15-10). The cerebral cortical sulci of the mesial hemisphere also fail to develop normally and appear to radiate like spokes of a wheel from the third ventricle (Fig. 15-11). Normally these sulci run anterior to posterior in the cingulated cortex. This defect is usually partial with the rostrum, genu and anterior portion of the corpus callosum being preserved and the caudal portion and splenium being absent. Agenesis of the corpus callosum can be asymptomatic or associated with mental retardation and seizures.

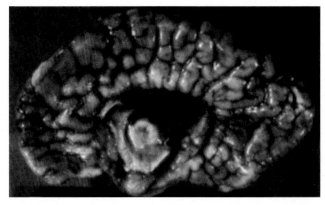

FIGURE 15-11. Agenesis of the corpus callosum with radial cingulate gyrus sulci.

Defects in Cortical Development

- Schizencephaly – focal loss of germinal matrix
  - Spatial destiny – specific regions of the germinal matrix provide cells that populate specific regions of the cerebral cortex
  - If a region of germinal matrix is damaged, the region of the cerebral cortex destined to arise from that region fails to develop
- Porencephaly – focal loss of previously formed cortex
- Hydranencephaly – global destruction of previously formed cortex

FIGURE 15-12. Defects of cortical development.

This malformation may be associated with midline lipomas or ependymal cysts. Some regard this malformation as being a telencephalic cleavage defect while others view it as a failure of axonal pathfinding.

Lissencephaly or "smooth brain" is a severe malformation in which the brain lacks sulci and gyri due to failure to populate the cerebral cortex with neurons. The condition may arise from failure of neuronal proliferation or migration (Figs. 15-12 and 15-13). This malformation is clinically accompanied by severe mental retardation and seizures. Karyotypic defects of chromosome 17 are seen in hereditary forms of lissencephaly.

In the double cortex syndrome or cortical heterotopia, groups of neurons fail to migrate all the way out to the neocortex and establish residence in the white matter. These neurons may be sufficiently numerous to form "bands" resembling the basal ganglionic or claustral nuclei. The "band" heterotopias do not appear to participate in normal cortical information processing and the afflicted individuals may be mentally retarded. The heterotopias may disrupt physiological suppression of cortical epileptiform activity or possibly even spawn convulsive activity, so affected persons may have seizures (sometimes very severe). Paradoxically, some individuals will reach adulthood and attain significant educational milestones only to be thwarted by the sudden onset of increasingly severe and uncontrollable seizures. This tragic evolution has been described particularly frequently in X-linked dominant double cortex where a protein doublecortin carried on the X chromosome is mutated. This mutation is presumed to be lethal in males, but in females there is random inactivation of one member of each X chromosome pair in each cell (Lyonization). If a neu-

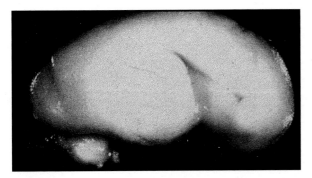

FIGURE 15-13. Lissencephaly or "smooth brain" due to failure to populate the cortex and form sulci. (Courtesy of Dr. S.Z. Powell, Baylor College of Medicine.)

ron has inactivation of the mutated chromosome, that neuron migrates to neocortex normally. In contrast, if the neuron has inactivation of the normal chromosome, that neuron fails to migrate properly and congregates with other similarly dysfunctional neurons to form a band heterotopia.

Localized regions of the developing neocortex are populated by neurons and glia arising from specific localized zones of the germinal matrix. If one of these discrete areas of the germinal matrix is destroyed, the missing region will not spawn the cellular constituents destined to form a specific region of the cortex leaving a "hole" in the cortex. The remaining germinal matrix will populate the cortex normally so that there is a sunken defect in the cerebral hemisphere called "schizencephaly" ("split or fissured" brain). The defect tends to be in the insular region and may be unilateral or bilateral. Such individuals are mentally retarded and have seizures.

Polymicrogyria is a milder defect of neocortical formation in which numerous small abnormal gyri with tiny shallow sulci with abnormal cortical cellular layering develop rather than the normal smooth gyri with deep sulci. The defect may be localized or pervasive, and is associated with mental retardation and seizures.

INTRAUTERINE AND PERINATAL CATASTROPHES

Several malformations of the brain actually reflect intrauterine catastrophic events that destroy previously properly formed structures. Hydranencephaly is such a condition in which the cerebral hemispheres appear to form and then are destroyed by vascular or infectious processes. The cerebral hemispheres are replaced by sacs consisting of leptomeninges and glial sheets devoid of ependyma. The skull is normally formed and may even be of relatively normal size, but on transillumination is hollow and glows like a grotesque jack-o'-lantern. The basal ganglia, brainstem and cerebellum are usually preserved. The cerebral hemisphere destruction leading to hydranencephaly may occur at any time from the 12th week of gestation to the immediate postgestational period (Fig. 15-14).

Porencephaly is a more focal form of cerebral cortical destruction leading to intracerebral hemispheric cysts composed of glial sheets and meninges without ependyma. Porencephaly can be grossly difficult to distinguish from schizencephaly.

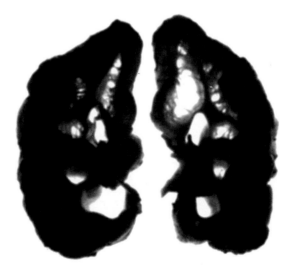

FIGURE 15-14. Multicystic leukoencephalopathy with glial strands bespeaking a perinatal catastrophe. (Courtesy of Dr. Hannes Vogel, Baylor College of Medicine.)

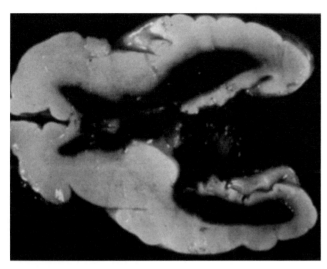

FIGURE 15-15. Germinal matrix hemorrhage in a premature. (Courtesy of Dr. S.Z. Powell, Baylor College of Medicine.)

The germinal matrix is still very active in the premature infant and this highly vascular tissue may hemorrhage forming subependymal matrix hemorrhages that range in severity from massive panventricular hematomas to small intramatrix hemorrhages that are eventually resorbed (Fig. 15-15). The vascular disturbance leading to hemorrhage may also result in ischemia of the matrix, subependymal region and periventricular white matter leading to periventricular leukomalacia that may calcify giving periventricular mineralization. While the premature is particularly susceptible to deep brain vascular catastrophes, the term infant is more prone to neocortical ischemic damage more akin to that seen in adults. This damage is similar to watershed infarcts in adults and results in narrow gliotic gyri in a condition called "ulegyria."

Developmental neurobiology is one of the most active areas of scientific investigation in modern neuroscience. This field encapsulates all of the basic neurochemical, neurogenetic, and physiological processes at work in the normal as well as the diseased nervous system. Fundamental insights into the pathophysiological processes underlying neoplasia, degeneration and cellular reaction to stress will continue to be gleaned from study of how the most complex biological system known self-assembles and matures.

16

THE TEN MOST COMMON PITFALLS IN SURGICAL NEUROPATHOLOGY

As illustrated in Chapter 2, the CNS is a wonderfully complex organ composed of a wide variety of distinctive cellular constituents. This heterogeneity conveys susceptibility to a large number of disease processes, many of which are unique to the nervous system. The combination of morphologic complexity and special nosologic vulnerabilities imparts the possibility of diagnostic error stemming from a large number of sources. In the following section, we will simplify and delineate the major underlying principles, cite specific examples of each, and suggest appropriate strategies for averting diagnostic misadventure. It is hoped that this brief discussion will convey the basic principles underlying the various sources of diagnostic error and enable the reader to recognize many of the most common specific situations in which diagnostic difficulty is likely to occur, and, by actively applying the strategies discussed, avoid the more common pitfalls.

CLINICAL INFORMATION IS CRITICAL!

Rule One is that a knowledge of the patient's clinical information is *absolutely essential* to avoid the disastrous consequences of misdiagnosis! Essential features that must be known are the patient's age, the anatomic location of the lesion, the magnetic resonance imaging (MRI) and/or computed tomography (CT) scan characteristics, and the duration and nature of the presenting signs and symptoms. The latter often falls into a simple dichotomy of either "of recent onset" or "of longstanding duration." In general, a long clinical history, particularly of seizures, suggests an indolent disease process or a low-grade neoplasm. Throughout the following discussion, we will repeatedly emphasize the central importance of an awareness of the patient's age, anatomic location and MRI features of the lesion, and duration and nature of the presenting symptoms.

TEN PRINCIPLES

Virtually all of the more common diagnostic mistakes made in surgical neuropathology can be grouped under one (or more) of 10 types of error. Following are listed the 10 principal categories of error and a specific example of each:

1. Mistaking normal structures for pathological processes
2. Mistaking nonneoplastic diseases for tumor
3. Mistaking of one tumor type for another
4. Unfamiliarity with rare tumor types

5. Failure to recognize common tumors in uncommon sites
6. Unfamiliarity with recently described disease entities
7. Misleading artifacts
8. Failure to recognize an inadequate or non-representative biopsy
9. Failure to perform appropriate diagnostic procedures
10. Failure to formulate an appropriate differential diagnosis

NORMAL STRUCTURES MISTAKEN FOR PATHOLOGICAL PROCESSES

Glioma Infiltrating Cortex Mistaken for Ganglioglioma

Astrocytomas, oligodendrogliomas, and mixed oligoastrocytomas commonly invade and diffusely infiltrate the cerebral cortex. In such situations, intrinsic cortical neurons are often surrounded and engulfed by dense swaths of infiltrating tumor cells. Such "entrapped" normal neurons can be mistaken for neoplastic ganglion cells. This pitfall can be avoided by an awareness of the innately infiltrative nature of gliomas and also by looking for the presence of other characteristic morphologic features of gangliogliomas before rendering a diagnosis. The ganglion cells of gangliogliomas are often abnormally clustered and haphazardly arranged, and binucleate or multinucleated forms are commonly seen. Gangliogliomas also often exhibit prominent numbers of eosinophilic granular bodies (EGBs), perivascular lymphocytic cuffing, and a glial component that is often composed of highly spindled astrocytes with a pilocytic morphology. In the absence of these supporting features, a diagnosis of ganglion cell tumor should be made only with extreme caution. In cases of doubt, it is a sign of intelligence to submit the case to an oncologic neuropathologist for an expert opinion!

Leptomeningeal Melanocytes Mistaken for Siderophages or Melanoma

Melanocytes are normal cellular constituents of the leptomeninges and are typically found in the pia covering the brainstem, especially the medulla. The distribution area may extend in some individuals up the basal aspects of the brain as far rostrally as the gyri recti, which lie between the olfactory bulbs and tracts. When cut in cross section, melanocytes resemble hemosiderin-laden macrophages or melanoma cells. However, on longitudinal section, their "dendritic" character allows easy identification. An awareness of the presence and neuroanatomic distribution of leptomeningeal melanocytes and their morphologic features, combined with knowledge that a surgical biopsy has been taken from an area of the CNS where melanocytes are indigenous, will prevent misidentification!

NONNEOPLASTIC DISEASES MISTAKEN FOR TUMOR: DEMYELINATING DISEASE MISTAKEN FOR GLIOMA

Demyelinating diseases can mimic glioma in several respects. They are hypercellular (reactive astrocytes and macrophages) and mitotic figures are present (macrophages are highly mitotically active). The reactive astrocytes may suggest astrocytoma while the macrophages with their round nuclei and cleared cytoplasm may suggest oligodendroglioma. The combination of these cell types may suggest mixed glioma.

This pitfall can be avoided by maintaining a high index of suspicion for demyelinating disease and confirming the identity of the cellular constituents that contribute to hypercellular biopsies. In the case of demyelinating diseases, a suspicion that a subset of cells might be macrophages is easily tested by immunostaining with one of several excellent antibodies that are commercially available, such as HAM-56 or KP-1. An additional "red flag" that should suggest to the pathologist the possibility of demyelinating disease is the presence of "Creutzfeldt astrocytes." These cells are reactive astrocytes that have abundant eosinophilic cytoplasm and distinctive small chromatin bodies or "micronuclei." The Creutzfeldt astrocyte is not pathognomonic for demyelinating disease, but is strongly associated with many demyelinating diseases and the presence of these cells should raise demyelinating disease as a possibility in the mind of the pathologist.

The misdiagnosis of demyelinating disease for glioma is particularly likely to occur when the demyelinating disease presents as a solitary mass lesion that suggests high-grade glioma on CT or MRI scans. This type of clinical presentation can occur as the initial manifestation of multiple sclerosis or as an idiopathic, clinically monophasic demyelinating pseudotumor.

MISIDENTIFICATION OF ONE TUMOR TYPE FOR ANOTHER

Lymphoma Mistaken for Glioblastoma

In small tissue samples, such as those obtained by stereotactic biopsy, lymphoma may mimic high-grade glioma. Similarities include the presence of large atypical tumor cells, mitotic figures, necrosis, GFAP-positive astrocytic cells (reactive astrocytes in the case of lymphoma), and, uniquely, diffuse infiltration of brain parenchyma by neoplastic cells. In regard to the latter phenomenon, gliomas and lymphomas are the only two classes of neoplasm that routinely show diffuse infiltration of brain parenchyma. In a fully representative biopsy of CNS lymphoma, the characteristic concentration of lymphoma cells around and within blood vessel walls will be seen; however, this cardinal feature is often lacking or obscured in smaller biopsies and a correct diagnosis will depend on the pathologist's index of suspicion and the ability to recognize the difference between infiltrating atypical lymphoma cells, which lack appreciable cytoplasm, and the prominently intermixed reactive astrocytes.

Two additional caveats regarding CNS lymphoma warrant mention. First, most CNS lymphomas are exquisitely sensitive to steroid administration at initial clinical presentation. Thus, when biopsy is performed after steroids have been given to control brain edema, very few tumor cells may be present in the biopsy and the expected hypercellular angiocentric cuffs of lymphoma cells will not be seen. (The opposite side of this coin is that a dramatic reduction in lesion size following steroid therapy is very suggestive of lymphoma in the appropriate clinical setting and is thus of significant interest to the pathologist. Moral of the story? Get the clinical history and find out what the MRIs show!) The second caveat is that some CNS lymphomas show only a very weak or equivocal immunoreaction to leukocyte common antigen (CD45), but very robust labeling with the B-cell marker CD20 (L26). Thus, if lymphoma is a consideration in the differential diagnosis, it is advisable to perform a full panel of three markers (CD45, CD20, and CD3), rather than CD45 alone.

Central Neurocytoma Mistaken for Oligodendroglioma

The H&E features of oligodendroglioma and central neurocytoma are virtually identical: small tumor cells with regular, round nuclei that are often surrounded by cleared cytoplasm ("perinuclear halos" or "fried egg" appearance). Central neurocytomas can also show a delicately branching vasculature that is characteristic of oligodendrogliomas ("chicken-wire" vascular pattern) as well as the scattered microcalcifications. Despite this exquisite mimicry of oligodendroglioma by central neurocytoma, the diagnosis is in fact a *very easy* one to make and should never be missed by the pathologist. Why? Because central neurocytomas are intraventricular tumors whereas the vast majority of oligodendrogliomas are intraparenchymal tumors! The pathologist must know the clinical history, which includes the neuroimaging (MRI/CT) features! An intraventricular tumor that looks like an oligodendroglioma is a central neurocytoma until proven otherwise. Because very rare examples of intraventricular oligodendrogliomas do exist, the diagnosis of central neurocytoma must be confirmed by demonstrating immunopositivity for neuronal markers (synaptophysin or NeuN). GFAP is negative in the neurocytoma cells and labels only scattered entrapped reactive astrocytes.

Hemangiopericytoma Mistaken for Meningioma

Hemangiopericytomas are dura-based tumors that can exhibit some similarities to meningioma, including gentle whorls; however, they must be distinguished from ordinary meningiomas because of their more aggressive behavior.

Subependymal Giant Cell Astrocytoma Mistaken for Gemistocytic Astrocytoma

Subependymal giant cell astrocytomas (SEGAs) are typically composed of plump tumor cells with abundant eosinophilic cytoplasm closely resembling gemistocytic astrocytes. Prominent central nucleoli may also be present and suggest ganglion cell tumor. Other areas may be more spindled and fibrillary. Thus, SEGAs closely mimic diffuse astrocytoma. However, as with central neurocytoma and oligodendroglioma discussed above, the diagnosis of subependymal giant cell astrocytoma should *never be missed* because SEGAs are intraventricular in location, whereas fibrillary astrocytomas, including gemistocytic astrocytomas, and gangliogliomas are intraparenchymal tumors! A quick glance at a pre-operative MRI scan or report, or a brief conversation with the neurosurgeon or radiologist, can give the pathologist invaluable information! One additional caveat: although SEGAs are associated with tuberous sclerosis (TS), not infrequently the tumor is the initial and sole presenting feature of the disease and in such cases there will be no history of TS at the time of intraoperative frozen section. It is incumbent upon the pathologist to find out the location of the lesion for all CNS biopsies!

Pilocytic Astrocytoma Mistaken for Anaplastic Astrocytoma

Pilocytic astrocytomas (PAs) exhibit three morphologic features that may cause them to be mistaken for a high-grade diffuse astrocytoma: (1) pleomorphism, (2) microvascular proliferation, and (3) invasion of the overlying leptomeninges and subarachnoid space. None of these features is a negative prognostic factor.

Pleomorphism and local invasion of the subarachnoid space are also commonly seen in several other types of low-grade brain tumors, including pleomorphic xanthoastrocytoma, ganglioglioma, and superficial cerebral astrocytoma of infancy.

Pleomorphic Xanthoastrocytoma Mistaken for Anaplastic Astrocytoma

As the name implies, pleomorphic xanthoastrocytomas (PXAs) are strikingly pleomorphic, so much so that the initial impression may be that of a high-grade diffuse astrocytoma or giant cell glioblastoma. However, on closer inspection, there is usually no necrosis or microvascular proliferation, as would be seen in high-grade astrocytomas, and mitotic figures are rarer than in typical high-grade astrocytoma. In addition, PXAs have abundant eosinophilic granular bodies (EGBs).

EGBs are typically seen in several types of low-grade tumors, most notably pilocytic astrocytoma, pleomorphic xanthoastrocytoma, and ganglioglioma. The presence of EGBs should serve as a "red flag" to alert the pathologist to consider these three entities high in the differential diagnosis. The biopsy can then be examined closely for the presence or absence of other specific features associated with each of these tumors (such as Rosenthal fibers in pilocytic astrocytomas or ganglion cells in ganglioglioma).

UNFAMILIARITY WITH RARE TUMORS

Paraganglioma of the Filum Terminale

If you have never seen, or even heard of, a particular tumor, it is difficult to diagnose it. One moderately rare tumor that is often not recognized by surgical pathologists is paraganglioma of the filum terminale (PFT). This distinctive lesion arises from the filum terminale or conus medullaris of the spinal cord in the lumbar cistern. The morphologic features of PFT mimic those of classical ependymoma, with prominent perivascular pseudorosettes as the dominant architectural feature. *The most common misdiagnosis for PFT is ependymoma.* However, whereas ependymomas are positive for the glial markers S-100 protein and GFAP, paragangliomas, similar to their systemic counterparts, are strongly reactive for neuroendocrine markers such as synaptophysin and chromogranin. Synaptophysin immunoreactivity is often stronger and more reliably positive than chromogranin in PFTs. PFTs also frequently show reactivity for cytokeratins. Thus, if the pathologist is not aware of the existence of this tumor and its immunophenotypic expressions, a misdiagnosis of metastatic carcinoma or neuroendocrine carcinoma may be rendered.

Ultrastructurally, paragangliomas show the expected features of neuroendocrine differentiation, including dense core (neurosecretory-type) granules, rather than the intercellular lumina with microvilli and cilia, and the surrounding intercellular junctional complexes that are characteristic of ependymoma.

Dysplastic Gangliocytoma of the Cerebellum (Lhermitte–Duclos Disease)

Another tumor that sometimes causes diagnostic problems is dysplastic gangliocytoma of the cerebellum (more commonly referred to eponymically as Lhermitte–Duclos disease). This quasi-hamartomatous lesion of the cerebellum expands the folia, producing a "hypertrophic" appearance. This distinctive feature can usually be clearly seen on MRI scans; hence, again, the importance of familiarity with the clinical information!

For both paraganglioma of the filum terminale (discussed above) and Lhermitte-Duclos disease, once you have seen one case it is very unlikely that you will forget either of these comparatively rare but distinctive entities!

FAILURE TO RECOGNIZE COMMON TUMORS IN UNCOMMON SITES: SUBEPENDYMOMA OF THE SPINAL CORD

Subependymomas are benign tumors that occasionally are found incidentally in the floor of the fourth ventricle at autopsy. More importantly, they may reach sufficient size to occlude either the interventricular foramen of Monro or the outlet foramina of the fourth ventricle, resulting in obstructive hydrocephalus. The treatment is surgical resection. Thus, subependymomas are commonly thought of as intraventricular tumors, and in fact most of them are; however, they can also arise within the parenchyma of the spinal cord, at which site they can cause considerable diagnostic confusion. The morphologic features of spinal cord subependymomas are identical to those of their intraventricular counterparts: lobulated clusters of benign-appearing glial cells within an abundant, fibrillary matrix. The key to avoiding diagnostic difficulty is simply an awareness that subependymomas can arise within the spinal cord, which everyone reading this book now has!

UNFAMILIARITY WITH RECENTLY DESCRIBED ENTITIES

Dysembryoplastic Neuroepithelial Tumor

Dysembryoplastic neuroepithelial tumors (DNETs) are intracortical lesions that are typically associated with a history of seizures in a child. Histologically, multiple intracortical nodules are seen, which are composed of "oligodendroglia-like cells" together with "floating neurons" in a loose, mucinous matrix. In the past, DNETs were misdiagnosed as low-grade oligodendrogliomas. Surgical resection is curative in most cases.

Chordoid Glioma of the Third Ventricle

Chordoid glioma (CG) of the third ventricle has recently been recognized as a distinct clinicopathologic entity and is codified in the most recent World Health Organization Classification of Brain Tumors. CGs are characterized by a constant neuroanatomic origin from the rostral wall of the third ventricle. Distinctive features include chords and nests of benign-appearing cells within a prominent mucinous matrix. Chronic inflammatory cell infiltrates, usually including a plasma cell component, have been described in all cases reported to date. Chordoid gliomas are strongly positive for GFAP. Although CGs have low-grade histologic features, they arise in a difficult region for complete surgical resection. Significant morbidity from surgical complications and recurrence of subtotally resected tumors have been reported.

MISLEADING ARTIFACTS

Collapsed Leptomeningeal Blood Vessels Mistaken for Vascular Malformation

There are many types of artifacts that may plague neurosurgical biopsy specimens; most are easily recognized. One artifact that occasionally misleads the unwary is artifactually collapsed and compressed leptomeningeal blood vessels that superficially mimic a vascular malformation. Avoidance of this pitfall depends on awareness of the artifact. An additional clue that one is dealing with an artifact rather than a genuine vascular malformation is provided by an examination of the adjacent brain parenchyma, which in the case of artifactually collapsed vessels will not show the characteristic histologic features associated with true CNS vascular malformations, such as astrogliosis with Rosenthal fiber formation, granular bodies, and hemosiderin deposition. It is exceptionally rare to have a vascular malformation that has no effect on the surrounding brain or spinal cord parenchyma!

Oligodendroglioma Mistaken for Astrocytoma on Frozen Section

Oligodendrogliomas are distinguished histologically by their regular round nuclei and surrounding perinuclear halos ("fried egg" appearance); however, both of these features are not typically present in intraoperative frozen sections. The freezing process distorts the round oligo nuclei to make them appear more pleomorphic, and the perinuclear halos, which form secondary to hydropic swelling of the cell cytoplasm during delayed formalin fixation, are not seen on frozen sections. The end result is to significantly increase the resemblance of oligodendroglioma to astrocytoma, and that misdiagnosis is often rendered at the time of intraoperative frozen section only to be reversed once the permanent sections are viewed. There are several ways to deal with this issue. One is to simply render a frozen section diagnosis of "infiltrating glioma" and defer more specific subclassification until the paraffin sections have been reviewed. This diagnosis is generally sufficient to guide the surgeon. Alternatively, a diagnosis of "infiltrating glioma, favor oligodendroglioma" can sometimes be made if a cytologic preparation (smear or squash prep) is performed in conjunction with the frozen section. Because freezing is not involved, the smear preparation will reveal the exquisitely round nuclei and scant to non-detectable cytoplasm of the oligodendroglioma; in contrast, astrocytomas and mixed gliomas will show astrocytic features on squash preps: abundant eosinophilic cytoplasm with elongated fibrillary processes.

FAILURE TO RECOGNIZE AN INADEQUATE OR NONREPRESENTATIVE BIOPSY

High-Grade Astrocytoma Misdiagnosed as Low-Grade Astrocytoma

High-grade fibrillary astrocytomas typically have epicenters of dense hypercellularity surrounded by an infiltrating margin of variable extent that gradually decreases in cellularity with increasing distance from the epicenter. The features that are used to grade the diffuse astrocytomas, such as the presence of necrosis, microvascular proliferation, and mitotic figures, also show a decreasing presence with increasing distance from the tumor epicenter. Because the fibrillary astrocytomas are graded based on the highest grade tumor present in a surgical specimen, a biopsy that misses the epicenter region of the tumor and samples only the infiltrating margin likely will not accurately reflect the grade of the tumor. In such cases, the pathologist must guard against rendering a misleading and incorrect diagnosis of "low-grade astrocytoma." How is the pathologist to know that the tumor being biopsied is not a low-grade astrocytoma even though that is exactly what the tissue section appears to show? *Familiarity with the clinical information!* If the MRI shows a classic "butterfly" lesion of the corpus callosum with central necrosis in a 65-year-old man, the diagnosis is not likely to be low-grade astrocytoma! So what is the pathologist to do in this situation? One possibility is to render a diagnosis of "infiltrating astrocytoma" and communicate to the surgeon that the features seen in the biopsy do not reflect the changes seen on the MRI scans and the biopsy is therefore likely not fully representative of the pathologic process. The surgeon can then obtain additional tissue for evaluation.

Metastatic Carcinoma Misdiagnosed as Glioblastoma

Another type of inadequate biopsy that can mislead the pathologist is failure to sample the brain-tumor interface of a metastasis. Metastases typically have a sharp, circumscribed margin (as mentioned before, the only two classes of tumors that diffusely infiltrate brain parenchyma are gliomas and lymphomas). Thus, regardless of the specific histologic features or quality of preservation of the tumor, a sharp interface with the surrounding parenchyma is strongly suggestive of metastasis. Contributing to the potential for diagnostic error is the frequent immunopositivity of glioblastomas for commonly used keratin antibodies.

FAILURE TO PERFORM THE APPROPRIATE DIAGNOSTIC PROCEDURE

Touch Preparation for Pituitary Adenoma

The evaluation of most surgical specimens submitted for intraoperative frozen section diagnosis is facilitated by performing a cytologic preparation (touch, smear, or scrape) in conjunction with the frozen section; for pituitary biopsies this procedure is essential. Pituitary microadenomas can be so small that it is possible to lose the adenoma during the initial facing of the frozen section tissue block; it is therefore highly prudent to perform a "touch" preparation on all transphenoidal pituitary biopsy specimens. Pituitary adenomas will shed profusely on touch preparations; in contrast, normal adenohypophysis sheds only very scant cells. There is a simple morphological basis for this difference in cell shedding. Normal anterior pituitary tissue is tightly parceled into acini by connective tissue septa; this is particularly well visualized with a reticulin stain. This packaging prevents copious cell shedding on the touch preparation. In contrast, with the monoclonal expansion of a pituitary adenoma there is loss of the normal acinar architecture and attendant fibrovascular parcellation; the very loosely cohesive adenoma cells thus freely shed onto the glass slide.

Spinal Cord Ependymoma Diagnosed as "Glioma"

Biopsies of spinal cord tumors are necessarily quite small (neurosurgeons simply cannot be persuaded to provide the pathologist with a full thickness cross section of spinal cord). Consequently, the limited tissue available for examination is usually superficial and may not contain the morphologic features that would otherwise permit an easy diagnosis in a larger specimen. The two most common primary spinal cord tumors are ependymoma and astrocytoma. Ependymomas are usually more circumscribed on MRI scans compared to the diffusely infiltrative astrocytomas; however, not every case is unequivocal on imaging studies and biopsy is usually performed for diagnosis. The perivascular pseudorosettes characteristic of ependymoma may not be present in tiny biopsy specimens. How can the diagnosis be more precisely determined to facilitate prognosis and treatment decisions? By immunohistochemistry? No, because both ependymomas and astrocytomas are positive for GFAP and S-100 protein, and there are currently no specific markers for ependymoma. The answer is electron microscopy. If the tumor is an ependymoma, the ultrastructural hallmarks will be seen in a majority of cases: intra- and intercellular lumina filled with microvilli and occasional cilia, with surrounding prominent intercellular junctional complexes. Astrocytomas, oligodendrogliomas, and mixed oligoastrocytomas do not exhibit these ultrastructural features.

The differential diagnosis between ependymoma and astrocytoma represents one of a relatively few remaining diagnostic dilemmas in surgical pathology in which electron microscopy has not been supplanted by immunohistochemistry! The pathologist should be aware of this.

FORMULATION OF AN APPROPRIATE DIFFERENTIAL DIAGNOSIS

Formulation of an appropriate differential diagnosis, which is an integral part of minimizing the chances of diagnostic difficulty, is dependent on a knowledge of the anatomic localization of a lesion as revealed by MRI or CT. Two good examples are provided by the differential diagnoses for an intraventricular mass and for a solitary lumbar cistern mass.

17

LEXICON OF NEUROPATHOLOGY

NEURONAL ALTERATIONS

"Ischemic change"/"red neuron"—Shrunken, angular, brightly eosinophilic perikaryon and pyknotic nucleus; hypoxia/ischemia 12–18 h prior to death.

"Blue neuron"—Artifactual shrinkage and angularity like in "red neuron," except cytoplasm is basophilic; seen at edge of biopsies; trap for the novice.

Neuromelanin—The pigment of pigmented (catecholaminergic) neurons; catecholaminergic neurons with neuromelanin are found in the locus ceruleus, substantia nigra, the dorsal motor nucleus of the vagus, and in several other smaller nuclear groups scattered throughout the brainstem. Discernible pigment accumulation begins about age 5 years and reaches adult appearance by age 20 years.

Ferrugination—Neuronal perikarya (and occasionally axons) adjacent to or within injured brain (especially old infarcts) may be encrusted with calcium salts and iron.

Central chromatolysis—Enlarged globular perikaryon with dispersion of rough endoplasmic reticulum (Nissl granules) and nuclear displacement peripherally, most commonly observed in the setting of axonal injury; attempted cellular repair; seen also in pellagra.

Neuronal achromasia—Ballooned neurons devoid of Nissl are seen in corticobasal ganglionic degeneration; neuronal loss and gliosis is common in this condition.

Spheroids—Local axonal dilatations, "red balls"; seen adjacent to injury of any cause and in axonal dystrophies; may be seen in diffuse axonal injury following trauma; a few can usually be demonstrated with increasing age in the fasciculus gracilis at the level of the nucleus gracilis.

Neurofibrillary tangles—Intracytoplasmic intraneuronal condensation of insoluble filamentous proteins probably related to neurofilaments; paired helical filaments, not "twisted tubules"; seen in old age, Alzheimer's disease, postencephalitic Parkinsonism, PSP, Down's syndrome (trisomy 21), dementia pugilistica, ALS/parkinsonism/dementia complex of Guam; stain strongly with silver stains.

Granulovacuolar degeneration (of Simchowicz)—Intracytoplasmic intraneuronal small vacuole with central granule, usually multiple; seen in hippocampal pyramidal cells in Alzheimer's disease and in old age. May be seen in brainstem nuclei in progressive supranuclear palsy.

Pick bodies—Intracytoplasmic intraneuronal argyrophilic round bodies seen in swollen neuron bodies in Pick's disease. (Note that Pick's disease is pathologically distinctive from Alzheimer's disease; in Pick's, there are swollen neurons with Pick's bodies + gliosis but no tangles or plaques.)

Bunina bodies—Intracytoplasmic intraneuronal small eosinophilic inclusions sometimes seen in amyotrophic lateral sclerosis in spinal neurons, but most commonly nonspecific finding (cousin of Hirano body).

Hirano bodies—Intracytoplasmic proximal dendritic eosinophilic inclusions made up of actin, seen in Alzheimer's disease and nonspecifically; may bespeak chronic neuronal degeneration.

Lewy bodies—Intracytoplasmic, spherical, sometimes laminated, eosinophilic structures seen in substantia nigra, locus ceruleus, and dorsal motor nucleus of X in idiopathic Parkinson's disease; may be seen in much more widespread distribution including cortex in Lewy body dementia.

Lafora bodies—Variable-sized spherical blue intracytoplasmic intradendritic inclusions (PAS+ carbohydrate polymers) in hereditary myoclonic epilepsy (biochemically similar to corpora amylacea but corpora are in astrocytes).

Marinesco bodies—Small acidophilic intranuclear inclusions seen predominately in pigmented neurons of brain stem; increase with age; no proven pathological significance.

Negri (lyssa) bodies—Irregular intensely eosinophilic intracytoplasmic inclusions in rabies.

Cowdry A inclusions—Intranuclear solitary large viral inclusions with surrounding halo resulting from margination of chromatin; seen in herpes simplex, herpes simiae, varicella zoster, cytomegalovirus, and with measles virus in subacute sclerosing panencephalitis. (Rarely seen with JC virus in progressive multifocal leukoencephalopathy.)

Cowdry B inclusions—Small multiple intranuclear inclusions without halos; may be seen nonspecifically and in viral infections, especially in acute stage of poliomyelitis. Marinesco bodies of the substantia nigra pigmented neurons provide a nonviral example.

Simple atrophy—Neuron degenerates and disappears without inciting inflammation, but some gliosis may occur; abiotrophy.

Transsynaptic (transneuronal) degeneration—Death or injury of one system of neurons may lead to degeneration of neurons on which initial system synapses; for example, degeneration of lateral geniculate nucleus neurons following orbital exenteration.

Olivary transneuronal hypertrophy—Usually seen following massive deafferentation of the olives (generally, loss of central tegmental tract input); olivary neurons hypertrophy, with cytoplasmic vacuolation; followed in months by gliosis and eventual neuronal atrophy; palatal myoclonus.

Neuronal intranuclear inclusions—Intranuclear inclusions seen in Huntington's disease and other CAG/polyglutamine expansion (trinucleotide repeat) diseases.

GLIAL CELLULAR CHANGES

Glia: "proletarians of the CNS society, providing shelter and maintenance for the aristocratic neurons" (James H. Morris, *Robbin's Pathological Basis of Disease*, 1989): Astrocytes (osmotic and neurochemical sinks and storehouses, repair, and reaction); Oligodendroglia (makers of myelin); Ependyma (makers of canals); and Microglia (resident tissue representatives of the reticuloendothelial system in the brain; reactive to injury).

Astrocytes—Rich in cytoplasmic intermediate filaments (glial fibrillary acidic protein—GFAP—identifies members of this clan); also stain with PTAH and Holzer; extend processes to vessels and surround neurons and synapses. Skinny (fibrous), Fat (protoplasmic), and Grossly Stuffed (gemistocytic) varieties. Reactive multiplication and/or cytoplasmic enlargement constitutes "gliosis" or "astrogliosis."

Bergmann glia—Layer of fibrillary astrocytes with cell bodies occupying the same plane as those of the Purkinje cells; reactive hyperplastic thickening of this layer is often referred to as "Bergmann gliosis." Another name for the Bergmann glia still occasionally encountered in the literature: "Golgi epithelial cells."

Alzheimer type II astrocytes—Astrocytes with large vesicular watery nucleus, sometimes with glycogen dot, and no conspicuous cytoplasm; seen in hyperammonemic states.

Opalski cells—Astrocytes with small nuclei and abundant foamy or granular cytoplasm; seen in basal ganglia in hyperammonemic states. (Note: some authorities believe these cells are degenerating neurons; others favor macrophage theory, but most accept the reported GFAP-immunopositivity as convincing evidence of astrocytic origin.)

Rosenthal fibers—Elongated, eosinophilic, irregularly nodular enlargements of astrocytic processes resulting from accumulation of filaments and granular material which is PTAH-positive but GFAP-negative (except at periphery); seen in pilocytic astrocytomas, Alexander's disease, and in a wide variety of conditions associated with long-standing gliosis (including pineal cysts).

Satellitosis—Normally a few oligos (and probably astrocytes and microglia as well) cluster about larger neuronal perikarya; increased numbers of satellite cells is a nonspecific change which may be seen with aging, seizure disorders, and in a variety of neurodegenerative disorders. Malignant glial cells (both oligos and astrocytes) often exhibit a similar propensity ("neoplastic satellitosis"—one of the "secondary Scherer structures").

Corpora amylacea—Amorphous, basophilic, spherical PAS-positive intracytoplasmic astrocytic inclusions. Nonspecific alteration. Similar in morphology to Lafora bodies.

Glial cytoplasmic inclusions—These are seen in oligodendroglia and to a lesser degree astrocytes in multiple system atrophy.

Microglia—Derived from blood-borne monocytes and are an intrinsic cellular population in the brain. In response to injury they elongate their processes, becoming "rod cells" and as they clear debris from damaged tissue they become lipid macrophages ("Gitter cells"). They often ingest iron pigments from blood breakdown ("siderophages").

Microglial nodule or star—A collection of microglia and astrocytes. Sometimes seen surrounding an expired neuron (termed a "glial shrub" when found around degenerating Purkinje cell dendritic arbors). Neuronophagia is the ingestion by these cells of such mortally wounded neurons. Nonspecific, may be seen in ischemia, trauma, or infection. Also known as Babes' nodes.

Granular ependymitis—Small piled-up collections of subependymal astrocytes in any of a variety of irritative processes.

OUTMODED TERMS

There are a large number of interesting and colorful old terms that have disappeared entirely from our modern scientific vocabulary such as, for example reticulum cell sarcoma (old term for primary CNS lymphoma). However, a few of these terms continue to surface occasionally in the professional literature. Their continued use is to be strongly discouraged. This list is provided to inform the reader of the more frequently encountered of these terms and the reasons why other terms are preferred.

Pinealoma—This term was coined prior to the recognition of a distinction between the pineal parenchymal tumors (PPTs: pineocytoma, pineoblastoma, mixed pineoblastoma-pineocytoma, pineal parenchymal tumor of intermediate differentiation) and germinoma of the pineal gland. Because the biology, clinical features, and treatment of PPTs and germinoma clearly differ, use of the inclusive and ambiguous term pinealoma should be avoided.

Angioblastic meningioma—This old term was used for all vascular meningeal tumors, that often (but not invariably) exhibited aggressive clinical behavior. We now separate this heterogeneous group into angiomatous (vascular) meningiomas, hemangiopericytomas, and hemangioblastomas. The hemangiopericytomas, in particular, must be correctly identified as they behave more aggressively than benign angiomatous meningiomas.

Malignant schwannoma—This superannuated term implies that malignant peripheral nerve sheath tumors (MPNSTs) arise by anaplastic progression from benign schwannomas. In fact, MPNSTs arising from preexisting schwannomas are exceptionally rare and the vast majority of MPNSTs arise either *de novo* or from neurofibromas.

Purkinjeoma—Old term for dysplastic gangliocytoma of the cerebellum (Lhermitte-Duclos disease), which erroneously assumed origin from Purkinje cells. Contemporary studies indicate that the abnormal neurons are more closely related to the granular cells.

STAINS USED IN NEUROHISTOLOGY

Hematoxylin and eosin (H&E)—This is the workhorse stain of diagnostic pathology, staining the cytoplasm red (eosinophilic) and nucleus dark blue (basophilic). This stain can be used to recognize the cellular constituents under view by nuclear and cytoplasmic morphology. The identity of cells, their number, and degree of pleomorphism can be accurately and quickly assessed.

Nissl stain—This stain is usually applied to sections that are thicker than the routine 5–10-μm-thick sections used in routine histology processing, and show neuronal cell bodies. They are often used when quantifying neuronal populations.

Luxol fast blue—This stains myelin deep blue and can be used to assess demyelination. Intracytoplasmic neuronal lipid deposits in ceroid lipofuscinosis and Fabry's disease can also be detected using this stain.

Myelin hematoxylin—Myelin can be stained selectively and with great sensitivity using hematoxylin in recipes named after their inventors including the Woelke, Weigert, and Weil stains.

Sudan black stains—These lipid-soluble stains can be used to demonstrate free lipid in myelin breakdown products and may be used to detect fat emboli. These stains must be performed on cryostat sections since normal paraffin embedding will remove all tissue lipids.

Oil red O stain—This lipid stain can be used in cryostat sections to show neutral lipid. This is used to show lipid droplets in skeletal muscle where lipid accumulation will occur in certain metabolic myopathies. Lipid in hemangioblastomas can also be demonstrated using this stain.

Reticulin—This technically easy silver stain shows fibroconnective tissue particularly in blood vessels and can be used to analyze vascular tumors, vascular malformations, fibrovascular septa effacement in pituitary adenomas and vascular proliferation in tumors. The peculiar vascular proliferation seen in primary CNS lymphoma stains as concentric arrays of reticulin fibers around blood vessels, and this appearance lead to early theories that this tumor was a "reticulum cell sarcoma."

Verhoeff's elastin stain—Elastic fibers in blood vessels can be seen using this technique, which is particularly useful for larger vessels.

Perl stain—This sodium ferrocyanide reaction shows tissue iron in brilliant blue staining. This technique can be used on gross tissue as well as tissue sections.

Von Kossa's stain—This tinctorial method shows tissue deposits of calcium phosphate seen in dystrophic calcification.

Fontana silver stain—This relatively straightforward silver stain shows true melanin and neuromelanin as dark black intracytoplasmic granules. HMB45 immunohistochemistry is more commonly and specifically used to demonstrate melanin-producing cells.

Neuronal silver stains (Bodian or Bielschowsky)—These technically difficult and expensive stains highlight axonal cytoskeletal proteins and intracytoplasmic neurofibrils. They have historically been used to detect neurofibrillary tangles and senile plaques. While they are still widely employed, immunohistochemical stains are gradually replacing them.

Phosphotungstic acid hematoxylin (PTAH)—This procedure stains glial processes and has historically been used to detect astrogliosis. Blepharoplasts (cilia basal bodies) can also be discerned using this stain. Glial fibrillary acidic protein (GFAP) immunohistochemistry has largely replaced this stain for detecting gliosis.

Congo red—This stain intercalates into the beta-pleated sheets of polymerized proteins forming amyloid. By light microscopy Congo red deposits appear as eosinophilic homogeneous accumulations that exhibit yellow-green birefringence under polarized light.

Thioflavin S—This technically easy and inexpensive stain provides a highly sensitive method for detecting amyloid. It is considerably more sensitive than Congo red but requires fluorescent microscopy. The thioflavin S stain can also be used to detect senile plaques and neurofibrillary tangles.

Periodic acid–Schiff–hematoxylin (PAS)—This stain demonstrates carbohydrate (glycogen) deposits. It also stains glycoproteins and carbohydrates in fungi, parasites and senile plaques. Glycogen deposits in glycogen storage diseases also can be seen with this stain. Some tumor types are rich in glycogen and this feature can be detected with this stain. Diastase digestion will obliterate PAS staining by destroying glycogen, so slides can be stained with PAS with and without diastase digestion to prove the chemical identity of the PAS positive material.

Alcian blue—This stain can be used to show acid mucopolysaccharides and highlights the capsules of cryptococci.

Gomori methenamine silver (GMS)—This stain stains fungal yeast and hyphae very well in tissue sections and can permit morphological provisional identification of these organisms. When used in the central nervous system, however, fine intracytoplasmic granular staining is normally seen in neurons and must not be mistaken for fungi. These granules are very tiny and are even smaller than histoplasmosis organisms.

Gram stain—Bacteria can be seen with this stain and characterized according to Gram positivity or negativity. In tissue sections this differentiation is not always reliable and organisms can be very difficult to discern, especially in necrotic tissue. The tissue stains for organisms are relatively insensitive and culture or PCR confirmation is always highly desirable.

Acid fast bacteria (AFB) stains—These stains are used to stain mycobacteria. The Ziehl–Neelsen stain uses carbol fuchsin methylene blue; organisms stain as dark red elongate spicules against a blue green background. The Fite–Faraco stain is an acid fast stain used to detect lepra bacilli.

INDEX

A

Abscesses
  amebic brain, 216
  bacterial brain, 204, 206, 207
  biopsy with, 223
  with Candida, 214
  with Cryptococcosis, 209
  of the muscle, 301
  spinal, 10
Acanthamoeba, 216
Acanthocytosis, 246
Acetylcholine (ACh), 83, 85–88, 296
Achromasia, 192, 199, 325
Acidophiles, 65
Aciduria, 246, 248
Actin, 76
Action conduction velocity, 77
Action potential, 79–82
Acute disseminated encephalomyelitis, 195–196, 201
Acute hemorrhagic leukoencephalopathy, 196
Acute idiopathic polyneuritis. *See* Guillain-Barré syndrome
Acute multiple sclerosis, 201
AD. *See* Alzheimer's disease
ADC (amylotrophy-dementia complex), 268
Adenohypophysis, 64, 65–66
Adenoma, 65, 171–174, 323
Adhalin, 297
Adipocytes, 61–62
Adrenoleukodystrophy, 198, 199, 201
Adrenomyeloneuropathy, 199–200
AFP (alpha fetoprotein), 171
Aging changes, 11–14, 15, 25–27, 41–42, 48–51. *See also* Apoptosis
AICA (anterior inferior cerebellar artery syndrome), 118–119
AIDS, 166, 196, 208, 214, 218–219, 220, 223
Alcohol, 127, 246, 249–253, 303
Alexander's disease, 34, 35, 199, 200–201
Alexia, 126
Alopecia, 246, 255
Alpha fetoprotein (AFP), 171
Alphamethyl-DOPA, 88
Alphazalone, 95
Alzheimer's disease (AD), 261–265
  cholinergic system with, 87–88
  clinical features, 269
  evolution of diagnosis, 264
  fibrillogenesis, 259

genetic aspects, 103
  neurons with, 13–14, 15, 20
  spongiform change, 221
  treatment, 87–88
Alzheimer Type I astrocytosis, 31, 32
Alzheimer Type II astrocytosis, 29, 30–33, 249, 327
Amino acids, 92–97
Aminogycoside antibiotics, 87
4-Aminopyridine (4AP), 80
Amitriptyline, 92
Ammonia, 31
AMPA receptor, 95
Amphetamine, 89, 90, 91
Amphotericin, 197
β-Amyloidopathies, 259, 261, 263, 265
Amyotrophic lateral sclerosis (ALS), 275, 276, 277
Amyotrophic lateral sclerosis-Parkinsonism-dementia of Guam, 277
Amyotrophy-dementia complex (ADC), 268
Anatomy, variants and incidental autopsy findings, 132–134, 142
Anencephaly, 307
Anesthetics, 80
Aneurysms, 176, 238, 240–241, 244
Angiitis, 237
Anoxia, 142, 221
Anterior inferior cerebellar artery syndrome (AICA), 118–119
Anterior spinal artery syndrome, 114
Anterior spinal cord syndrome, 107–108
Antibodies, 95, 221, 277, 318
Anticonvulsants, 95
Antidepressants. *See* Tricyclic antidepressants
Antifreeze, 252
Antioncogenes, 4, 148
Antiprolactin antibodies, 68
Antipsychotics, 92
Anti-tRNA synthetase syndrome, 301
Anxiolytics, 95
AP5-7, 94
Aphasia, 126, 261, 269
Apnea test, 142
Apoptosis, 1, 2, 3, 4–5, 6, 230
Arachnoid barrier cell layer, 56, 57–59, 69
Arachnoid cells, 63, 71
Arachnoid cyst, 133, 176
Arachnoid plaques, 132
Arboviruses, 218
Area postrema, 68

Arms. *See* Extremities
Arsenic intoxication, 254
Artane, 87
Arteriovenous malformations (AVM), 242, 243
Arteritis, 211, 235
Arylsulfatase A, 199
Aseptic viral meningitis, 216, 218
Aspartate, 83, 93, 228
Aspartylacyclase, 200
Aspergillosis, 208, 209, 212, 213, 214
Astroblastoma, 163
Astrocytes, 24–35
  aging changes, 25–27
  Creutzfeldt, 32–33, 318
  effects of ischemia, 234
  function, 27, 74, 77, 78
  immunohistochemistry, 24–25, 77, 326
  light microscopy, 24
  in microglial nodule, 327
  pathologic reactions, 27–35
  physiology, 24–25, 77
  in the pineal gland, 63, 169–170
  specialized spindled, 68
  types, 24
  ultrastructure, 25, 77
  vs. oligodendroglia, 38
Astrocytoma, 33, 34, 111
  anaplastic, 152, 161, 319–320
  biopsy, 322
  chromosomal alterations, 187
  circumscribed, 154–156
  classification, 146, 149, 150
  desmoplastic cerebral, of infancy, 156, 157, 165
  diffuse, 150–154
  fibrillary brainstem, 123
  infiltration into cortex, 317
  juvenile pilocytic, 123
  low-grade, 152
  pilocytic, 155–156, 319
  subependymal giant cell, 156, 179
  vs. oligodendroglioma, 322
Astrogliosis, 29, 30, 193
Ataxia
  with cerebellum lesions, 112
  episodic, 237
  Friedreich's, 102, 103, 109, 271, 274–275
  ipsilateral appendicular, 122
  sensory, 246
  spinocerebellar, 99, 103, 270, 271
  truncal, 249